D1416506

Giving Drugs by Advanced Techniques

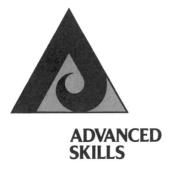

**ADVANCED
SKILLS**

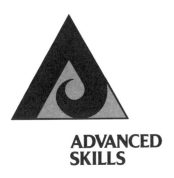

**ADVANCED
SKILLS**

Giving Drugs by Advanced Techniques

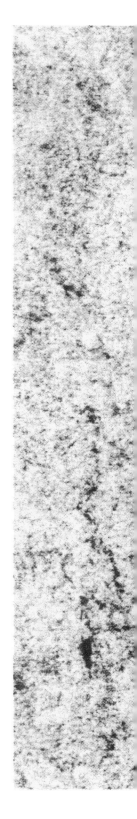

Springhouse Corporation
Springhouse, Pennsylvania

Staff

Executive Director, Editorial
Stanley Loeb

Senior Publisher
Matthew Cahill

Art Director
John Hubbard

Senior Editor
Stephen Daly

Clinical Project Director
Patricia Dwyer Schull, RN, MSN

Editors
Elizabeth Weinstein, Marylou Ambrose, Jody Charnow, Margaret Eckman, Kathy Goldberg, Elizabeth Mauro, Gale Sloan

Clinical Editors
Tina R. Dietrich, RN, BSN, CCRN; Kimberly McKelvey Jack, RN; Mary Jane McDevitt, RN, BS; Sandra M. Nettina, RN,C, BSN, MSN, CRNP

Copy Editors
Cynthia Breuninger and Jane V. Cray *(supervisors)*, Christina P. Ponczek, Nancy Papsin, Doris Weinstock

Designers
Stephanie Peters *(associate art director)*, Matie Patterson *(senior designer)*, Linda Franklin, Joseph Laufer

Illustrators
Jean Gardner, Linda Gist, Jackie Facciola, Bob Jackson, Robert Neumann, Judy Newhouse

Art Production
Robert Wieder

Typography
David Kosten *(director)*, Diane Paluba *(manager)*, Elizabeth Bergman, Joyce Rossi Biletz, Phyllis Marron, Robin Mayer, Valerie Rosenberger

Manufacturing
Deborah Meiris *(manager)*, Anna Brindisi, T.A. Landis

Production Coordination
Patricia W. McCloskey

Editorial Assistants
Maree DeRosa, Beverly Lane, Mary Madden, Margaret Rastiello

Library of Congress Cataloging-in-Publication Data
Giving drugs by advanced technique.
   p.   cm. — (Advanced skills)
  Includes bibliographical references and index.
   1. Drugs—Administration. 2. Nursing.
I. Springhouse Corporation. II. Series.
  [DNLM: 1. Drug Therapy—methods—nurses's instruction. WB 330 G539]
RM147.G57 1993
615'.6—dc20
DNLM/DLC   92-49089
ISBN 0-87434-553-7   CIP

Contents

Advisory board

At the time of publication, the advisors
held the following positions.

Cecelia Gatson Grindel, RN, PhD
Assistant Professor
Villanova University
College of Nursing
Villanova, Pa.

Judith Ski Lower, RN, MSN, CCRN, CNRN
Nurse Manager, Neurology Critical Care Unit
The Johns Hopkins Hospital
Baltimore

Kathleen M. Malloch, RN, BSN, MBA, CNA
Clinical Nursing Administrator
Maryvale Samaritan Medical Center
Phoenix, Ariz.

Marguerite K. Schlag, RN, MSN, EdD
Director, Nursing Education and Development
Robert Wood Johnson University Hospital
New Brunswick, N.J.

Karen Then, RN, MN
Assistant Professor, Faculty of Nursing
University of Calgary, Alberta

Contributors and consultants

At the time of publication, the contributors held the following positions.

Georgia M. Bosserman, RN
Coordinator, Parenteral Therapy
VAD Specialist
The Johns Hopkins Hospital
Baltimore

Deborah L. Dalrymple, RN, MSN, CRNI
Associate Professor
Montgomery County Community College
Blue Bell, Pa.
Staff IV Nurse
Doylestown (Pa.) Hospital

Sandra L. Dearholt, RN, MS, CCRN
Nurse Manager, Oncology
The Johns Hopkins Hospital
Oncology Nursing Administration
Baltimore

Mary Collins Derivan, RN, MSN, OCN
Clinical Nurse Educator
Fitzgerald Mercy Division
Mercy Catholic Medical Center
Darby, Pa.

Tina R. Dietrich, RN, BSN, CCRN
Nurse Consultant
Bethlehem, Pa.

Christine Ferrante, RN, BSN
Nurse Manager, Oncology Unit
Fitzgerald Mercy Division
Mercy Catholic Medical Center
Darby, Pa.

Karin C. Hehlinger, RN, BSN
CCU Cardiac Care Nurse
Albert Einstein Medical Center
Philadelphia

Sharon Lehman, RN, MSc, CCRN, CNSN
Metabolic Nurse Consultant
Nutrition Support Service Team
Staff Nurse, Surgical ICU
University of Minnesota Hospital
Minneapolis

Mary Jane McDevitt, RN, BS
Staff Nurse, Oncology Unit
Fitzgerald Mercy Division
Mercy Catholic Medical Center
Darby, Pa.

Sandra M. Nettina, RN,C, MSN, CRNP
Adult Nurse Practitioner
Mercy Primary Care Group
Mercy Medical Center
Baltimore

Marian Newton, RN, MN, PhD
Clinical Nurse Specialist
Outpatient Psychiatry
Samuel S. Stratton
Veterans Affairs Medical Center
Albany, N.Y.

Elizabeth G. Osborne, RN, PHN, PNS
Director of Nursing
California Infusion Services
Sausalito, Ca.

Joan Priddy-Southern, RN, BSN
Clinical Nurse Specialist in Pain Management
Bowman Gray School of Medicine
Pain Control Center
Winston-Salem, N.C.

Linda Roy, RN, MSN, CCRN
Clinical Instructor
Doylestown (Pa.) Hospital

At the time of publication, the consultants held the following positions.

Tess Angeles, BSN
Vice President
Perivascular Nurse Consultants, Inc.
Rockledge, Pa.

Jean Krajicek Bartek, RN, PhD, CARN
Assistant Professor
Department of Adult Health and Illness
University of Nebraska Medical Center
College of Nursing
Omaha

Charles W. Heckenberger, RRT, AS, CRTT
Staff Respiratory Therapist
Inservice Coordinator
Doylestown (Pa.) Hospital

Sue Masoorli, RN
CEO and President
Perivascular Nurse Consultants, Inc.
Rockledge, Pa.

FOREWORD

Giving injections, setting up I.V. lines, and dispensing pills—that's probably what you picture when you think of drug administration. But today, as your role in drug therapy continues to expand, you face greater challenges than ever before. Not only are you expected to understand the benefits and drawbacks of an ever-increasing number of drugs, but you must also be familiar with the latest administration techniques, such as transdermal patches, subcutaneous implants, and central venous infusion.

To master these administration skills and understand these new drugs—many of which have been developed through biotechnology—you need a reliable guide that covers all aspects of drug delivery, but also one that focuses on the most advanced administration methods. Fortunately, *Giving Drugs by Advanced Techniques*, the latest book in the Advanced Skills series, does just that. Fully illustrated, with dozens of helpful charts, illustrations, and instructional photographs, the book tells you in straightforward language everything you need to know and do to perform advanced drug administration with skill and confidence.

The book consists of nine chapters. In the first chapter, you'll find an overview of pharmacologic principles and a broad-ranging discussion of the various advanced administration techniques. The chapter describes how biotechnology has changed drug administration, as well as the risks and benefits of different administration techniques.

Chapters 2 through 8 cover various drug administration routes, highlighting the more advanced methods for delivering drugs by each route. For instance, Chapters 2 and 3 cover peripheral and central venous therapy, and include sections on administering drugs using advanced equipment, such as implantable vascular access ports. Chapter 4 examines parenteral nutrition, with an emphasis on the complications you need to watch for, and Chapter 5 covers the latest techniques in chemotherapy.

Chapter 6 discusses how drugs reach and affect the central nervous system; it contains detailed sections on epidural and intrathecal administration. Chapter 7 deals with techniques for respiratory drug delivery and includes the latest information on metered-dose inhalers, nebulizers, and endotracheal drug administration. Chapter 8 covers transdermal and subdermal administration, and the final chapter discusses other important delivery techniques, among them intrapleural, intraosseous, and intra-articular administration.

To save you time, Chapters 2 through 8 follow the same format. Each begins with an overview of the drug delivery method. A discussion of the pharmacologic principles of the method follows, describing how that particular method affects drug absorption. A detailed anatomic illustration shows the drug's route, and a helpful chart provides guidelines for administering common drugs.

Next come separate entries, each covering a different method or technique used to administer drugs through that route. Each entry includes sections on the equipment you'll be working with and a step-by-step guide to drug administration. The entry also covers complications that may arise and how to intervene when they do, nursing considerations to keep in mind, and patient teaching.

Throughout the book you'll find logos— graphic devices that alert you to key information. The *Advanced equipment* logo signals a detailed look at the newest type of equipment you'll be working with. The *Troubleshooting* logo highlights information on detecting and correcting problems with equipment. The *Home care* logo accompanies important information on providing the special care patients need at home. And the *Complications* logo alerts you to the steps you can take to recognize and treat adverse reactions to therapy.

You'll also find many helpful illustrations and photographs throughout the book. For example, in Chapter 3, which covers central venous therapy, you'll find a step-by-step photographic guide to administering drugs using a peripherally inserted central catheter, a procedure that more and more nurses are being trained to perform.

At the back of the book, you'll find an *Advanced skilltest,* a multiple-choice self-test that lets you evaluate what you've learned. The answers, along with complete rationales, immediately follow the test.

I know you'll find *Giving Drugs by Advanced Techiques* an indispensable aid to your nursing practice. Whether you're a new or experienced nurse, the pressure to understand the latest administration techniques can be intense, the amount of information you're expected to know at times overwhelming. *Giving Drugs by Advanced Techniques* will help you meet the challenges of advanced drug administration, bolstering your skills while boosting your confidence. I highly recommend it.

Marian Newton, RN, MN, PhD

Clinical Specialist in Psychiatry
Samuel S. Stratton Veterans Affairs Medical Center
Albany, New York

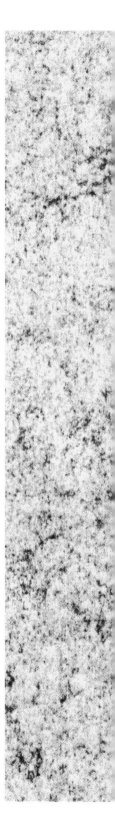

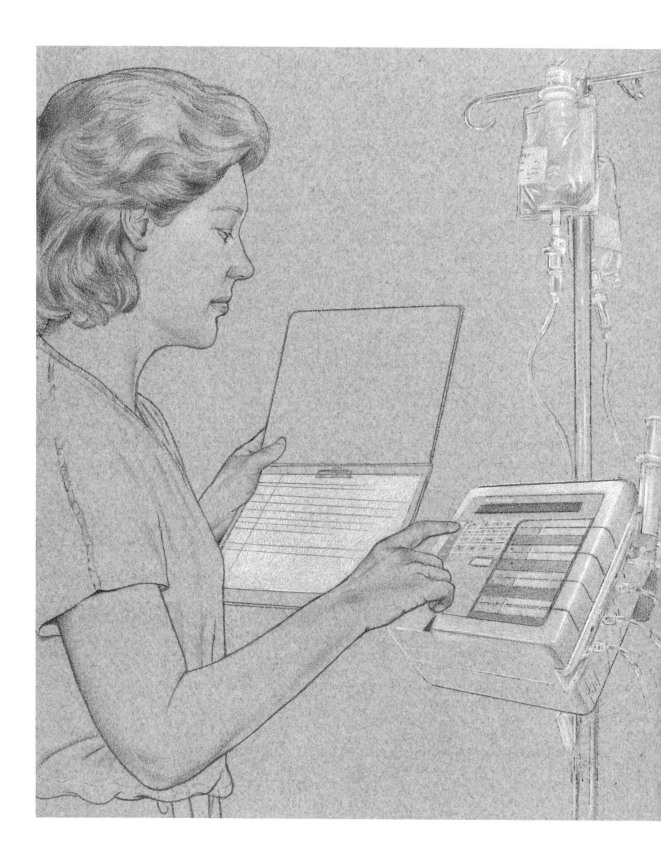

CHAPTER 1

Understanding advanced drug delivery

Drug administration poses a greater challenge today than ever before. Dramatic advances in the development of drugs and drug delivery systems have improved the quality of patient care. But they've also brought with them increased responsibilities and the expectation that as a nurse you're capable of administering drugs using the latest techniques.

To do this, not only must you exercise technical competence, sound judgment, and meticulous attention to detail, but you also must stay abreast of the newest developments in pharmacology and drug administration. If your nursing education and experience haven't prepared you for these added responsibilities, you may feel uneasy when a doctor prescribes a new drug or an advanced administration method for your patient. This chapter and the others in this book will help give you the knowledge, skill, and confidence you'll need to effectively use the most sophisticated drug delivery systems.

Guidelines for safe drug administration

To administer drugs safely and accurately, you need to know the latest information about the drug you're about to give and you need to follow safe procedures. You should also be aware that the law requires you to know the goals of your patient's drug regimen, the drug's mechanism of action, expected and unusual drug effects, dosage, proper administration methods, contraindications, and possible interactions with food or other drugs.

Measures to remember
To ensure safe and accurate drug administration, follow these guidelines:
• When you receive a new medication order, evaluate it carefully. If any part of the order seems unusual, don't carry it out until you've clarified the problem with the doctor.
• Assess your patient regularly to help identify potential adverse reactions. As part of your assessment, consider the patient's laboratory test results, other prescribed medications, medical history, and pertinent psychosocial factors.
• If you believe your patient's expected or potential response to a drug requires nursing intervention, formulate appropriate nursing diagnoses.
• Administer the right drug, to the right patient, in the right amount, at the right time, and by the right route.
• Assess your patient's responses to drug therapy, staying alert for both therapeutic and adverse effects.
• If your patient has adverse reactions or if you must deviate from the prescribed drug regimen, notify the doctor.
• Teach the patient how to take the medication safely.
• Evaluate the effectiveness of any nursing interventions.

This chapter provides an overview of various advanced drug delivery systems and reviews important pharmacologic principles, explaining how different drugs move through the body and exert their effects. You'll learn how administration routes affect drug absorption, how technologic advances have helped regulate the absorption rate, and how diseases affect drug distribution and metabolism.

New drug delivery systems

Researchers have developed drug delivery systems that can control the rate, duration, or tissue site of drug release. Some systems combine one drug with another or use a specific delivery device or process. Others release a drug in response to a certain physiologic condition, such as a high glucose level.

Advanced drug delivery systems have many advantages over conventional ones. They can deliver drugs produced by the new biotechnologies, and by carrying drugs more directly to target tissues, such as tumors, they can help limit drug toxicity and increase efficacy. These advanced delivery systems also allow smaller or less frequent doses by supplying a drug exactly where and when it's needed. For instance, an implantable pump can be programmed to administer a drug into the epidural or pleural space, the spinal canal, a joint, a bone, or the peritoneal cavity.

The new systems also produce fewer toxic metabolites, keep blood drug levels more constant, and are less likely to cause adverse effects. They can avoid obstacles posed by physiologic barriers, such as the skin and the blood-brain barrier. By reducing the risk of unpleasant GI effects and simplifying drug therapy, they also improve patient compliance.

With these new methods come new nursing responsibilities. When the doctor selects an advanced drug delivery system for your patient, you'll need to learn how to use the equipment, following strict aseptic technique to avoid infection and other complications. As with any drug you administer, you'll want to know if the patient is receiving the dosage he needs or if he's at risk for toxicity. You'll also need to understand the drug's mechanism of action and learn how to observe for both therapeutic and adverse effects. And, of course, you'll want to teach the patient about his drug regimen. (See *Guidelines for safe drug administration.*)

Topical administration

In the past, topical drugs exerted only short-term, local effects. But today, many new topical drugs have a long duration, and some of them act systemically. Topical administration methods now include transdermal patches, ocular inserts, and collagen shields.

Transdermal patches
These patches are used to administer such drugs as antihypertensives, analgesics, estrogen, nitroglycerin, scopolamine (to prevent motion sickness), and nicotine (to help people quit smoking). A transdermally administered drug diffuses through the skin into the bloodstream at a steady rate, so its plasma concentration remains stable. Bypassing the GI tract, the drug avoids uneven absorption and first-pass metabolism (which can cause too-rapid drug clearance) and reduces adverse GI effects. Because the patches are easy to use, they promote patient compliance. Patients change them only once daily or, with some drugs, weekly.

Nevertheless, transdermal patches do have certain drawbacks. At present, they can deliver only nonirritating, lipophilic drugs with a low molecular weight, and they're also more expensive than drugs taken orally.

Intraocular inserts
These inserts deliver drugs to the eye. For instance, Ocusert Pilo supplies pilocarpine to the ciliary muscles to treat glaucoma. The prolonged effect of an eye medication disk, which sustains drug release for an entire week, is an important benefit over eyedrops. However, intraocular inserts cost much more than eyedrops and may cause eye discomfort. Also, systemic drug absorption may occur, causing adverse effects.

Collagen shields
Presoaked in a drug solution, collagen shields are applied to the eye to treat corneal ulcers and severe iridocyclitis. Although they have not yet been approved by the Food and Drug Administration, collagen shields may prove more effective than injecting collagen beneath the conjunctiva, where it's poorly absorbed.

Intradermal implants

Inserted beneath the skin, intradermal implants are pellets or capsules containing small amounts of medication. From the dermis, the medication seeps slowly into the tissues. Goserelin, one such implant, is inserted into the upper abdominal wall to manage advanced prostate cancer. With the female contraceptive Norplant, another type of intradermal implant, six silicone capsules containing levonorgestrel are inserted beneath the skin of the upper arm. They provide contraception for 5 years.

Because intradermal implants require no patient action once they're in place, they eliminate the problem of noncompliance. Their major drawback is the need for minor surgery to insert or remove them.

Pharmacokinetics

Increasing your knowledge of pharmacokinetics — the movement of a drug through the body — can help you predict your patient's response to a particular regimen and anticipate potential problems.

Pharmacokinetics encompasses four basic processes — absorption, distribution, metabolism, and excretion. (See *Phases of drug disposition,* page 4.) You should be aware, though, that the new biotechnologic drugs may have more complex pharmacokinetics than conventional drugs. In addition, some drug delivery systems may not release these new drugs as readily.

Absorption

Before a drug can act, it must be absorbed into the bloodstream. Absorption takes the

Phases of drug disposition

Drug disposition begins once a medication is given to the patient. Next, the medication proceeds through pharmacokinetic, pharmacodynamic, and pharmacotherapeutic phases. The chart at right shows these various phases, the activities that occur during them, and the factors that influence those activities.

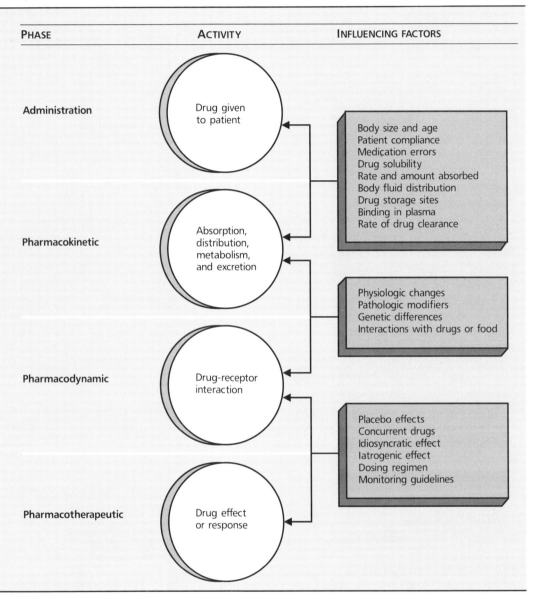

PHASE	ACTIVITY	INFLUENCING FACTORS
Administration	Drug given to patient	Body size and age Patient compliance Medication errors Drug solubility Rate and amount absorbed Body fluid distribution Drug storage sites Binding in plasma Rate of drug clearance
Pharmacokinetic	Absorption, distribution, metabolism, and excretion	Physiologic changes Pathologic modifiers Genetic differences Interactions with drugs or food
Pharmacodynamic	Drug-receptor interaction	Placebo effects Concurrent drugs Idiosyncratic effect Iatrogenic effect Dosing regimen Monitoring guidelines
Pharmacotherapeutic	Drug effect or response	

drug from the administration site to the circulatory system. (I.V. drugs, however, enter the bloodstream directly.) To enter the circulation, a drug must cross cell barriers by means of passive diffusion or active transport.

Passive diffusion
This mechanism occurs by means of concentration gradients. Consider, for instance, what happens when you administer an oral drug to your patient. Because the drug has a higher concentration in the GI tract than in the bloodstream, it will penetrate the GI membrane and enter the bloodstream until drug concentrations are equal on both sides of the membrane. If the drug is lipid-soluble (which

most drugs are), passive diffusion requires no cellular energy because the drug simply moves from a high- to a low-concentration area.

Passive diffusion typically occurs through diffusion of small molecules across membranes or, to a lesser degree, through pores. Drugs with larger molecules also cross membranes, although more slowly.

With some drugs, passive diffusion takes place with the aid of a carrier. In *carrier-mediated diffusion* (also called *facilitated diffusion*), substances with low lipid solubility penetrate cell membranes by combining with carrier substances and moving across membranes with the concentration gradient.

Absorption of vitamin B_{12} is a classic example of carrier-mediated diffusion. After administration, it binds with the intrinsic factor, a substance produced by the stomach wall. The complex then selectively but passively moves to an area of lower concentration in the gut lumen. Many new biotechnologic drugs undergo carrier-mediated diffusion rather than passive diffusion because of their molecular size and their electrical attractions to other molecules due to their polar nature.

In *convective absorption,* a minor passive transport process, small drug molecules accompany fluid through the pores in cell walls. Some electrolytes are absorbed this way.

Active transport

This transport mechanism works against the concentration gradient. Combining with a carrier, the drug moves from a low-concentration area to a high-concentration area, then dissociates from the carrier. Sodium, potassium, and a few drugs, such as the antiparkinsonian agent levodopa, are absorbed by active transport.

In *pinocytosis,* a form of active transport, a cell forms a vacuole or vesicle around an undissolved drug particle, then carries the particle across the cell membrane. The fat-soluble vitamins A, D, E, and K are absorbed this way.

Factors affecting absorption

How well a patient's body absorbs a drug depends on various factors, including the absorbing surface and the administration route.

Absorbing surface

The site and condition of the absorbing surface affect both the rate of drug absorption and the amount of drug absorbed. For instance, if you give a topical agent to a patient who has psoriasis with open lesions, you can expect the drug to be absorbed quickly and in large amounts. Conversely, if a patient has had a bowel resection, you should anticipate slow absorption of any oral drug you administer.

Administration route

The route used to administer a drug plays a key role in how much and how quickly the drug is absorbed.

Oral route. An orally administered drug has the most variable absorption. Changes in the pH of the GI tract or in intestinal membrane permeability, fluctuations in GI motility or blood flow, and the presence of food or other drugs in the GI tract can alter the amount of drug available to the systemic circulation. The oral route also moves drugs through the liver, where an elaborate enzyme system may inactivate them before they can pass into the systemic circulation.

Intraosseous route. The rich vascular network of the long bones ensures rapid absorption of intraosseous drugs. When administered into a bone, a drug works its way through a dense network of sinusoids in the bone marrow until it exits the bone and enters the systemic circulation. Drugs and solutions administered through the bone marrow are absorbed as rapidly as those administered I.V.

Intrapleural route. A drug administered intrapleurally crosses the pleural membrane and enters the pleural cavity, where it works locally at the disease site.

Intraperitoneal route. After intraperitoneal administration, a drug crosses the peritoneal membrane and enters the peritoneal cavity, where it works locally.

I.V. route. A drug administered I.V. enters the bloodstream directly. Because the drug is absorbed immediately and completely, the patient's response is rapid.

Epidural route. With epidural administration, a drug is absorbed into the cerebrospinal fluid, where it works directly on the central nervous system.

Inhalation and intratracheal routes. A drug administered by one of these routes is absorbed into the bloodstream from alveolar sacs. The bronchial tree's large surface area provides an extensive, highly perfused region for enhanced absorption.

Topical route. A topical drug is absorbed into subcutaneous sites. The greater the skin hydration, the faster the drug's absorbed. Applying a physical barrier, such as plastic wrap or an occlusive bandage, over the drug enhances skin hydration. Another way to enhance absorption is to increase drug concentration in the patch or disc or the surface area over which the preparation is applied.

Until recently, drug absorption through the skin has been variable and hard to control. However, the transdermal patch now provides controlled, consistent drug delivery. (See *Transdermal drug absorption.*)

Although a drug may be applied to a patient's mucous membranes strictly for its local effect, some drugs applied to the mucosa of the mouth, nose, eye, vagina, or rectum can be absorbed systemically. The highly vascular nasal mucosa, for instance, allows systemic absorption while avoiding hepatic first-pass metabolism. Researchers are investigating intranasal delivery of insulin and contraceptives as well as rectal delivery of proteins and peptides and contraceptive delivery through the uterus and vagina.

Advances in controlling drug absorption

Scientists have developed new techniques to control the rate of drug absorption. To sustain a drug's release, they can coat oral medications with a matrix barrier or an ion exchange resin; the coating delays absorption until the drug reaches a specific environment. To achieve tighter control of the release of drugs, they've developed delivery systems, such as putting drugs in liposomes, that release a drug only when a specific osmotic pressure occurs.

Distribution

Once a drug enters the bloodstream, it's distributed to body tissues and fluids through the circulatory system. Consequently, highly perfused tissues, such as the heart, liver, kidneys, and brain, receive the drug before less vascular tissues, such as the skin, fat, muscle, and viscera.

Distribution depends partly on a drug's ability to cross lipid membranes. Some drugs can't cross certain cell membranes and thus have limited distribution. For instance, antibiotics have trouble permeating the prostate gland, abscesses, and exudates.

Certain diseases impede drug distribution by altering the *volume of distribution* — the total amount of drug in the body relative to the amount of drug in the plasma. Usually constant during therapy, the volume of distribution can be altered by such conditions as congestive heart failure (CHF), dehydration, and burns. If your patient has CHF, expect to increase the dosage, as the drug must be distributed to a larger volume. On the other hand, if your patient's dehydrated, you'll probably decrease the dosage because the drug will be distributed to a much smaller volume.

Plasma-protein binding

After absorption, some drug molecules move to receptor sites, the parts of the cell membrane that interact with a drug to produce a therapeutic effect. But other molecules bind with plasma proteins. The percentage of molecules that bind with plasma proteins varies among drugs. With highly protein-bound drugs, little drug remains available to exert a pharmacologic effect.

Once the unbound, or free, drug acts on surrounding cells, the level of unbound drug in the plasma drops. In response, some plasma proteins release more of the drug. This can cause problems if your patient has a low

Transdermal drug absorption

Where you place a transdermal patch on your patient's body can affect the amount of drug that's absorbed. The graph below shows how transdermal absorption varies at different skin sites.

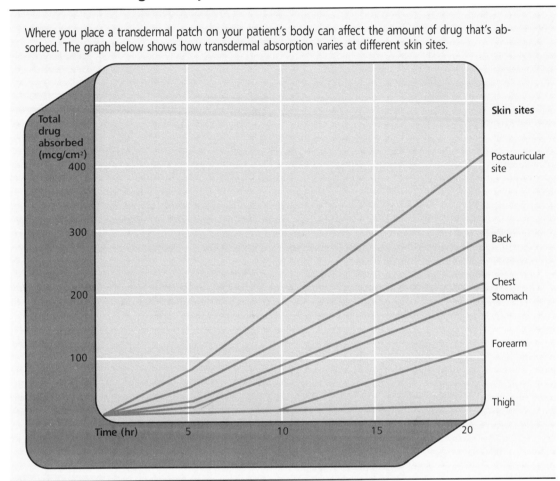

plasma protein level, such as from malnutrition, kidney disease, or reduced hepatic synthesis. If he receives a standard dose of a highly protein-bound drug, more of the drug will remain available to exert a pharmacologic effect, possibly causing a toxic reaction.

Compartmentalization
To better understand drug distribution, think of the body as a system of physiologic compartments based on blood flow. The bloodstream and highly perfused organs make up the central compartment. Less perfused areas form the peripheral compartment, which is subdivided into the tissue compartment (consisting of muscle and skin) and the deep compartment (consisting of fat and bone). Each compartment stores portions of an administered drug, releasing its store as plasma drug concentrations decline. (See *Understanding compartmentalization,* page 8.)

Metabolism

Metabolism, or biotransformation, is the chemical conversion of a drug into a form the body can eliminate. Metabolism reduces a drug's ability to cross semipermeable membranes. This makes the drug more likely to remain in the

Understanding compartmentalization

The body can store a drug in fat, bone, or skin. Using the blood as a compartment, it can transfer a drug to a fetus or across the blood-brain barrier. Knowing the characteristics of each drug storage compartment will help you understand how distribution can affect a drug's duration of action.

Fat storage
A drug that dissolves easily in lipids migrates to adipose tissue. Because this tissue lacks receptors for drug action, the drug remains inactive there. Eventually, it's released by fat cells to exert its pharmacologic effect. With some drugs, this slow, prolonged action is an advantage. For instance, slow release of anesthetic barbiturates provides effective anesthesia during surgery. With other drugs, such prolonged action can be dangerous.

Bone storage
Bone acts as a storage compartment for certain drugs. Tetracycline, for example, distributes throughout bone and may eventually crystallize there. In a growing child, this can cause tooth discoloration. Lead and certain chemicals can also accumulate in bone, resulting in prolonged, harmful exposure to these toxins.

Skin storage
Storage of drugs in the skin typically causes photosensitivity. Tetracycline is an example.

Fetal transfer
A drug administered to a pregnant patient may cross the placental membrane by passive diffusion or active transport and enter the fetal circulation. This can lead to teratogenic effects in utero, especially during the first and third trimesters.

Blood-brain barrier
The blood-brain barrier consists of specialized capillary walls in the central nervous system (CNS) and surrounding glial membranes. Separating the CNS from the systemic circulation, it allows only nonionized drugs to enter the CNS. Although protective, the blood-brain barrier complicates treatment of CNS disorders. To circumvent the barrier, some medications may be given by intrathecal injection.

plasma and undergo filtration by the kidneys.

In the liver, the site of most metabolism, drugs are broken down by enzymes. This increases their water solubility, promoting their excretion. However, metabolism increases the fat solubility of certain drugs, which are then excreted through the biliary system.

Metabolites
The end products of metabolism, metabolites typically are inactive forms of the original drug, with no pharmacologic effect. However, metabolites of some drugs remain active and can cause a reaction. Imipramine, an antidepressant agent, has an active metabolite, desipramine, in addition to several inactive metabolites.

In a few cases, metabolism converts an inactive drug into an active metabolite. Levodopa, for instance, is metabolized after crossing the blood-brain barrier. The resulting metabolite, dopamine, counteracts symptoms of Parkinson's disease.

Variations in drug metabolism
The body doesn't metabolize all drugs to the same degree or by the same mechanisms. And it doesn't metabolize certain drugs at all. Unmetabolized drugs, such as aminoglycosides, pass through the body unchanged.

At the other extreme are drugs that stimulate their own metabolism. Barbiturates, for example, use a process called autoinduction to reduce the concentration of active drug in the body. In foreign induction, a related process, one drug stimulates another's metabolism. Foreign induction occurs with phenobarbital, which induces enzyme activity that stimulates theophylline metabolism.

Some drugs inhibit enzyme metabolism. This can cause a drug administered concurrently to accumulate in the body, increasing the risk of toxicity or an adverse reaction. For instance, if your patient received cimetidine and theophylline concurrently, theophylline would accumulate in his bloodstream because cimetidine inhibits its metabolism.

A disease can affect drug metabolism as well, by interfering with hepatic blood flow or transport of drugs to the liver. A drug given to a patient with end-stage cirrhosis, for instance, might not reach metabolic sites because the disease reduces blood flow to the liver. Likewise, in patients with CHF, retained fluid impedes transport of drugs to metabolic sites.

Age, life-style, diet, and genetic factors also play a role in drug metabolism. Infants and elderly patients typically metabolize drugs more slowly than adults, so they're more vulnerable to drug accumulation and toxicity. Drug metabolism may be faster in smokers than in nonsmokers because cigarette smoke contains substances that induce production of hepatic enzymes. A diet high in fat or carbohydrates may slow the metabolism of certain drugs, whereas a high-protein diet may speed metabolism.

Excretion

The body excretes most drugs through the kidneys. However, some drugs are excreted hepatically, via the bile into the feces, and a few drugs leave the body by minor routes, including lung exhalations, saliva, sweat, and breast milk. When natural excretion mechanisms fail, such as from drug overdose or renal dysfunction, drugs can be removed through dialysis.

Renal excretion
For excretion by the kidneys, a drug usually must undergo glomerular filtration. In this process, endothelial pores in glomerular capillaries filter unbound drug particles. Most drugs are reabsorbed passively in the proximal and distal tubules, then return to the bloodstream where they continue to exert an effect.

Large-molecular-weight compounds, such as the plasma protein albumin, do not undergo glomerular filtration. Highly protein-bound drugs are secreted actively into the urine.

When considering a drug's renal excretion, you must take into account your patient's sex, age, and renal status. Typically, females, elderly patients, and those with renal disorders excrete drugs more slowly and thus are more vulnerable to drug accumulation and toxicity. Also, the kidneys excrete ionized, water-soluble drugs and metabolites more effectively than nonionized, lipid-soluble substances.

Hepatic excretion
Highly ionized drugs and metabolites with a large molecular weight may be extracted by the liver from the bloodstream and secreted into the bile. Because bile enters the duodenum, such substances commonly end up in the feces. However, intestinal pH or flora may convert a metabolite back into a nonionized, lipid-soluble form, returning it to the bloodstream and prolonging its action.

Other factors affecting drug action

A drug's blood concentration level, half-life, accumulation, and clearance affect its action.

Blood level
You're probably aware that the drug's blood level plays an important role in a patient's response to therapy. In fact, by knowing the blood level, you can help determine if your patient is achieving the goals of his medication regimen. Factors that influence the blood level include the amount of drug absorbed, the rate of absorption, the drug's distribution, the process and timing of drug metabolism, and the rate and route of excretion.

A drug's therapeutic range extends from the minimum effective concentration (the minimum amount that must be present in the blood to produce a therapeutic effect) to the minimum toxic concentration (the minimum amount causing toxic effects). The duration of a drug's action is the time its blood level remains between these values.

Drugs that take a long time to reach the therapeutic range have limitations. For example, the cardiac glycoside digoxin may take 8 days to reach its therapeutic range when administered in maintenance doses. Obviously, this delay is unacceptable if your patient has a life-threatening arrhythmia. So you'd expect to administer a large initial dose, or loading dose, to rapidly bring the blood level to the desired range. After that, you'd give smaller daily doses to maintain this level.

Importance of half-life

Your patient's drug dosage depends on half-life — the time it takes for a drug's blood level to fall to half its peak amount. This diagram shows the time required (2½ hours) for the blood level of gentamicin, given by I.V. injection, to fall to 3 mcg/ml — one-half its peak level of 6 mcg/ml.

Determining half-life
Blood samples taken at specific intervals can reveal how much of the drug remains in the patient's bloodstream. This information helps to establish how much of a drug to give — and how often — to maintain a therapeutic blood level. Some drugs have a half-life of 30 minutes or less; others, 8 hours or more.

When half-life lengthens
A drug may have a prolonged half-life when given to a patient who has trouble metabolizing or excreting drugs. For example, a patient with hepatic or renal disease may retain a drug in the bloodstream or tissues for a prolonged period, extending the drug's half-life. In this case, expect to adjust the dose or the frequency, or both, to prevent drug accumulation and toxicity.

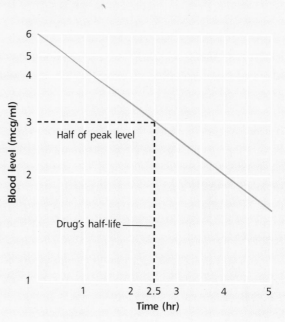

Drug half-life
Knowing a drug's half-life — the time it takes for the peak blood level to drop by half — helps establish the optimum dosage regimen. For most drugs, half-life correlates roughly with the duration of effective action. Most drugs given in a single dose are eliminated from the body completely after five half-lives. (See *Importance of half-life.*)

Many new recombinant protein drugs have very short half-lives. For this reason, they must be administered at their site of action so that they won't be metabolized before they can exert their therapeutic effect.

Drug accumulation
If each successive dose of a drug is given before the previous dose has been completely excreted, the drug will accumulate. This process will continue until the dose the patient is receiving equals the amount he's excreting. At this point, blood drug levels reach a *steady state.*

Once a steady state has been achieved, the blood level will remain within a therapeutic range. However, it won't remain static but will increase, peak, and decline within this range.

Drug clearance
Clearance, or the time needed to eliminate a drug from the body, can have important implications for drug therapy. The more rapidly a drug is eliminated, the higher its clearance rate. When administering a drug with a high clearance rate, you may need to give it more frequently and in larger doses. On the other hand, when administering a drug with a low clearance rate, you must use caution to prevent toxicity from drug accumulation.

Pharmacodynamics

After absorption, drug molecules migrate to target tissues or organs, interacting with receptors to cause the *drug action*. A series of complex physical or chemical reactions, the drug action in turn alters the function of the target cell, causing the *drug effect*. The drug effect may be the desired therapeutic response — or it may be an adverse reaction.

The entire process, encompassing both drug action and drug effect, is called the pharmacodynamic phase. The study of the interactions between drugs and living tissues, pharmacodynamics serves as the basis of drug treatment.

Drug-receptor interactions

Drug-receptor interactions hinge on the concept that each drug is selectively active and attracted to a specific receptor. A certain portion of the drug molecule interacts selectively or combines with a receptor to produce a pharmacologic effect. Although a drug can't force a cell or tissue to assume a new function, it can modify the cell's function or environment in a way that interrupts, replaces, or potentiates a physiologic process.

When a drug modifies cell function
Some drugs interact with receptors or enzymes to alter cell function. A drug can be an agonist or antagonist in the way it works at a receptor site. An agonist mimics the activity of the hormone or other natural chemical that normally binds to the receptor site. This triggers *intrinsic activity,* a response that enhances the receptor's functional properties.

In contrast, an antagonist blocks the action of the agonist drug or the natural substance that normally acts on the receptor. An antagonist may compete directly with an agonist or it may be drawn to the same receptors. In either case, binding of an antagonist with a receptor stops the agonist from binding, preventing the intrinsic activity.

A drug may also interact with enzymes to stimulate or depress certain biochemical reac-

tions. For example, neostigmine, used to treat myasthenia gravis, interacts with the enzyme acetylcholinesterase to prevent acetylcholine destruction. This causes acetylcholine to accumulate in the tissues, resulting in enhanced cell activity that increases gastric contractions and gastric acid secretion.

When a drug modifies cell environment
Some drugs lack structural specificity, acting through general effects on cellular membranes and processes. By penetrating cells or accumulating in cell membranes, these drugs interfere physically or chemically with a cell function or basic metabolic process. Typically, such drugs alter a cell's physical or chemical environment to produce a systemic effect.

For instance, if you administer sodium bicarbonate I.V. to a patient with severe diabetic ketoacidosis, the drug will alter the cell environment by restoring normal pH. This change, in turn, will improve cell function. Other drugs that act nonspecifically on the cell environment include osmotic diuretics, stool softeners, skin protectants, cathartics, plasma expanders, and chemical antidotes.

Outcome of drug action

Both the location and function of a drug's receptors determine the outcome of drug action. Drugs that interact with common receptors throughout the body, such as chemotherapeutic drugs, have widespread effects. Obviously, this poses a danger if the drug causes a toxic reaction.

On the other hand, drugs that interact with specific receptors in highly differentiated cells cause a safe, predictable response. For example, controlled doses of radioactive iodine, which has a strong affinity for receptor sites in the thyroid gland, effectively treat hyperthyroidism.

The outcome of drug action also depends on whether the drug affects target organs and tissues directly or indirectly. Theophylline, used to treat asthma, directly modifies bronchodilator receptors in the lungs to improve ventilation. Such a direct effect promotes a rapid clinical response. (Theophylline also appears in the peripheral circulation, so the doctor can use the drug's blood levels to determine the correct dosage.)

In contrast, levodopa exerts an indirect action on tissues. A dopamine precursor, it breaks down into dopamine after crossing the blood-brain barrier. To slow peripheral breakdown of levodopa and increase its availability for transport to the brain, the doctor may prescribe it in combination with carbidopa. Although effective, this approach produces a slower therapeutic response than if dopamine could be supplied directly.

Dose-response relationship

Drug concentration at the receptor site also affects the outcome of drug action. The patient's response to a drug reflects the size of the administered dose. Typically, as the dose increases, the pharmacologic response increases gradually and continuously until receptor sites become fully occupied with the drug. At this point, increasing the dose won't enhance the response, but it will increase the risk for adverse reactions. A dose-response curve illustrates the relationship between dose and response.

Because all drugs elicit more than one response, the dose-response relationship isn't an absolute. In small doses, for example, morphine may calm an irritable bowel. But in larger doses, it acts as a narcotic analgesic. Furthermore, an adverse reaction can occur when administering therapeutic doses. For instance, in some patients, morphine can cause respiratory depression when given in doses needed to effectively control pain.

Drug potency and efficacy

A drug's action also depends on its potency and efficacy. *Potency* refers to the amount of drug needed to produce a desired response. By comparing the required doses of two comparable drugs, you can determine which one is more potent. For example, when giving tetracycline, you need to administer 1,000 to 2,000 mg/day to achieve a therapeutic effect, compared with just 100 to 200 mg/day of

doxycycline. Because doxycycline achieves comparable effects at a lower dosage, it's considered more potent.

Efficacy refers to the effect achieved when the dose-response curve reaches its plateau. For example, at its plateau, morphine relieves a greater degree of pain than aspirin. But to assess a drug's efficacy, you must also consider the incidence and severity of adverse reactions. A drug that's likely to cause severe adverse reactions before reaching its plateau has reduced efficacy. Efficacy also decreases if the plateau falls short of the maximal drug amount needed for effective treatment.

Adverse reactions

An undesirable or harmful response to a drug, an adverse reaction can occur in any patient. It can range from a mild reaction that disappears when the drug is withdrawn to a severe reaction that progresses to a chronic, debilitating disease. The patient's response to a given drug and his risk for adverse reactions depend on many factors. (See *Predicting a patient's response to drug therapy.*)

Adverse reactions can be predictable or unpredictable. Predictable reactions are usually dose related, whereas unpredictable reactions typically result from patient sensitivity. Although some predictable reactions can be prevented, others can't be prevented because they're closely tied to the drug's therapeutic effects.

Predictable reactions

Administering an excessive dose can cause two types of predictable reactions—an excessive therapeutic effect or drug accumulation. An excessive therapeutic effect most commonly occurs with drugs requiring precise, individualized dose calculation. For example, a diabetic patient who receives too much insulin will suffer an excessive blood glucose decrease.

Accumulation can occur with certain chemotherapeutic drugs. If these drugs accumulate around hair follicles, they can damage the follicles, causing alopecia.

Giving a drug too rapidly can also cause a predictable adverse reaction. For example, rapid administration of I.V. aminophylline can cause hypotension and circulatory collapse.

Most drugs produce a secondary pharmacologic action in addition to a therapeutic effect. In some cases, this secondary action is an undesirable but predictable adverse reaction. For example, morphine may help control a patient's pain but may also cause constipation and respiratory depression. Occasionally, though, a doctor will prescribe a drug specifically for its secondary action. For example, minoxidil is used mainly as an antihypertensive, but it may be prescribed in topical form to treat alopecia.

Unpredictable reactions

Upon first exposure to a drug, a patient's immune system may identify the drug, its metabolite, or a drug contaminant as a dangerous foreign substance that must be neutralized or destroyed. This initial exposure sensitizes the immune system, which then mobilizes to fight the drug if the patient receives a subsequent dose of the same or a similar substance. Called a hypersensitivity reaction, this unpredictable adverse reaction is a type of allergic reaction.

Allergic reactions range in severity from mild (type IV hypersensitivity) to life-threatening (type I hypersensitivity). Mild allergic reactions include contact dermatitis, such as from a topical medication; life-threatening reactions include anaphylactic shock, such as from penicillin.

Another type of unpredictable reaction occurs in patients who are highly susceptible to a drug's primary or secondary actions. (Such increased susceptibility may stem from altered pharmacokinetics leading to an excessively high serum concentration level or increased receptor sensitivity.) In these patients, even a normal therapeutic dose may trigger an adverse reaction.

Idiosyncratic reactions are also unpredictable. For example, phenobarbital, a sedative-

---

Predicting a patient's response to drug therapy

Because no two patients are identical, the response to a given drug may vary greatly. To help predict how your patient will respond to a particular drug regimen, consider the following factors:

Patient factors
• Age
• Albumin concentration
• Body mass
• Body rhythm variations
• Disease
• Environmental factors
• Fever
• General physiologic status (including cardiovascular, GI, hepatic, immunologic, and renal function)
• Genetic constitution
• Immunization status
• Infection
• Lactation
• Life-style (including diet, alcohol intake, exercise, and smoking)
• Occupational exposures
• Pregnancy
• Starvation
• Stress
• Trauma

Drug factors
• Additives
• Administration route
• Administration technique
• Dosage
• Expiration date
• Number of drugs administered
• Variation among brands

---

hypnotic agent, may cause nervousness and excitability in some patients. Idiosyncratic reactions may have a genetic cause.

Iatrogenic reactions

Sometimes, a drug produces an iatrogenic reaction — a pathologic disorder unrelated to the condition for which the drug was given. The reaction may be predictable or unpredictable. Typically, it manifests as a blood dyscrasia, liver or kidney dysfunction, or a skin condition. In a pregnant patient, it may cause teratogenic effects.

Misdiagnosis is a potentially serious consequence of an iatrogenic reaction. Confronted with the pathologic disorder, the doctor may mistakenly treat the disorder instead of discontinuing the drug.

Drug interactions

Some drugs interact when given together, neutralizing their therapeutic effects or causing an adverse reaction. Other drugs can interact with certain foods or alter the results of laboratory tests, whereas I.V. drug interactions can present their own unique problems.

To reduce the risk of interactions, find out if your patient is receiving any other drugs, either prescribed or over-the-counter, before giving any new one. Be especially careful when caring for elderly patients. Many are receiving multiple drugs, and their age makes them more sensitive to drug effects. As a safeguard, make it a habit during the initial health history to ask your patient which drugs he's taking.

Interactions between drugs

An interaction between drugs can cause one of several effects. Both drugs may simply promote the action of the most active component of the combination. Called *indifference,* this is the most common type of interaction. Indifference doesn't alter the therapeutic effects of either drug or produce unpredictable adverse reactions.

In an *additive interaction,* the total effect of the two drugs together equals the sum of the drugs' separate effects. Sometimes, additive interactions are intended and desirable—for instance, aspirin and codeine are often prescribed together to enhance pain relief. But an unplanned additive interaction can

have adverse effects, causing extreme sedation or other dangerous conditions.

In a *synergistic interaction,* one drug multiplies the other's effects, causing a total effect greater than the sum of the drugs' separate effects. Like an additive interaction, synergism can be beneficial or harmful.

In an *antagonistic interaction,* one drug interferes with the other's actions, negating its therapeutic value. Suppose, for example, you administer levodopa and pyridoxine (vitamin B_6) to your patient at the same time. Normally, levodopa reduces stiffness, rigidity, and other symptoms of Parkinson's disease. However, because pyridoxine antagonizes levodopa, your patient may not experience levodopa's therapeutic actions.

Interactions with food

Food can delay or reduce absorption of an oral medication, reducing the drug's therapeutic effects. With an acidic drug, however, food enhances absorption by stimulating gastric acid secretion.

By the same token, some drugs can alter the metabolism of nutrients in food. A drug taken with a certain food may bind with the food, for instance, impairing vitamin and mineral absorption. And certain drugs can interfere with the body's vitamin supply even when given alone. Broad-spectrum antibiotics, for instance, alter the intestinal flora that produce vitamin K, impeding synthesis of this vitamin.

Interference with laboratory tests

Certain drugs can cause misleading laboratory test results. For example, the calorimetric method used to measure serum creatinine levels can't differentiate between creatinine and a noncreatinine chromogen contained in many cephalosporins, such as cefazolin and cefoxitin. Therefore, if your patient is receiving a cephalosporin, you should stay alert for a falsely elevated creatinine level. Similarly, iron supplements can skew the results of stool guaiac tests, and ascorbic acid can lead to inaccurate urine glucose test results.

Some drugs can alter your patient's electrocardiogram (ECG) pattern, possibly causing incorrect assessment. For example, quinidine, an antiarrhythmic, can widen the QRS complex and prolong the QT interval. If you saw these features on your patient's ECG strip without checking his medication record, you might suspect he has a cardiac conduction problem.

I.V. drug incompatibility

Administering incompatible I.V. drugs or solutions to your patient at the same time can cause an undesired physical or chemical reaction. One drug may inactivate the other; or, worse yet, the drugs may interact in a way that harms the patient.

Mixing physically incompatible I.V. drugs causes a reaction that can interfere with the pharmacologic action of one or both drugs. Color changes, gas formation, cloudiness, or precipitation can result. Suppose, for example, the doctor prescribes I.V. phenytoin to control your patient's seizures. In 0.9% sodium chloride solution, phenytoin remains stable. But when the drug is placed in an I.V. line containing dextrose, a cloudy white precipitate will form. Infusing a precipitate can cause pain, thrombophlebitis, or an embolism. That's why you must always flush the line with 0.9% sodium chloride solution before and after infusing phenytoin.

I.V. penicillin and aminoglycoside antibiotics (such as amikacin, gentamicin, and tobramycin) are also incompatible. Prolonged contact — either in an I.V. solution or in the body of a patient who has severe renal failure — can inactivate the aminoglycoside. This can cause problems, particularly if you're trying to monitor the serum aminoglycoside level of a patient with renal failure. Because the penicillin in a blood sample will continue to neutralize the aminoglycoside, the aminoglycoside level may be falsely decreased unless the laboratory measures the drug's blood level promptly.

Adsorption
Some I.V. drugs adhere to plastic containers, syringes, and administration sets. This adherence, known as adsorption, can reduce drug availability or cause a precipitate to form. Diazepam, for instance, forms a precipitate after prolonged contact with plastic. For this reason, you should administer I.V. diazepam by slow injection *directly* into a large vein. If this isn't possible, you may inject it into an existing I.V. line. However, be sure to flush the line with dextrose 5% in water beforehand, then inject the drug as close to the I.V. insertion site as possible.

You should also be aware that some biotechnologic drugs, such as interleukins, interferons, and colony-stimulating factors, adhere to I.V. bags, bottles, syringes, and tubing. To prevent this problem, these items should be coated with human serum albumin before you use them.

Photolysis
Some I.V. drugs become discolored on exposure to light. Discoloration may or may not indicate chemical breakdown. Nevertheless, you should consult the pharmacist before administering a drug that's changed color.

Preventing incompatibility
To avoid I.V. drug incompatibility, don't combine any drugs if you're unsure of their compatibility. Also, before administering an unfamiliar drug or drug combination, consult the pharmacist or the manufacturer's recommendations. For general guidelines, you can use a drug compatibility chart. As a further precaution, never combine more than two drugs in the same syringe.

If your patient's I.V. fluid contains multivitamins or other additives, confirm compatibility before administering other drugs through the same line. If you can't easily access the patient's peripheral veins, consider asking the doctor to place a central line or replace the peripheral line with a multilumen catheter so you can administer incompatible drugs simultaneously.

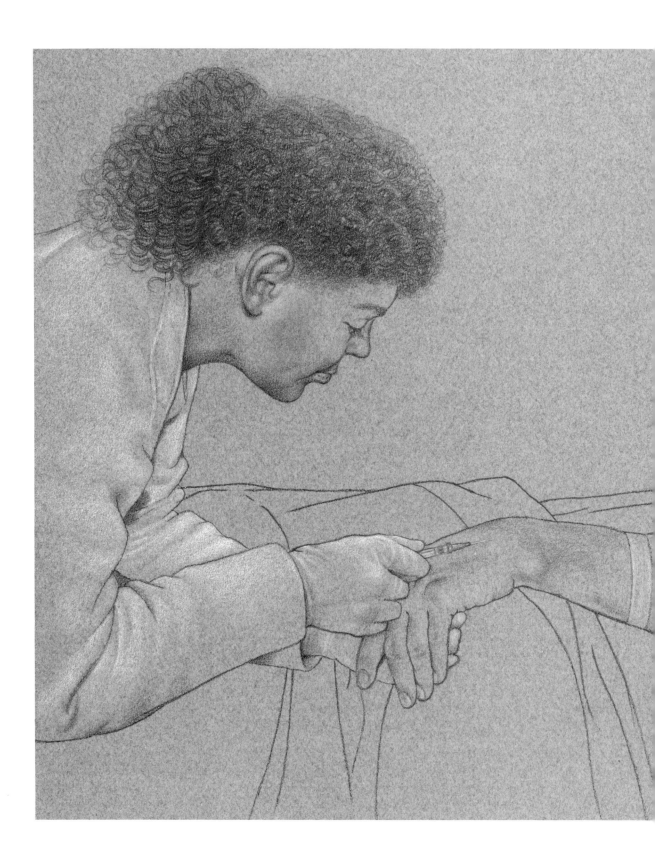

CHAPTER 2

Giving drugs through peripheral veins

So many patients receive some form of I.V. therapy as part of their care that you may consider it routine. Still, continual advances in each kind of I.V. therapy make it a challenge. Depending on the type of therapy chosen for your patient, you may both insert and maintain your patient's I.V. line. You're also responsible for teaching patients how various I.V. methods work and, in the case of some home care patients, how to maintain the lines themselves.

This chapter covers the principles, equipment, and methods used in peripheral venous therapy. By presenting detailed information about the newest, most advanced I.V. therapy techniques and equipment, the chapter helps you keep current with this changing field.

The chapter focuses on giving both drugs and blood products via peripheral veins. The first major section covers peripheral venous therapy, including how to give bolus doses, intermittent infusions, and continuous infusions.

Peripheral veins and drug delivery

This illustration shows the location of the veins most often used in peripheral venous therapy. The inset shows a catheter in place, delivering the drug directly into the circulation.

Catheter in vein

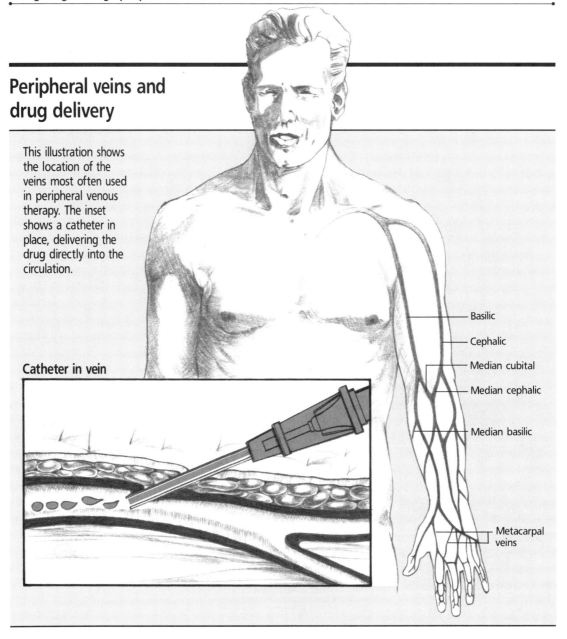

- Basilic
- Cephalic
- Median cubital
- Median cephalic
- Median basilic
- Metacarpal veins

Next, comes a section on transfusing blood products. The chapter then closes with explanations of how to use patient-controlled analgesia and infusion pumps and controllers.

For your convenience, each section follows the same format. After a brief overview, you'll find a discussion of the necessary equipment, administration guidelines, complications, and nursing considerations, including patient teaching.

Before reading these major sections of the chapter, however, you should review the advantages and disadvantages of peripheral venous therapy. As you'll see, these advantages and disadvantages relate directly to the pharmacokinetics of this delivery method.

Advantages

Peripheral venous delivery of drugs has distinct advantages over other methods, such as oral, subcutaneous, and I.M. delivery. When a drug is given through the peripheral veins, the entire drug reaches the systemic circulation immediately. Thus, I.V. drugs begin to act almost instantly. By contrast, oral drugs must be absorbed into the bloodstream before they can take effect. Some oral drugs are unstable in gastric juices and digestive enzymes or irritate gastric mucosa. With subcutaneous and I.M. delivery, absorption may be erratic if the patient has impaired tissue perfusion or excessive fat tissue. Plus, with other methods, less than 100% of the drug reaches the systemic circulation. Certain oral drugs, for instance, must first pass through the liver, where significant amounts are lost before they reach the bloodstream. (See *Peripheral veins and drug delivery.*)

I.V. drug delivery also allows more accurate dosing than other methods. Because delivery is immediate, an effective dose can be administered by adjusting the concentration and flow rate of the I.V. solution.

And I.V. drug delivery causes less discomfort than either I.M. or subcutaneous injection. That's because veins have a higher pain threshold than muscle or subcutaneous tissue. When venous irritation does occur, the I.V. solution or concentration can be changed or the rate slowed, or the I.V. site could be changed.

Disadvantages
As with any invasive procedure, the peripheral I.V. method carries associated risks, including infection and bleeding. Plus, if the drug causes adverse effects, they may be immediate and severe.

Incompatibility—both pharmaceutical and therapeutic—can be a drawback. When two drugs or I.V. solutions can't be mixed with each other, they are considered pharmaceutically incompatible. When two drugs negate each other's actions, they are therapeutically incompatible.

Giving drugs I.V. is impossible with some patients. If a patient's veins are in poor condition or if they've collapsed from hypovolemia or vasoconstriction, they won't be accessible.

Finally, the peripheral venous method is more costly than the oral, subcutaneous, and I.M. methods. (See *Administering common I.V. drugs,* pages 20 to 25.)

Peripheral venous therapy

You'll use peripheral I.V. therapy when a patient needs surgery, or when a patient faces a life-threatening situation and needs immediate drug intervention. You'll also administer peripheral I.V. therapy to critically ill patients who require constant titration of medications. To give drugs in large doses or drugs that can cause subcutaneous or I.M. damage, you'll typically use I.V. therapy. And certain medications can only be given I.V.—dopamine, for example.

Drugs may be given I.V. using one of three methods: bolus injection, intermittent infusion, or continuous infusion.

Your role includes inserting the I.V. needle or catheter, initiating the therapy, caring for the site during therapy, and discontinuing therapy. When I.V. therapy has been ordered, you'll need to select the proper equipment and prepare it for use. Then you must choose the best possible venipuncture site and device for the patient's needs.

Equipment
Before peripheral I.V. therapy, you'll decide which type of venipuncture device is best for your patient and the kind of infusion you're using. You'll also determine whether an in-line filter or a filter needle is needed, according to the policy of your health care facility.

Selecting a venipuncture device
The venipuncture device you choose hinges on several factors, including your patient's age, weight, and condition. A rule of thumb is to select the device with the shortest length and the smallest diameter that allows for proper administration of the solution. Selection also depends on the type of solution to be used, the frequency and duration of the infusion, and the types of veins available.

You'll choose from among three types of venipuncture devices: a winged infusion set, an over-the-needle catheter, and a through-the-needle catheter. (See *Choosing a venipuncture device,* page 26.)

(Text continues on page 25.)

Administering common I.V. drugs

DRUG	I.V. PUSH	INTERMITTENT INFUSION	CONTINUOUS INFUSION	COMPATIBILITY
acyclovir	Not recommended.	5 mg/kg every 8 hr (15 mg/kg daily) diluted with 50 to 125 ml dextrose 5% in water (D₅W), maximum concentration of 7 mg/ml, and infused over at least 1 hr; maximum dosage is 30 mg/kg daily.	5 mg/kg every 8 hr diluted with 50 to 125 ml D₅W and infused over 1 to 3 hr.	D₅W
aminophylline	Give undiluted loading dose (25 mg/ml) slowly, not exceeding 25 mg/min; don't give through a central venous catheter; rapid injection can be fatal.	Not recommended.	For maintenance therapy, administer desired dose in a large volume (500 to 1,000 ml) of compatible solution; adjust infusion rate to deliver prescribed amount each hour.	D₅W, 0.9% sodium chloride solution, lactated Ringer's (LR) solution, dextrose 5% in LR (D₅LR), and other common I.V. solutions
ampicillin	Inject reconstituted drug into large vein or catheter over 10 to 15 min; after injection, flush catheter with 0.9% sodium chloride solution.	Give diluted solution through I.V. piggyback or catheter over 30 to 60 min.	Not recommended.	D₅W, 0.9% sodium chloride solution
atropine sulfate	300 to 500 mcg initially; repeat every 3 to 5 min, if needed, up to 2 mg total; subsequent doses of 300 mcg to 1mg every 4 to 6 hr may be administered.	Not recommended.	Not recommended.	Doesn't require dilution
calcium chloride	200 mg/min; maximum dose is 1 g; wait about 2 hr before repeating.	Dilute 1 g in at least 100 ml, and administer over 30 min (preferably longer), using an infusion control device; up to 2 g daily may be administered.	Dilute 1 g in 1,000 ml and administer over at least 8 hr.	D₅W, 0.9% sodium chloride solution, and other common I.V. solutions
cefazolin	Inject the solution into a vein over 3 to 5 min or into I.V. tubing containing a free-flowing compatible solution.	Insert a 21G or 23G needle into the port of primary tubing, and infuse 50 to 100 ml of solution over 30 min.	Not recommended.	D₅W, 0.9% sodium chloride solution, and other common I.V. solutions
cefoxitin	Inject diluted drug over 3 to 5 min directly into vein through an intermittent infusion device or into an I.V. line containing a free-flowing, compatible solution.	Give 50 to 100 ml solution through a butterfly or scalp vein needle, an intermittent infusion device, or a patent I.V. line at the ordered flow rate; interrupt primary solution during cefoxitin infusion; administer over 15 to 30 min.	Infuse up to 1 liter of solution over the prescribed time.	D₅W, 0.9% sodium chloride solution, and other common I.V. solutions

Administering common I.V. drugs *(continued)*

DRUG	I.V. PUSH	INTERMITTENT INFUSION	CONTINUOUS INFUSION	COMPATIBILITY
cimetidine	Inject diluted drug over at least 2 min directly into vein or through an I.V. line containing free-flowing, compatible solution; rapid injection may increase the risk of arrhythmias and hypotension.	Give 50 to 100 ml of diluted drug over 15 to 20 min, using an intermittent infusion device or infused into an I.V. line containing a free-flowing, compatible solution.	Dilute 900 mg of drug in 100 to 1,000 ml of compatible solution; using an infusion pump, give no more than 37.5 mg/hr; total dosage: not to exceed 900 mg daily.	D_5W, 0.9% sodium chloride solution, D_5LR, and other common I.V. solutions
clindamycin	Not recommended.	Usually 300 mg but up to 600 mg every 6 hr; may also be administered at a dose of 600 to 900 mg every 8 hr; concentration should not exceed 6 mg/ml; infuse no faster than 300 mg/15 min.	Not recommended.	D_5W, 0.9% sodium chloride solution, D_5LR, and other common I.V. solutions
dexamethasone	0.5 to 100 mg in one dose; up to 200 mg daily in divided doses.	0.5 to 100 mg daily in divided doses administered every 4 to 6 hr; dilute each dose in 25 to 50 ml, and administer over 15 to 30 min.	Not recommended.	D_5W, 0.9% sodium chloride solution
diazepam	*For a patient not on a ventilator:* up to 20 mg every 4 hr; administer no faster than 2 mg/min; must be given with doctor present. *For a patient on a ventilator:* 5 to 10 mg.	Not recommended.	Not recommended.	Doesn't require dilution
digoxin	Rapid digitalization: 6 to 12 mcg/kg, with an initial dose of 0.25 to 0.5 mg followed at 4- to 6-hr interval with additional dose; maintenance dose is usually 0.125 to 0.25 mg up to 1 mg daily; administer each dose over at least 1 min.	Not recommended.	Not recommended.	Doesn't require dilution
diphenhydramine	Up to 50 mg four times a day; administer each dose over 1 min.	Dilute each dose in at least 25 ml, and administer over 15 to 30 min.	Not recommended.	D_5W, 0.9% sodium chloride solution, dextrose 5% in 0.9% sodium chloride solution, LR
dobutamine	Not recommended.	Not recommended.	Usually 2.5 to 10 mcg/kg/min but up to 40 mcg/kg/min; dilute each 250-mg dose in 50 ml (preferably more); use infusion control device.	D_5W, 0:9% sodium chloride solution

(continued)

Administering common I.V. drugs (continued)

DRUG	I.V. PUSH	INTERMITTENT INFUSION	CONTINUOUS INFUSION	COMPATIBILITY
dopamine	Not recommended.	Not recommended.	Usually 5 to 20 mcg/kg/min, but up to 50 mcg/kg/min; dilute each 200-mg dose in 250 ml or more; use infusion control device.	D₅W, 0.9% sodium chloride solution, LR
epinephrine hydrochloride	Slowly inject drug directly into vein or into an I.V. line containing a free-flowing, compatible solution.	Using an appropriately diluted concentration, piggyback drug into a compatible I.V. solution and infuse 1 to 4 mcg/min.	Not recommended; use infusion control device.	D₅W, 0.9% sodium chloride solution, LR, D₅W in 0.9% sodium chloride solution
erythromycin	Not recommended.	Infuse diluted solution through a patent I.V. line over 20 to 60 min.	Infuse diluted solution over 4 to 8 hr; longer infusion risks loss of patency.	0.9% sodium chloride solution
famotidine	Inject 5 or 10 ml of reconstituted drug over at least 2 min.	Infuse drug diluted in 100 ml over 15 to 30 min.	Not recommended.	D₅W, 0.9% sodium chloride solution, LR, dextrose 10% in water (D₁₀W)
furosemide	20 to 100 mg maximum, administered in a single dose at a rate not to exceed 20 mg/min; maximum daily dosage is 500 mg.	20 to 200 mg at a rate not to exceed 4 mg/min; dilute each 100-mg dose in at least 25 ml or 5 mg/ml (preferable 50 ml or 2 mg/ml); maximum dosage is 4 g/24 hr.	1 g diluted in suitable volume (250 ml) and administered no faster than 4 mg/min; maximum daily dosage: 4 g; maximum concentration: 5 mg/ml; use infusion control device.	D₅W, 0.9% sodium chloride solution, LR
gentamicin sulfate	Not recommended.	Usually 2 mg/kg/day but up to 5 mg/kg/day administered in divided doses every 6 to 8 hr; dilute 1 mg in 1 ml, and administer each dose over 30 to 60 min.	Not recommended.	D₅W, 0.9% sodium chloride solution, LR, and other common I.V. solutions
heparin sodium	Usually 1,000 to 10,000 units every 4 to 6 hr; administer each dose over 1 to 2 min.	Usually 1,000 to 10,000 units every 4 to 6 hr; dilute each dose in at least 25 ml, and administer over 15 to 30 min.	Daily dosage: up to 30,000 units added to a suitable volume of I.V. fluid and administered over 24 hr; use infusion control device.	D₅W, 0.9% sodium chloride solution
hydrocortisone sodium succinate	Up to 1 g daily in a single or divided dose; administer 1 g over 5 min.	Usually 100 to 200 mg every 4 to 12 hr or 500 mg twice a day, or 1 g daily, diluted to 1 mg/ml; administer each dose over 15 to 30 min.	Up to 1 g diluted in a suitable volume no more concentrated than 1 mg/ml and administered continuously; use infusion control device.	D₅W, 0.9% sodium chloride solution, amino acids
insulin (regular)	Up to 15 units.	Dose must be individualized; dilute each dose to 20 ml or more, and administer over 15 to 20 min.	Initial rate: 0.1 unit/kg/hr; rate of infusion is titrated upward according to patient's metabolic response; maximum infusion rate is 0.5 unit/kg/hr; dilute to 0.2 unit/ml; use infusion control device.	D₅W, 0.9% sodium chloride solution, amino acids, dextrose 5% in 0.45% sodium chloride solution

Administering common I.V. drugs (continued)

DRUG	I.V. PUSH	INTERMITTENT INFUSION	CONTINUOUS INFUSION	COMPATIBILITY
magnesium sulfate	Inject directly into vein, not exceeding 150 mg/min.	Administer diluted drug over 1 to 3 hr.	Give by infusion pump, not exceeding 150 mg/min (1.2 mEq/min).	D_5W, 0.9% sodium chloride solution, total parenteral nutrition
mannitol	12.5 to 200 g daily in divided doses; administer 50 g over 3 to 5 min.	Dosage range is 12.5 to 200 g daily; dilute each 12.5-g dose in 50 ml or more of solution, and administer over at least 5 min; larger daily dosages are administered in divided doses at equal intervals.	12.5 to 50 g in 250 to 500 ml administered continuously; use infusion control device.	D_5W, 0.9% sodium chloride solution
meperidine	Usually 25 to 50 mg but up to 100 mg every 4 to 6 hr; concentration should not exceed 10 mg/ml; administer each 25-mg dose no faster than over 3 min.	Not recommended.	Not recommended.	D_5W, 0.9% sodium chloride solution
methylprednisolone sodium succinate	10 mg to 2 g in a single dose; up to 8 g daily in divided doses; dilute each gram in at least 50 ml; administer each dose over 1 to 5 min.	Dilute each gram in 50 ml or more, and administer over 15 to 30 min.	Not recommended.	D_5W, 0.9% sodium chloride solution
metronidazole	Not recommended.	Loading dose is 15 mg/kg diluted to a concentration of 8 mg/ml in 0.9% sodium chloride solution and infused over 1 hr; maintenance dosage is 7.5 mg/kg every 6 hr, diluted to a concentration of 8 mg/ml in 0.9% sodium chloride solution and infused over 1 hr.	7.5 mg/kg every 6 hr, diluted to a concentration of 2 to 8 mg/ml in 0.9% sodium chloride solution and infused over 1 to 3 hr.	D_5W, 0.9% sodium chloride solution
morphine	*For patients on a ventilator:* 5 to 10 mg, not to exceed 200 mg/24 hr. *For patients not on a ventilator:* usually 2 to 5 mg but up to 20 mg in 4 hr; dilute each dose to 1 mg/ml, and administer over 3 to 5 min.	Not recommended.	Initial dose is 1 to 10 mg (usually 5 mg); dose adjustments: 0.5 to 4 mg/hr increments; use infusion control device; doctor must be present for first 10 minutes of initial dose.	D_5W, 0.9% sodium chloride solution, LR, D_5LR
nafcillin	500 mg to 2 g every 4 hr; dilute each dose to 15 to 30 ml, and inject over 5 to 10 min through a running I.V. line.	Dilute each gram in 50 to 100 ml or more, and administer each dose over 30 to 60 min.	Not recommended.	D_5W, 0.9% sodium chloride solution, LR, D_5LR, and other common I.V. solutions

(continued)

Administering common I.V. drugs *(continued)*

DRUG	I.V. PUSH	INTERMITTENT INFUSION	CONTINUOUS INFUSION	COMPATIBILITY
nitroglycerin	Not recommended.	Not recommended.	Initial dose of 6.6 mcg, followed by a double dose every 3 to 5 min (for example, 6.6 to 13.2 mcg, 26.4 to 52.8 mcg) until patient is free of chest pain and desired blood pressure has been obtained; nitroglycerin must be administered via an infusion control device, and patient must be on an electrocardiogram (ECG) monitor; maximum dose is 226 mcg/min.	D_5W, 0.9% sodium chloride solution
nitroprusside sodium	Not recommended.	Not recommended.	Using an infusion control device, administer diluted solution at a rate that maintains desired hypotensive effect.	D_5W and use infusion control device
penicillin G potassium or penicillin G sodium	Not recommended.	Daily dosage range is 1 to 40 million units divided into equal daily doses.	Not recommended.	D_5W, 0.9% sodium chloride solution
phenobarbital	Usually 100 to 300 mg in a single dose; maximum loading dose is 15 mg/kg; administer at a rate not exceeding 50 mg/min.	Not recommended.	Up to 1 mg/kg/hr for 16 hr; maximum dilution is 1.25 mg/ml.	D_5W, 0.9% sodium chloride solution
phenytoin	100 to 300 mg daily in a single or divided dose; administer at a rate not exceeding 50 mg/min.	15 to 18 mg/kg/day in three to four equal divided doses; administer at a rate not exceeding 25 to 50 mg/min (up to a maximum of 1 g/24 hr) diluted to 1,000 ml in 0.9% sodium chloride solution (1 mg/ml).	Not recommended.	0.9% sodium chloride solution
potassium chloride	Not recommended or used.	Not recommended or used.	Infuse diluted solution slowly, not exceeding 20 mEq/hr; infusing too rapidly can cause fatal hyperkalemia; infusion rate shouldn't exceed 1 mEq/min for adults or 0.02 mEq/kg/min for children.	D_5W, 0.9% sodium chloride solution, and use infusion control device
propranolol	1 to 5 mg administered at 1 mg/min; dose may be repeated once within 24 hr.	0.5 to 2 mg diluted in 20 to 50 ml and administered over at least 10 min; dose may be administered over at least 10 min and may be repeated every 4 hr.	Not recommended.	D_5W, 0.9% sodium chloride solution
quinidine gluconate	Not recommended.	Infuse solution through I.V. line over prescribed duration.	Infusion solution through I.V. line initially at 1 ml/min; then adjust rate to control arrhythmias.	D_5W

Administering common I.V. drugs *(continued)*

DRUG	I.V. PUSH	INTERMITTENT INFUSION	CONTINUOUS INFUSION	COMPATIBILITY
ranitidine	Inject drug into a patent I.V. line over at least 5 min.	Infuse diluted drug into patent I.V. line through a piggyback set over 15 to 20 min.	Infuse 150 mg in 1,000 ml of a compatible solution over 24 hr at a rate of 6.25 mg/hr; no loading dose required.	0.9% sodium chloride solution, D_5W, $D_{10}W$, LR
sodium bicarbonate	One ampule (44 to 50 mEq) every 5 to 10 min according to arterial blood gas results.	Not recommended.	2 to 5 mEq/kg infused over 4 to 8 hr; maximum concentration: 180 mEq/liter.	D_5W, 0.9% sodium chloride solution, LR
thiamine	Not recommended.	Administer ordered amount at a rate not exceeding 20 mg/min; use infusion control device.	Add ordered dose to maintenance I.V. fluids and infuse at a rate not exceeding 20 mg/min.	D_5W, 0.9% sodium chloride solution, LR, amino acids
tobramycin	Not recommended.	Usually 1 mg/kg every 8 hr but up to 5 mg/kg/day in three or four divided doses (every 6 to 8 hr); dilute each dose in 50 to 100 ml, and administer over 20 to 60 min.	Not recommended.	D_5W, 0.9% sodium chloride solution, LR, and other common I.V. solutions
vancomycin	Not recommended.	15 to 30 mg/kg/day in four divided doses; dilute each 500 to 1,000 mg in 150 to 300 ml; infuse over 45 to 60 min every 6 to 12 hr.	1 to 2 g in 500 to 1,000 ml administered over 24 hr.	D_5W, 0.9% sodium chloride solution, LR
verapamil	Range: 0.075 to 0.15 mg/kg; maximum: 10 mg I.V. bolus (under ECG and blood pressure control) given over a 1-min period; repeat in 15 min if necessary; first dose must be administered with doctor present.	Not recommended.	0.005 mg/kg/min; first dose must be administered with doctor present.	D_5W, 0.9% sodium chloride solution

Winged infusion set. The winged infusion set, sometimes called a butterfly needle, has a steel needle. It comes in many gauges (16G to 27G) and is ¾″ (2 cm) long. Because this needle is extremely sharp, it's easy to insert. The winged infusion set may be used for short-term therapy or for a one-time I.V. push injection, as in chemotherapy. You may use a winged infusion set with a stable, cooperative patient as well as with an infant or a child or an elderly patient who has fragile or sclerotic veins. But the rigid catheter may produce infiltration more frequently than a flexible catheter would.

Over-the-needle catheter. This type of venipuncture device is used for long-term therapy and is suitable for most patients. A flexible, plastic catheter that's left in the vein, this device is less likely, once inserted, to puncture the vein than a rigid needle. Once in place, an over-the-needle catheter is more comfortable for the patient than a winged infusion set. The catheter contains radiopaque threads so it can be easily located. Some catheters have an attached syringe so that you can easily check for blood return. Some have wings for easier anchoring, and one (Intina) has wings to hold during insertion.

Choosing a venipuncture device

The illustrations below show the three types of venipuncture devices used for I.V. infusions.

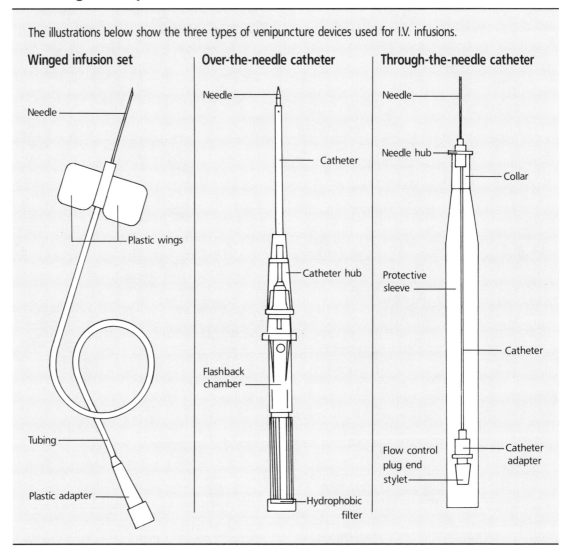

Winged infusion set

Needle

Plastic wings

Tubing

Plastic adapter

Over-the-needle catheter

Needle

Catheter

Catheter hub

Flashback chamber

Hydrophobic filter

Through-the-needle catheter

Needle

Needle hub

Collar

Protective sleeve

Catheter

Flow control plug end stylet

Catheter adapter

Through-the-needle catheter. Also called an inside-the-needle catheter, this device can be used in long arm veins. One type combines an 8″ to 12″ (20 to 30.5 cm) catheter with a 1½″ to 2″ (4 to 5 cm) introducer needle, which must be guarded by an enclosed shield after insertion. Patients using this device seldom require an armboard.

This longer catheter decreases the risk of infiltration, but leakage at the insertion site may occur because the needle produces a skin puncture that's larger than the catheter. This device is used occasionally when venous access is poor or when administering caustic drugs or hypertonic solutions.

In-line I.V. filters and filter needles
Using an in-line filter helps reduce the risk of phlebitis by removing impurities from the I.V. solution. But because in-line filters are expensive and their installation cumbersome and time-consuming, they're not routinely used.

Many health care facilities require a filter only for administering an admixture. If you're unsure of whether to use a filter, check the policy of your health care facility. You can expect to use an in-line I.V. filter when:
• administering solutions to an immunodeficient patient
• administering total parenteral nutrition
• using additives comprising many separate particles, such as antibiotics requiring reconstitution, or when administering several additives
• repeatedly using rubber injection sites or plastic diaphragms
• phlebitis is likely to occur.

Be sure to change the in-line filter according to the manufacturer's recommendations (typically every 24 to 96 hours). If you don't, bacteria trapped in the filter release an endotoxin, a pyrogen small enough to pass through the filter into the bloodstream.

When infusing lipid emulsions and albumin mixed with nutritional solutions, use an add-on filter with a larger pore size (1 to 2 microns).

Don't use an in-line filter when:
• administering solutions with large particles that will clog a filter—for example, blood and its components, suspensions, lipid emulsions, and high-molecular-volume plasma expanders
• administering 5 mg or less of a drug (because the filter may absorb the drug).

You'll use a filter needle when removing drugs from a glass ampule and when mixing and drawing up drugs in powder form. If the top of an ampule breaks off, microscopic slivers of glass could fall into the drug solution. So before withdrawing the drug from an ampule, place the filter needle on the syringe. Remove and discard it before injecting the drug into the diluent.

When removing a reconstituted drug from a vial, use a filter needle to filter out any glass or undissolved particles. Injecting foreign particles into a patient's peripheral vein could cause an embolism.

Gathering supplies
Make sure you have alcohol sponges, povidone-iodine sponges and, if your health care facility requires it, antiseptic ointment or solution. You'll need gloves, a tourniquet (rubber tubing or a blood pressure cuff), gauze pads or a transparent semipermeable dressing, and nonallergenic tape.

Obtain the I.V. solution you need and an attached and primed administration set. (Your choice of administration set depends on whether you'll give the drug by the bolus, intermittent, or infusion method.) You may also need an I.V. pole, a sharps container, an armboard, roller gauze, tube gauze, warm packs, a local anesthetic (such as 1% lidocaine without epinephrine), a U-100 insulin syringe with a 27G needle, and gloves.

Insertion of the device
Once you've selected the venipuncture device and gathered the rest of the supplies, you're ready to set up the equipment, select a site, apply the tourniquet, prepare the site, and perform the venipuncture.

Setting up
Check the information on the label of the I.V. solution container including the patient's name and room number, the type of solution, the time and date of preparation, the preparer's name, and the ordered infusion rate. Compare the doctor's orders with the label to verify that the solution is correct. Then select the smallest gauge needle or catheter that will deliver the solution (unless subsequent therapy will require a larger one). Smaller gauges cause less trauma to veins, allow greater blood flow around their tips, and reduce the clotting risk.

If you're using a steel-winged infusion set, connect the adapter to the administration set, and unclamp the line until fluid flows from the open end of the needle with a protective cover. Then close the clamp and place the needle on a sterile surface, such as the inside of its packaging.

If you're using a catheter, open the package to allow easy access.

If you're inserting an intermittent infusion device (heparin lock), remove the set from the packaging, wipe the port with an alcohol sponge, and inject a dilute heparin solution or 0.9% sodium chloride solution to fill the tub-

Applying a tourniquet

Place the tourniquet under the patient's arm, about 6″ (15 cm) above the venipuncture site. Position the arm on the middle of the tourniquet, as shown.

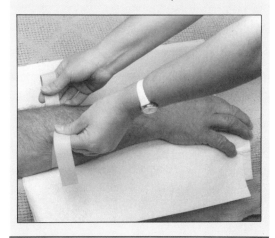

ing and 25G needle. (This removes air from the system, preventing formation of an air embolus.)

If you're using an I.V. pole, place it in the proper slot in the bed frame. If you're using a portable I.V. pole, position it close to the patient. Hang the I.V. solution with the attached, primed administration set on the I.V. pole. Verify the patient's identity by comparing the information on the solution container with his wristband.

Wash your hands thoroughly to avoid spreading microorganisms. Then explain the procedure to the patient to ensure his cooperation and help him relax. Anxiety can cause a vasomotor response, resulting in venous constriction.

Selecting a site
Typically, you'll choose a vein in the patient's nondominant arm or hand. The most favorable venipuncture sites are the cephalic and basilic veins in the lower arm and the veins in the dorsum of the hand. Leg and foot veins are considered least favorable because of the increased risk of thrombophlebitis.

Choose a small vein unless a large vein will be needed for later therapy; this leaves the large veins available for an emergency infusion. If long-term therapy is planned, start with a vein at the most distal site so you can move proximally as needed for subsequent I.V. insertion sites. For an infusion of an irritating medication, choose a large vein distal to any nearby joint. Be sure the vein can accommodate the catheter used.

Antecubital veins can be used if no other veins are available. They may also be used to accommodate a large-bore needle or to administer drugs requiring large volume dilution.

Don't insert a line in a sclerotic vein, an edematous or impaired arm or hand, or near burns or an arteriovenous fistula.

Place the patient's arm in a dependent position to increase capillary fill of the lower arm and hand. If the patient's skin is cold, warm it by rubbing and stroking the arm, or try covering the entire arm with warm packs for 5 to 10 minutes.

Applying the tourniquet
To dilate the vein, apply the tourniquet about 6″ (15 cm) above the intended puncture site. Check the distal pulse. If it's not present, release the tourniquet and reapply it with less tension to prevent arterial occlusion. (See *Applying a tourniquet.*)

Lightly palpate the vein with your index and middle fingers, while stretching it with your opposite hand to prevent rolling. The vein should feel soft and elastic. If the vein feels hard or ropelike, select another.

If the vein is easily palpable but not sufficiently dilated, try one or more of the following techniques:
• Flick the skin over the vein with one or two sharp snaps of your finger.
• Place the patient's arm or leg in a dependent position for several seconds.
• Rub or stroke the skin upward toward the tourniquet.
• If you have selected a vein in the arm or hand, tell the patient to open and close his fist several times.

If you're still having trouble, you may be able to locate a vein using transillumination.

ADVANCED EQUIPMENT

Using a vein light

To locate hard-to-find peripheral veins, try using a transillumination device such as the Landry vein light. This device uses bright light from a pair of adjustable fiber-optic arms to reveal the blood vessels.

With the attached Velcro strap, secure the vein light to the patient's limb. Dim the room lights. With the device on its brightest setting, scan the limb distal to the tourniquet for a vein. The vein absorbs the light and appears as a dark line, while the surrounding subcutaneous tissue appears pink.

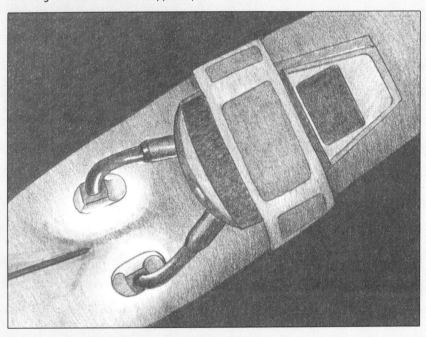

Using a vein light not only makes seeing the vein easier, it also helps prevent the vein from rolling. (See *Using a vein light*.)

Leave the tourniquet in place for no more than 2 minutes. If you can't find a suitable vein and prepare the site in that time, release the tourniquet for a few minutes; then reapply it and continue the procedure.

Preparing the site
When you're ready to prepare the site for venipuncture, put on gloves. Clip the hair around the insertion site, if necessary, and clean the site with one of the following antiseptic solu-

tions: 70% alcohol, povidone-iodine, tincture of iodine, or chlorhexidine. Don't apply alcohol after an iodophor because alcohol negates its effects. Work in a circular motion outward from the site to a diameter of 2" to 4" (5 to 10 cm) to remove flora that would otherwise be introduced into the vascular system with the venipuncture. Let the antiseptic solution dry.

If ordered, administer a local anesthetic. Make sure the patient isn't allergic to lidocaine, a commonly used anesthetic.

Performing the venipuncture
If you're using a winged infusion set or an

Inserting the venipuncture device

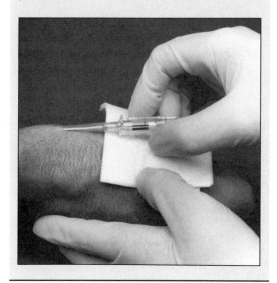

When inserting the venipuncture device, lower the needle to a 15- to 20-degree angle and slowly pierce the vein.

over-the-needle catheter with wings, hold the short edges of the wings (with the needle bevel facing upward) between the thumb and forefinger of your dominant hand. Then squeeze the wings together.

With an over-the-needle catheter, grasp the plastic hub with your dominant hand, remove the cover, and examine the catheter tip. If the edge isn't smooth, discard and replace the device.

If you're using a through-the-needle catheter, grasp the needle hub with one hand, and unsnap the needle cover. Then rotate the catheter until the bevel faces upward.

Using the thumb of your opposite hand, stretch the skin taut below the puncture site to stabilize the vein. Lightly press the vein with a fingertip of your dominant hand about 1½" (4 cm) from the intended insertion site. The vein should feel round, firm, fully engorged, and resilient.

Be sure to tell the patient when you're

about to insert the device. He won't feel the insertion if lidocaine has been used. (See *Inserting the venipuncture device.*)

For the direct approach, hold the needle bevel up and enter the skin directly over the vein at a 30- to 45-degree angle. For the indirect approach, enter the skin slightly adjacent to the vein. With this second approach, you'll direct the catheter into the side of the vein wall.

Advance the catheter steadily until you meet resistance. Don't penetrate the vein. Lower the catheter to a 15- to 20-degree angle, and slowly pierce the vein. Sometimes, but not always, you'll feel the catheter enter the vein.

When you observe blood flashback in the hub, tilt the catheter slightly upward and advance it farther into the vein to prevent puncture of the posterior vein wall. (You may not see blood return with a small vein.)

If you're using a winged infusion set, advance the needle fully, if possible, and hold it in place. Release the tourniquet, open the administration set clamp slightly, and check for free flow or infiltration.

If you're using an over-the-needle catheter, advance the device to at least half its length to ensure that the catheter itself, not just the introducer needle, has entered the vein. Then remove the tourniquet. Grasp the catheter hub to hold it in place in the vein, and withdraw the inner needle.

Advance the catheter up to the hub or until you meet resistance. To advance the catheter while infusing I.V. solution, release the tourniquet and remove the inner needle. Using aseptic technique, attach the I.V. tubing and begin the infusion. While stabilizing the vein with one hand, use the other to advance the catheter into the vein. When the catheter is advanced, decrease the I.V. flow rate. This method reduces the risk of puncturing the vein's opposite wall because the catheter is advanced without the steel needle and because the rapid flow dilates the vein.

To advance the catheter before starting the infusion, first release the tourniquet. While stabilizing the vein with one hand, use the other hand to advance the catheter up to the hub.

Next, remove the inner needle and, using aseptic technique, quickly attach the I.V. tubing. This method often causes less blood to spill.

If you're using a through-the-needle catheter, remove the tourniquet, hold the needle in place with one hand and, with your opposite hand, grasp the catheter through the protective sleeve. Then, slowly thread the catheter through the needle until the hub is within the needle collar. Never pull back on the catheter without pulling back on the needle to avoid severing and releasing the catheter into the circulation, causing an embolism. If you feel resistance from a valve, withdraw the catheter and needle slightly and reinsert them, rotating the catheter as you pass the valve. Then withdraw the metal needle and cover it with the protector. Remove the stylet and protective sleeve, and attach the administration set to the catheter hub. Open the administration set clamp slightly, and check for free flow or infiltration.

Dressing the site
After you've inserted the venipuncture device, clean the skin completely. If necessary, place the inner needle in a sharps container. Then regulate the flow rate (if necessary). You may use a transparent semipermeable dressing to secure the device.

If you don't use a transparent dressing, apply antiseptic ointment at the insertion site, according to the policy of your health care facility; cover the site with a sterile gauze or a small adhesive bandage.

Loop the I.V. tubing on the patient's limb and secure the loop with tape. This helps prevent accidental dislodgment of the catheter. Many health care facilities use a small piece of extension tubing for the loop. It's attached to the end of the I.V. tubing and to the catheter hub. On a piece of tape, note the type and gauge of your needle or catheter, the date and time of insertion, and your initials. Adjust the flow rate, as ordered.

Drug administration
You can give I.V. medications using one of three methods: direct or bolus, intermittent or piggyback, and continuous. The bolus method delivers a one-time dose of a drug whereas the intermittent and continuous methods deliver the necessary dose over a given period. The pharmacy at your health care facility may mix the I.V. solutions and drugs for you, or you may need to mix them yourself.

Preparation
Before reconstituting a drug powder, verify the compatibility of the medication and the diluent. Most doses are mixed in the I.V. bag using 0.9% sodium chloride, sterile water, or dextrose 5% in water (D_5W). Before adding medication to any solution, check for particles in the minibag and for cloudiness in the solution. If you see any evidence of either, discard the solution.

To reconstitute a drug powder, draw up the amount and type of diluent recommended by the drug manufacturer. Wipe the rubber stopper of the drug vial with an alcohol sponge. Insert the needle on the syringe containing the diluent and inject the diluent into the vial. Mix gently until the drug dissolves.

Once the drug has dissolved, aspirate the solution into a syringe through a filter needle to isolate any particles of powder or rubber. Then dispose of the filter needle and replace it with a 20G needle. Wipe the injection port of the I.V. bag or bottle with an alcohol sponge and inject the medication into the bag. Gently invert the bag or bottle twice to mix the medication throughout the solution. Don't squeeze or shake the bag or bottle because this can produce tiny air bubbles.

If you need to add a medication to an I.V. bag or bottle, make sure the bag or bottle will be at least two-thirds full when you're finished. This provides adequate dilution for the medication. Clamp the I.V. tubing and take the bag down. Then wipe the administration port with an alcohol sponge and add the medication. Invert the bag twice to thoroughly distribute the medication. Hang the bag upright and open the roller clamp to adjust for the proper infusion rate.

Always label both the I.V. solution bag or bottle and the administration tubing. The I.V. bag should be labeled with the patient's name and room number, the date and time the bag was hung, the flow rate, and any medication that was added to the bag. Label the tubing with the date and time it was hung, the date and time it should be changed, and your initials.

Bolus administration

You'll give a bolus injection directly through a primary I.V. tubing or through a heparin lock. Because it allows the patient more freedom to move around, a heparin lock is used more often than a keep-vein-open line.

In preparation for giving a bolus injection, gather the supplies you'll need: three alcohol sponges, one needle (20G or smaller) with a syringe containing 0.9% sodium chloride solution, a syringe containing the drug you're giving, a saline- or heparin-filled syringe for flushing, and tape. If the drug you're giving isn't compatible with the primary solution, you'll need another syringe filled with saline flush solution.

Now, recheck the dosage with the doctor's orders. Double-check the patient's identity by comparing his wristband with his chart. Tell him what the medication is and why it's being given.

If you're injecting the bolus into a primary I.V. line, follow these steps:
• Put on gloves.
• Close the flow clamp on the I.V. tubing and clean the port closest to the insertion site with an alcohol sponge.
• Puncture the center of the port with the needle attached to the medication syringe. Aspirate slightly to check for a blood return.
• Inject the medication slowly over the recommended time interval. Remove the syringe and the needle.
• Clean the port with an alcohol sponge. Then inject the contents of the saline-filled syringe to clear all the medication from the tubing, port, and catheter. Remove the syringe and needle.
• Clean the port with the third alcohol sponge.

If you're administering an I.V. bolus through a heparin lock, follow these steps:
• Put on gloves. Wipe the injection port of the heparin lock with an alcohol sponge and insert the needle attached to the saline-filled syringe.

• Check for a blood return. If no blood appears, apply a tourniquet tightly above the injection site, keep it in place for about 1 minute, and aspirate again. If blood still doesn't appear, remove the tourniquet and inject the saline solution slowly.
• If you feel resistance or see swelling, stop the injection immediately. Resistance indicates that the device is occluded; swelling indicates infiltration. If these occur, insert a new heparin lock.
• If you feel no resistance, watch for signs of infiltration while you slowly inject the saline solution. The signs are stiffness or pain at the injection site. If you note these signs, insert a new heparin lock.
• If you aspirate blood, slowly inject the saline solution and continue observing for signs of infiltration. The solution flushes out any residual heparin solution that may be incompatible with the medication.
• Withdraw the needle and the syringe.
• Insert the needle attached to the medication syringe.
• Inject the medication at the required rate. Then remove the needle from the injection port.
• Insert the needle of the remaining saline-filled syringe into the injection port and slowly inject the saline solution. This flushes all the medication through the device.
• Remove the needle and syringe, and insert and inject the heparin (or saline) flush solution to prevent clotting in the device.
• Discard all uncapped needles immediately to prevent needle sticks.

Intermittent administration

The most common and flexible method of administering I.V. drugs, intermittent infusion allows you to maintain therapeutic blood levels over short periods at varying intervals. You may deliver a small volume (25 to 250 ml) over several minutes or a few hours. You can deliver an intermittent infusion through a piggyback line or heparin lock, or through the primary line.

Intermittent administration entails certain risks. When you're giving a dose through the primary I.V. line, both drugs or solutions must

Avoiding needle sticks

Needle-stick injuries may be greatly reduced with a needleless system or a click-lock system. Both devices can be used to give piggyback infusions with a heparin lock.

Needleless systems
The needleless system consists of a blunt-tipped plastic insertion device and a rubber injection port. The port may be part of a special administration set or an adapter for existing administration sets. This rubber injection port has a preestablished slit that can open and reseal immediately.

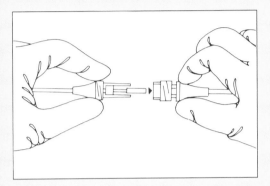

Click-lock system
You may also use a click-lock I.V. system with a heparin lock. The system has two components: a transparent housing that contains a recessed needle and a diaphragm-covered port on the heparin lock that fits into the needle housing. A locking device on the needle housing then clicks over a flange at the base of the port, securing the components as the needle pierces the diaphragm.

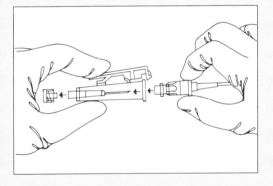

be compatible. Repeated needle sticks into the ports increases the risk of contamination of the tubing or the heparin lock cap.

To infuse a drug through a piggyback line, you'll need the medication in the piggyback minibag, piggyback tubing, a 20G (or smaller) needle or a recessed needle device, and a syringe filled with 1 ml of heparin or saline flush, two needles with syringes filled with 2 ml of 0.9% sodium chloride solution, three alcohol sponges, and an I.V. pole.

Your pharmacy may provide premixed minibags. If you get a minibag of diluent attached to a vial of undiluted medication, you'll need to remove the plug on the vial and mix the two solutions.

To give a piggyback infusion through a heparin lock, follow these steps:
• Check the medication dose in the minibag and make sure it matches the doctor's order. Double-check the patient's identity by comparing his wristband with his chart. Explain to the patient what the medication is and why it's being given.
• Remove the I.V. administration tubing from the box. Straighten the tubing and close the roller clamp. Remove the protective cap from the end and attach the 20G needle. You may also use a needleless system or a click-lock I.V. system. (See *Avoiding needle sticks.*)
• Remove the protective cap from the diaphragm of the minibag and remove the cap

from the I.V. tubing spike. Insert the spike into the diaphragm of the minibag. Hang the bag on the I.V. pole.

• Squeeze the drip chamber of the I.V. tubing and allow the chamber to fill halfway. Remove the cap from the needle, needleless, or recessed-needle system, and open the roller clamp to prime the tubing and needle. Close the roller clamp when the solution reaches the tip of the needle. Cover the needle with its protective cap.

• Clean the port on the heparin lock with an alcohol sponge. Remove the needle cap and insert the needle, needleless, or recessed-needle system into the heparin lock. Securely tape this connection to reduce the risk of needle dislodgment. Check the I.V. site for infiltration.

• Adjust the roller clamp to infuse the medication over the recommended time interval.

• When the infusion is completed, remove the needle or needleless system from the heparin lock. Clean the port of the heparin lock with an alcohol sponge and inject the saline solution. Follow with a heparin flush, if used.

• Dispose of any uncapped needles immediately to avoid needle sticks.

To administer a piggyback infusion of compatible medication into a primary I.V. line, follow these steps:

• Follow the first four steps for administering a piggyback infusion through a heparin lock.

• Using an alcohol sponge, clean the Y-port above the roller clamp of the primary I.V. tubing. Insert the needle or recessed-needle system of the piggyback tubing into the port. Tape this connection securely if a needle is used. Recessed needles don't require taping.

• Hold the primary I.V. bag or bottle lower than the minibag using the extension hook included in the piggyback tubing box.

• Open the roller clamp on the piggyback tubing. Adjust the roller clamp of the primary bag to set the infusion rate of the minibag. (While the minibag is infusing, the primary I.V. solution will not run.) When the minibag has finished infusing, the primary I.V. solution will resume infusing. You must readjust the roller clamp back to the rate of the primary I.V. solution.

If you need to give a secondary medication that isn't compatible with the primary I.V. solu-

tion, you can use either another heparin lock or a T-connector. This small piece of extension tubing has an injection port close to its luer-lock connection. This allows you to infuse a secondary medication with the primary I.V. without incompatibility problems. (See *Using a T-connector.*)

You can also deliver a secondary medication using a controlled-release infusion system (CRIS). The CRIS adapter lets you give a drug using a vial of reconstituted drug powder. With this system you must be sure that the medication in the vial is compatible with the primary I.V. solution.

Continuous administration
A continuous, or primary, I.V. infusion helps maintain a constant therapeutic drug level. This method may be least irritating to the patient. And it's probably more convenient for you because you'll spend less time mixing solutions and hanging bags than with the intermittent method. You'll also handle less tubing, thereby decreasing the risk of infection.

Continuous administration does have some disadvantages. If the drip rate isn't monitored, the I.V. fluid and medication may infuse too rapidly. You may also have trouble finding a suitable vein in a patient who's had previous long-term I.V. therapy. Finally, you must make sure that any drugs you give together are compatible.

To administer a continuous infusion, you'll need the prescribed medication in a container of I.V. solution, an administration set, and gloves. You may also need an infusion pump or a controller. If so, make sure you have the correct administration set for the pump or controller.

To give a drug by continuous infusion, follow these steps:

• Make sure the I.V. solution container is labeled with the name and dose of the medication.

• Attach the administration set to the solution container and prime the tubing with the I.V. solution. Attach the administration set to the pump or controller, if appropriate.

• Put on gloves and remove the protective cap at the end of the administration set. Then attach the set to the venipuncture device. If you're using luer-lock tubing, secure the luer connector to the catheter hub.

• Begin the infusion and regulate the flow for the ordered rate.

• Frequently monitor the patient and the flow rate.

Maintain accurate intake and output records and be alert for excessive fluid retention. When a patient receives small amounts hourly, an excessive total daily volume may not be obvious.

Remember too that giving a large volume of fluid can change a patient's electrolyte levels. Be sure to check the patient's laboratory results to make sure his electrolyte levels stay within normal limits.

The tubing used for continuous infusion lasts for 48 to 72 hours, but you'll need to change the bags every 24 hours. Check the drip rate at regular intervals to ensure delivery of the medication as ordered. At times, you'll need to regulate the infusion using the roller clamp. Calculate the drip rate in drops per minute, according to the calibration established by the manufacturer of the equipment you're using. (See *Calculating drip rates,* page 36.)

Complications

Peripheral venous therapy can produce both local and systemic complications. The following discussion covers the most common complications as well as the possible causes, signs and symptoms, nursing interventions, and prevention techniques.

Local complications

Common local complications include phlebitis, extravasation and infiltration, occlusion, venous irritation, severed catheter, hematoma, venous spasm, and thrombosis.

Phlebitis. You'll identify phlebitis by a redness at the catheter tip that continues up the vein. The patient may complain of tenderness along the catheter and above it. Plus, the vein may feel hard, and the surrounding tissue may be edematous and warm.

Possible causes of phlebitis include a clot at the tip of the catheter, catheter movement

Using a T-connector

The T-connector is a piece of small-bore extension tubing 3″ to 6″ (7.6 to 15 cm) long. It's fitted with an injection port near the luer-lock connection. With this additional injection site, you can simultaneously give drugs and fluids, a primary I.V. solution, or an incompatible drug.

To add the T-connector, wash your hands and don gloves to minimize exposure to body fluids. To reduce the patient's anxiety, explain what you are doing. Prime the tubing with I.V. fluid; then attach one end of the T-connector to the I.V. tubing.

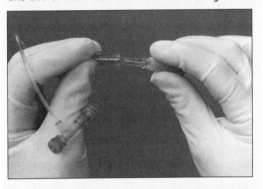

Open the slide clamp, purge the tubing, and close the clamp. Now you're ready to connect the luer-lock tip to the I.V. cannula. Remove the luer-lock tip-protector cap and carefully insert the tip into I.V. cannula. Open the clamp.

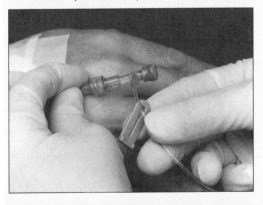

Secure this connector in place with tape. Another I.V. needle can be inserted into the latex injection cap.

Calculating drip rates

When calculating the flow rate of I.V. solutions, remember that the number of drops required to deliver 1 ml varies with the type of administration set you're using.

To calculate the drip rate, you must know the calibration of the drip rate for each manufacturer's product. As a quick guide, refer to the chart below. Use this formula to calculate specific drip rates:

$$\frac{\text{volume of infusion (in ml)}}{\text{time of infusion (in minutes)}} \times \text{drop factor (in drops/ml)} = \text{drops/minute}$$

ADMINISTRATION SET	DROPS/ ML	ORDERED VOLUME					
		500 ml/ 24 hr or 21 ml/hr	1,000 ml/ 24 hr or 42 ml/hr	1,000 ml/ 20 hr or 50 ml/hr	1,000 ml/ 10 hr or 100 ml/hr	1,000 ml/ 8 hr or 125 ml/hr	1,000 ml/ 6 hr or 166 ml/hr
		DROPS/MINUTE TO INFUSE					
Macrodrip							
Abbott	15	5	10	12	25	31	42
Baxter Healthcare	10	3	7	8	17	21	28
Cutter	20	7	14	17	34	42	56
IVAC	20	7	14	17	34	42	56
McGaw	15	5	10	12	25	31	42
Microdrip							
Various manufacturers	60	21	42	50	100	125	166

within the vessel, and poor blood flow around the catheter. Phlebitis may also result when a catheter is left in the vessel too long or when the infused solution has a particularly high or low pH or a high osmolarity.

To treat phlebitis, remove the catheter immediately and apply warm soaks to the affected area. If the patient develops a fever, notify his doctor.

To prevent phlebitis from occurring or reccurring, try one of these measures:
• When inserting a new catheter, use either a larger vein or a smaller gauge catheter to ensure adequate blood flow around it.
• Use a filter. This may prevent phlebitis by filtering out small particles that may cause irritation.

• Anchor the venipuncture device securely to avoid any irritating movement.
• Change the catheter site at routine intervals and at the first sign of vein tenderness or redness.

Extravasation and infiltration. Both common complications of I.V. therapy, extravasation is the leakage of a vesicant solution into the surrounding tissues, and infiltration is the leakage of a nonvesicant solution into the surrounding tissues.

You'll note swelling at and above the I.V. site, and decreased skin temperature and blanching around the site. The drip rate will slow considerably. If you're using a pump, the flow rate may continue despite an occlusion.

The patient may complain of burning, tightness, and pain at the I.V. site. Usually this is caused by the catheter's becoming dislodged from the vein. To prevent extravasation, check the I.V. site often, especially if an infusion pump is being used. Don't apply tape or tight restraints above the site. And tell the patient to report any discomfort, pain, or swelling as soon as possible. (See *Preventing and treating extravasation,* page 38.)

Besides catheter dislodgment, you may suspect partial retraction from the vein or infiltration into the surrounding tissues. If so, make sure the I.V. line isn't tangled in the patient's clothes or bed linen. If the I.V. solution hasn't infiltrated, retape the I.V. without pushing the catheter back into the vein. If the solution has infiltrated, remove the I.V. line and insert a new one. Make sure the I.V. catheter and tubing are securely taped to the patient.

Keep in mind that seeing a blood return in an I.V. catheter doesn't confirm that the catheter is in the vein. Similarly, if you don't see a blood return, you can't assume that the catheter is not in the vein. If the patient has low venous pressure, or if the catheter and vein are too small, the I.V. catheter may not show a blood return even if it is in the vein. Conversely, sometimes the I.V. solution may have infiltrated and you'll still see a blood return because the tip of the catheter is partially out of the vein.

Occlusion. Look for two indications of occlusion: a backflow of blood into the I.V. tubing and a flow rate that doesn't increase when the bag is elevated. Occlusion may result from an interruption of the I.V. flow rate during a piggyback infusion, from a heparin lock that's not flushed, or from a backflow of blood into the tubing when the patient moves around. If you observe an occlusion, aspirate and then flush the I.V. line using mild pressure. If this doesn't work, remove the line and restart it in a new site.

To prevent occlusion, check the I.V. line frequently and maintain the I.V. flow rate. Always flush a heparin lock after each drug adminis-

tration. And encourage the patient to walk with his arm across his chest to avoid a backflow of blood.

Venous irritation. Your patient may feel irritation or pain during an I.V. infusion. The site may blanch during a venous spasm, or the skin over the vein may turn red. This may be a preliminary sign of phlebitis. Certain I.V. solutions may also cause irritation, including potassium chloride, vancomycin, nafcillin, phenytoin, or any solution with a high or low pH or high osmolarity.

To relieve the patient's discomfort, slow the infusion rate and use an infusion pump to maintain a steady flow. The I.V. medication may be diluted in 250 ml of solution rather than 100 ml. Check with the doctor and pharmacist to see if the solution can be buffered with sodium bicarbonate. If the irritating solution is to be given over a long period, the doctor may recommend using a central I.V. line (see Chapter 3). Ice or heat over the I.V. site may alleviate discomfort during the infusion.

Severed catheter. If you notice solution leaking from the catheter, a severed catheter may be the cause. A catheter may be severed when accidentally cut with scissors, or when the needle is reinserted into the catheter.

If a catheter is severed, try to retrieve the broken part if it's visible. Otherwise, apply a tourniquet above the I.V. site.

To avoid this problem, don't use scissors while inserting a catheter and don't reinsert the needle into it. If you're unable to insert the catheter, remove the catheter and needle together.

Hematoma. A hematoma may result if the opposite vein wall is punctured during insertion or if infiltration causes blood leakage into the surrounding tissue. If the patient has a hematoma, you'll notice that you're unable to advance the catheter beyond a certain point. You may also notice a bruise around the insertion site, and the patient may complain of tenderness at the site.

If you notice a hematoma, remove the

(Text continues on page 40.)

Preventing and treating extravasation

Extravasation—the infiltration of a drug into the surrounding tissue—can result from a punctured vein or from leakage around an I.V. site. If vesicant (blistering) drugs or fluids extravasate, severe local tissue damage often results.

Prevention
To prevent extravasation when giving vesicants, use proper administration techniques and follow these guidelines:
• Don't use an existing I.V. line unless its patency is ensured. Perform a new venipuncture to ensure correct needle placement and vein patency.
• Select the site carefully. Use a distal vein that allows successive proximal venipunctures. To avoid tendon and nerve damage from extravasation, avoid using the hand's dorsal surface. Also avoid the wrist and fingers (they're hard to immobilize) and areas previously damaged or with compromised circulation.
• If you need to probe for a vein, you may cause trauma. Stop and begin again at another site.
• Start the infusion with dextrose 5% in water (D_5W) or 0.9% sodium chloride solution.
• Use a transparent semipermeable dressing to allow inspection of the site.
• Check for extravasation before starting the infusion. Apply a tourniquet above the needle to occlude the vein and see if the flow continues. If the flow stops, the solution isn't infiltrating. Another method is to lower the I.V. container and watch for blood backflow. This method is less reliable because the needle may have punctured the opposite vein wall yet still rest partially in the vein. Flush the needle with 0.9% sodium chloride solution to ensure patency. If swelling occurs at the I.V. site, the solution is infiltrating.
• Give vesicants by slow I.V. push through a free-flowing I.V. line or by a small-volume (50 to 100 ml) infusion.
• During administration, observe the infusion site for erythema or infiltration. Tell the patient to report burning, stinging, pain, pruritus, or temperature changes.

• After drug administration, instill several milliliters of D_5W or 0.9% sodium chloride solution to flush the drug from the vein and to prevent drug leakage when the needle is removed.
• Administer vesicants last when multiple drugs are ordered.
• If possible, avoid using an infusion pump to administer vesicants because a pump will continue the infusion after infiltration occurs.

Treatment
Extravasation of vesicants requires emergency treatment. Follow the policy of your health care facility. Essential steps should include the following:
• Stop the I.V. flow and remove the I.V. line, unless you need the needle to infiltrate the antidote.
• Estimate the amount of extravasated solution, and notify the doctor.
• Instill the appropriate antidote according to hospital protocol (see the chart opposite). Usually, you'll give an antidote for vesicant extravasation in one of two ways—either you'll instill it through an existing I.V. line to infiltrate the area or you'll inject small amounts subcutaneously in a circle around the infiltrated area, using a 1-ml syringe. With the latter method, you should change needles before each injection.
• Elevate the arm.
• Apply either ice packs or warm compresses to the affected area.
• If skin breakdown occurs, apply silver sulfadiazine cream and gauze dressings or wet-to-dry povidone-iodine dressings, as ordered.
• If severe debridement occurs, the patient may need surgery and physical therapy.
• Record the location of the extravasation site, the patient's symptoms, the estimated amount of infiltrated solution, and the treatment. Also record the time you notified the doctor and the doctor's name. Continue documenting the site's appearance and associated symptoms.

Antidotes to vesicant extravasation

The following chart lists common antidotes you may administer. Some will be used in combination with others.

ANTIDOTE	DOSE	EXTRAVASATED DRUG
ascorbic acid injection	50 mg	dactinomycin
edetate calcium disodium (calcium EDTA)	150 mg	cadmium copper manganese zinc
hyaluronidase 15 units/ml	Mix a 150-unit vial with 1 ml 0.9% sodium chloride solution for injection; withdraw 0.1 ml and dilute with 0.9 ml 0.9% sodium chloride solution to get 15 units/ml; give five 0.2 ml S.C. injections around site	aminophylline calcium solutions contrast media dextrose solutions (concentrations of 10% or more) nafcillin potassium solutions total parenteral nutrition solutions vinblastine vincristine vindesine
hydrocortisone sodium succinate 100 mg/ml Usually followed by topical application of 1% hydrocortisone cream	50 to 200 mg (25 to 50 mg/ml of extravasate)	doxorubicin vincristine
phentolamine mesylate	Dilute 5 to 10 mg with 10 ml of 0.9% sodium chloride solution for injection	dopamine epinephrine metaraminol norepinephrine
sodium bicarbonate 8.4%	5 ml	carmustine daunorubicin doxorubicin vinblastine vincristine
sodium thiosulfate 10%	Dilute 4 ml with 6 ml sterile water for injection; administer 10 ml	dactinomycin mechlorethamine mitomycin plicamycin

catheter and reinsert it at a new site. Apply pressure to the area and recheck periodically for bleeding. Once the bleeding has stopped, apply warm soaks.

Venous spasm. If the patient complains of pain along the vein, he may be experiencing venous spasm. You'll notice that the I.V. flow rate is sluggish even when the roller clamp is fully open. Venous spasm may result from solutions that irritate the vein, from the administration of cold medications, and from a rapid infusion rate.

To treat venous spasm, apply warm soaks over the area and slow the infusion rate. You can prevent venous spasm by allowing solutions to reach room temperature before giving.

Thrombosis. With thrombosis, the vein will be painful, reddened, and swollen. The I.V. flow rate will be sluggish or may have stopped completely. Thrombosis results from injury to the endothelial cells of the vein wall, allowing platelets to adhere and a thrombus to form.

In case of thrombosis, remove the I.V. line immediately and reinsert it in another limb, if possible. Apply warm soaks and monitor the site for infection.

Systemic complications

Four systemic complications may result from I.V. therapy: circulatory overload, systemic infection, speed shock, and allergic reaction.

Circulatory overload. In circulatory overload, the patient may show signs of congestive heart failure (CHF), increased blood pressure, crackles, neck vein distention, and shortness of breath. Typically caused by an increased flow rate over time, circulatory overload can be life-threatening.

Notify the doctor immediately. Raise the head of the patient's bed, then administer oxygen and medications, as ordered. To prevent circulatory overload, use a pump when administering I.V. therapy to patients who have problems eliminating fluids. Such patients include those with a history of CHF, decreased renal

function, and decreased cardiac output. Check and monitor the flow rate frequently.

Systemic infection. This complication may result from not using aseptic technique. It may also result from severe phlebitis, prolonged use of a venipuncture device, and poor taping that allows the catheter to slide back and forth within the vein when the patient moves, thus introducing skin microorganisms into the vein. With systemic infection, the patient has chills, fever, and malaise without an apparent cause.

Notify the doctor, obtain a culture of the infected site, and give any ordered medications. To prevent systemic infection, always use aseptic technique when inserting a new catheter. Change sites, tubing, and solutions when appropriate, and make sure all connections are secure.

Speed shock. This complication occurs when a medication is administered too quickly, causing plasma levels to reach the toxic level. Speed shock is more common with bolus injections than with other methods. The patient will have a headache, syncope, a flushed face, tightness in his chest, an irregular pulse and, possibly, shock and cardiac arrest.

If you suspect speed shock, discontinue the infusion immediately and notify the patient's doctor. You may give D₅W at a keep-vein-open rate. You can prevent speed shock by making sure you're familiar with the manufacturer's recommendations for administering a medication.

Allergic reaction. If your patient has an allergic reaction to a medication, you may note itching, bronchospasm, wheezing, urticaria, and edema at the I.V. site. If you detect these signs and symptoms, stop the infusion immediately and notify the patient's doctor. Help maintain the patient's cardiopulmonary status. If ordered, give corticosteroids, nonsteroidal anti-inflammatory drugs, and epinephrine. To prevent allergic reactions, you should know the patient's allergic history. Keep in mind that a delayed repeat allergic reaction can occur hours after an initial reaction.

Nursing considerations

• If the patient has a clotting disorder, use 1 to 2 ml of 0.9% sodium chloride solution instead of heparin flush.

• If you're giving a bolus injection of a drug that's incompatible with D_5W, such as diazepam (Valium) or phenytoin (Dilantin), flush the device with 0.9% sodium chloride solution.

• If the patient feels a burning sensation during the heparin injection, stop the injection and check needle placement. If the needle is in the vein, inject the heparin at a slower rate to minimize irritation. If the needle isn't in the vein, remove and discard the needle. Then select a new venipuncture site and, using fresh equipment, restart the procedure.

• Drugs administered by bolus injection produce an immediate effect. Be alert for signs of an acute allergic reaction or anaphylaxis, which can develop rapidly.

• If you're unable to rotate injection sites because the patient has fragile veins, document this in your notes.

• If you note problems with the flow rate, check your equipment. You may need to replace the container, straighten the tubing, or adjust the height of the container. Or the tubing may have an air bubble.

• Whenever you insert or remove a needle from a heparin lock, be sure to stabilize the device to prevent dislodging it from the vein.

• Change intermittent infusion devices regularly (usually every 48 to 72 hours), according to universal precaution guidelines and the policy of your health care facility.

• Change a sterile gauze dressing every 24 to 48 hours, or according to the policy of your health care facility. Change a heparin lock every 72 hours using a new venipuncture site. A transparent semipermeable dressing and a stretch net protective sleeve that covers the entire device give the patient more freedom and allow you better observation of the injection site.

• Document each procedure you perform. Make sure you document the gauge and length of the catheter, the date and time of insertion, and the number of attempts to insert it. You'll also document the insertion site as well as the types of I.V. solution and medi-cations given and the rates at which they're given. Document your patient teaching and describe the patient's comprehension. If you started the patient's therapy, initial his chart. On the dressing protecting the catheter site, indicate the catheter's length and gauge, time and date of insertion, and your initials.

Every 4 to 8 hours during therapy, document the status of the insertion site and dressing and any evidence of complications. In case of complications, indicate the interventions taken. When therapy is discontinued, document why and note if it was reinitiated.

Patient teaching

Many patients feel apprehensive about peripheral I.V. therapy. So before you begin, teach the patient what to expect before, during, and after the procedure. Thorough patient teaching can reduce anxiety, making therapy easier.

First describe the procedure. Tell the patient that *intravenous* means inside the vein and that a plastic catheter or needle will be placed in his vein. Explain that fluids containing certain nutrients or medications will flow from a bag or bottle, through a length of tubing, then through the plastic catheter or needle into his vein. Tell the patient about how long the catheter or needle will stay in place, and explain that his doctor will decide how much and what type of fluid he needs.

Tell the patient that although he may feel transient pain at the insertion site, the discomfort will stop once the catheter or needle is in place. Explain that the I.V. fluid may feel cold at first, but that this sensation should only last a few minutes.

Instruct the patient to report any discomfort after therapy begins. Also, explain any restrictions on his activity. If appropriate, tell the patient that he may be able to walk while receiving I.V. therapy. Depending on the insertion site and the device, he also may be able to shower or take a tub bath.

Make sure the patient knows not to put tension on the tubing, not to remove the container from the I.V. pole, and not to twist the tubing or lie on it. Instruct him to call a nurse if the flow rate suddenly slows down or speeds up.

Teaching I.V. therapy to patients

Candidates for home I.V. therapy should be selected carefully. The patient must be willing and able to administer I.V. solutions safely, learn the potential complications and interventions, understand the basics of asepsis, and obtain the necessary supplies. A patient who needs help must enlist a home caregiver, such as a family member or friend.

Home care patients may receive I.V. fluids or such I.V. medications as antibiotics, antifungals, antineoplastic agents, insulin, chelating agents, or analgesics. More recently, some blood products have been given at home following an initial transfusion at the health care facility.

Before discharge

Although most patients receiving I.V. therapy at home will have a central venous line, you may care for a patient who will be going home with a peripheral venous line. Teach the patient how to care for the I.V. site and how to identify complications. If he must observe movement restrictions, make sure he understands which movements to avoid.

What to watch for

Tell the patient to examine the site and to notify his doctor if the dressing becomes moist, if blood appears in the tubing, or if redness, swelling, or discomfort develops. Also tell the patient to report any problems with the I.V. line. He should always notify the doctor if the solution stops infusing, or if an alarm goes off on the infusion pump or controller.

Explain that the I.V. site will be changed at established intervals by a home care nurse. Make sure that the patient or caregiver knows how and when to flush the heparin lock.

How to use the equipment

Because the patient may have special drug delivery equipment that differs from the equipment in the health care facility, demonstrate it and ask him to perform a return demonstration.

Be sure to teach the patient what the settings on the equipment should be. If he notices that they're incorrect, he can report it before a problem develops. But make sure that any lock-out feature is activated so the patient can't inadvertently change the settings.

Before removing an I.V. line, tell the patient that it's a simple procedure. Reassure him that once the device is out and the bleeding stops, he'll be able to use the affected arm or leg as he did before therapy.

Since a growing number of patients are receiving I.V. therapy at home, you may also need to instruct home care patients. (See *Teaching I.V. therapy to patients*.)

Transfusions

Because blood plays such a fundamental role, the procedure of transfusing blood and blood products is as complex and demanding as giving I.V. drugs. Blood carries everything the tissues require for energy and synthesis and removes all cellular waste products. It supplies oxygen and nutrients for tissue maintenance, growth, and repair. It transports cellular waste, including carbon dioxide, to the elimination organs. Blood also provides a defense against infection by transporting antibodies. It regulates and equalizes body temperature and helps to maintain the acid-base balance and water and electrolyte content of body tissue.

Different blood components may be administered for different deficiencies. Although this section focuses on the transfusion of whole blood and packed red blood cells (RBCs), other blood products you may administer include platelets, fresh frozen plasma, and granulocytes. (See *Reviewing transfusion products*.)

Whole-blood transfusion replenishes both the volume and the oxygen-carrying capacity of the circulatory system. You'll give whole blood when a patient has massive blood loss, requiring replacement of the oxygen-carrying capacity of the RBCs and the volume expansion of the plasma. Whole blood is also given as an exchange transfusion in neonates. If the patient is actively bleeding, you may note a fluctuation in the hematocrit and hemoglobin due to the constant and rapid fluid shifts. In a stable, nonbleeding adult, the hematocrit rises by at least 3 percentage points and the hemoglobin rises by at least 1 g/dl after a unit of whole blood is given.

Reviewing transfusion products

Use this chart to review the types of blood products you may administer and the ways you'll use them.

PRODUCT	DESCRIPTION	NURSING CONSIDERATIONS
Whole blood	500-ml unit contains about 200 ml of red blood cells (RBCs) and about 300 ml of plasma.	• Indicated for massive blood loss and exchange transfusion in neonates. • Multiple-lead tubing (preferably a Y-type set) is recommended over piggybacking on a straight-line set. • Monitor vital signs frequently throughout transfusion. • Administer ABO group- and Rh type-specific product.
RBCs (packed)	350- to 400-ml unit contains about 200 to 250 ml of RBCs (with same amount of hemoglobin as whole blood) and 150 ml of plasma and additive solution (0.9% sodium chloride solution, adenine, glucose, or mannitol).	• Indicated for inadequate oxygen-carrying capacity. • A filter with larger surface area may be used to increase transfusion rate. • Administer ABO group- and Rh type-specific product, if possible. If not, group- and type-compatible product can be transfused safely. • A leukocyte removal filter may be ordered.
RBCs (deglycerol-ized or leuko-cyte-poor)	200-ml unit contains RBCs suspended in 50 ml of 0.9% sodium chloride solution, with virtually all leukocytes and plasma proteins removed. Deglycerolized RBCs, taken from donors with rare blood types, are first frozen (with glycerol added to preserve RBCs), then thawed and deglycerolized before transfusion. Leukocyte-poor RBCs aren't frozen.	• Same indications as for packed RBCs. Also used to prevent febrile reactions from leukocyte antibodies and to treat immunosuppressed patients. • All tubing should be rubber-free to prevent platelets from sticking. • Transfuse more rapidly than whole blood to prevent platelets from clumping and sticking to the side of the bag. • Administer ABO group- and Rh type-compatible product if possible. • Inspect unit for color. It should have a yellow tinge. • Agitate bag more often than other blood products because platelets tend to clump. • Adverse reactions are usually slight. • The American Red Cross recommends that units of platelet concentrates be pooled in blood bank into transfer packs, rather than administered as single-donor units. Expiration date is usually 2 to 5 days from date of collection.
Platelets	30- to 60-ml unit contains about half the number of platelets originally found in one unit of whole blood.	• Indicated to treat thrombocytopenia, acute leukemia, and bone marrow aplasia, and to restore platelet count preoperatively in a patient with a count of 100,000/mm³ or less. • ABO compatibility not necessary but recommended for repeated platelet transfusions. • Use a component drip administration set; infuse 100 ml over 15 minutes. • Patients with a history of platelet reaction require premedication with antipyretics and antihistamines. • Avoid administering when patient has a fever. • A leukocyte removal filter may be ordered.
Fresh frozen plasma	200- to 250-ml unit contains all coagulation factors and 250 mg of fibrinogen.	• Indicated to expand plasma volume, treat postoperative hemorrhage or shock, and correct coagulation factor deficiencies. • ABO compatibility not necessary. • Use a filtered straight-line set or Y-type set and administer rapidly. • Large volume transfusions may require correction for hypocalcemia.
Cryoprecipitated antihemophilic factor	Frozen 20-ml unit contains mostly coagulation factor VIII, plus 250 mg of fibrinogen.	• Indicated for hemophilia A, von Willebrand's disease, hypofibrinogenemia, and "fibrin glue." • Smaller needle or catheter size (22G or 23G for adults) may be used because product is not viscous. • Use component Y-type set if available. Tubing doesn't have to be rubber-free because product won't stick. • Transfuse more rapidly than whole blood because coagulation factors become unstable after thawing. • Administer ABO group-compatible product. • Patient usually receives multiple units. The American Red Cross recommends that they be pooled into transfer packs. Administer all units within 6 hours. • Because product has short half-life, transfusions may need to be repeated.

(continued)

Reviewing transfusion products *(continued)*

PRODUCT	DESCRIPTION	NURSING CONSIDERATIONS
Granulocytes	Unit volume varies (200 to 500 ml), but units contain mostly granulocytes (exact number depends on method of salvage) and RBCs, plasma, and platelets.	• Indicated in severe gram-negative infection or severe neutropenia unresponsive to routine forms of therapy in immunosuppressed patient. Also indicated in severe granulocyte dysfunction. • Microaggregate filter is contraindicated because it traps granulocytes. • Administer ABO group-compatible and, when possible, Rh type-compatible and human leukocyte antigen-compatible products. • For best results, administer as soon as possible after salvage. • Procedure must be repeated daily for 4 days or longer to be effective. • Because product consists of white blood cells, watch for chills and fever. Other adverse reactions include coughing and shortness of breath. Continue transfusion if possible but, if severe dyspnea develops, stop transfusion, keep vein open, and notify the doctor.
Serum albumin (5% and 25%) and plasma protein fraction (PPF)	25% albumin comes in 50-ml and 100-ml units. 5% albumin and PPF (essentially the same product) come in 250-ml units.	• Indicated in hypovolemia and hypoproteinemia (in burns, for example). • Because product comes in glass bottle, use administration set supplied with it. The set will have a filtered air inlet; 0.9% sodium chloride solution isn't needed as a starter. Product needs no blood filter. • 25% albumin is not usually given at more than 1 ml/min because of the danger of fluid overload. PPF given at over 10 ml/min may produce hypotension. • Compatibility testing isn't required because product contains no RBCs or plasma antibodies. • Product is free from human immunodeficiency and hepatitis viruses. • 25% albumin is used for patient with depleted vascular volume but extravascular fluid accumulation. • Because 25% albumin rapidly mobilizes large volumes of fluid into circulation, watch for pulmonary edema and other signs and symptoms of fluid overload. • Product is stored at room temperature and has an extremely long shelf life. Always check expiration date before administering.

Unlike whole-blood transfusion, transfusion of packed RBCs, from which 80% of the plasma has been removed, restores only the oxygen-carrying capacity. Administering packed RBCs instead of whole blood prevents fluid and circulatory overload. You don't give packed RBCs to increase a patient's overall well-being, for volume expansion, or to facilitate wound healing. Giving one unit of packed RBCs should have the same effect on the patient's hemoglobin and hematocrit as one unit of whole blood. Today, packed RBCs are given much more frequently than whole blood.

Equipment
You'll need tubing, a filter and, possibly, a pump for giving whole blood and packed RBCs. You should also have gloves, an I.V. pole, a 250-ml bag of 0.9% sodium chloride solution, and the unit of whole blood or blood product to be transfused.

Blood administration sets come with both straight sets and multiple-lead or Y-type tubing. Because it limits your ability to give other products or saline along with the blood, the straight-line set is usually not recommended.

A Y-type set minimizes the risk of contamination, especially when transfusing multiple units of blood. This set allows you to administer other blood products or volume expanders safely and easily; it also provides the option of adding saline solution to make the packed RBCs less viscous.

Use an in-line filter or I.V. tubing and a separate filter to remove any particles in the blood. The policy of your health care facility may require you to change the in-line filter or tubing with the filter after each unit of blood. The standard filter size is 170 microns.

You may also use a filter when you need

to remove specific blood components, most often leukocytes. Patients who require repeated transfusions sometimes develop antibodies against transfused leukocyte antigens. But they can still accept transfusions of leukocyte-poor RBCs or leukocyte-poor whole blood. You can clear the transfusion of 99% of the leukocytes by adding a leukocyte-removal filter to the blood bag.

If the patient needs large amounts of blood quickly, you may choose from three types of blood pumps: a pump built into the Y-type set, a pump that you slip over the blood bag, or an electronic infusion pump. You'll need to make sure that the pump's manufacturer recommends using it to administer blood. For information about electronic infusion pumps, see the discussion about using infusion controllers and pumps later in this chapter.

To use the pump built into a Y-type set, you'll squeeze the pump continuously while the blood is transfusing. The slip-on pump slips right over the blood bag. Air is pumped into the pump up to 300 mm Hg. If the pressure exceeds this, the RBCs may be damaged, the line may disconnect, or the bag may rupture. If the vein is too small to accommodate the blood under pressure, the blood may infiltrate the skin. (See *Transfusing blood under pressure: Using a slip-on blood pump,* page 46.)

Blood administration
Before starting a blood transfusion, you'll follow several precautionary measures to prevent the patient from receiving the wrong blood. You must get the patient's informed consent, obtain a baseline set of vital signs, and confirm his identity and the compatibility of the blood you're planning to administer. Then you're ready to gather your equipment and initiate the transfusion.

Preparation
First, take the patient's temperature. If he has a fever, notify his doctor because a fever can mask adverse reactions to the transfusion. If the patient has a history of allergic reactions to transfusions, the doctor may prescribe prophylactic medications, such as an antihistamine or acetaminophen. Also report any other abnormal vital signs.

Make sure you obtain the blood or blood product from the blood bank within 30 minutes of the transfusion start time. Check the expiration date on the blood bag, and observe the contents for abnormal color, RBC clumping, gas bubbles, and extraneous material that may indicate bacterial contamination. If you see any of these, return the bag to the blood bank.

Confirming the patient's identity. After obtaining blood from the blood bank and before hanging each unit, you and another nurse should identify the unit. Then verify the patient's identity. If he's alert, ask him to state his name, and check the name and identification number on his wristband. (When blood is drawn for typing and crossmatching, the patient receives an identification wristband that includes his full name, health care facility number, room number, the date and time the blood was drawn, the number of the blood component compatibility tag, and the name or initials of the person who performed the blood collection.) After confirming the patient's identity, you and the other nurse should examine the compatibility tag attached to the blood bag and the information printed on the bag. Make sure that the ABO group, Rh type, and unit number match. Report any discrepancies to the blood bank, and delay the transfusion until they're resolved.

Inserting the catheter. Now, insert an 18G or a 20G catheter into a large peripheral vein. Smaller catheters will inhibit flow rates.

Transfusing blood
Whether you're transfusing whole blood or packed RBCs, you'll start and monitor the transfusion the same way. First, put on gloves. Then open the box with the Y-type administration set and remove the tubing. (See *Do's and don'ts of blood administration,* page 47.)

Move the roller clamp on the main line directly under the drip chamber, and close the clamp. Also close the clamps on the 0.9% sodium chloride solution line and the blood line.

Transfusing blood under pressure: Using a slip-on blood pump

When you're using the slip-on pump for blood transfusion, you'll follow the steps described below. The pump slips right over the blood bag.

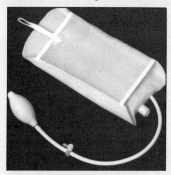

Insert the spike of the blood administration set into the blood bag and prime the tubing. Insert your hand into the pump envelope, and pull the blood bag up through the center opening. Grasp the pump envelope loops (used for hanging) and slip them through the blood bag loop, as shown below. Then, hang the set on an I.V. pole.

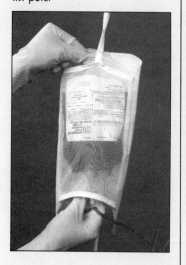

Turn the stopcock to the right, as shown.

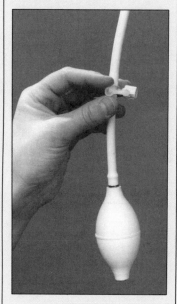

Connect the line to the venipuncture device and open the flow clamp on the administration set. Squeeze the bulb of the pump until you've reached the desired flow rate.

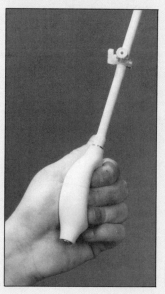

Don't let the pressure on the pump exceed 300 mm Hg. A pressure beyond that level may damage the red blood cells, cause the line to disconnect, or rupture the bag. Turn the stopcock to the OFF position to maintain a constant pressure rate.

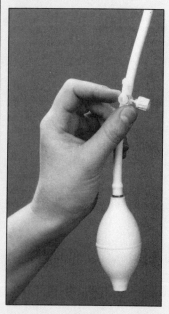

Repeat the procedure with each new blood bag. Remember that as the bag empties, pressure decreases. Check the flow rate and adjust the clamp, as necessary. Observe the site carefully. If the vein is too small to accept the blood under pressure, the blood may infiltrate the skin.

Do's and don'ts of blood administration

Administering a blood transfusion requires extreme care. Review the following tips on what to do and what not to do during a transfusion.

Do's
• Write the number of the blood bag on the intake-and-output flow sheet. That way, you'll have a backup in case the sticker falls off.
• Record vital signs before the transfusion, 15 minutes later, and after the transfusion (or more often, according to the policy of your health care facility). Most acute hemolytic reactions occur during the first 50 ml of the transfusion, so watch your patient carefully for the first half hour.
• Act promptly if the patient develops wheezing and bronchospasm. These reactions may indicate an allergic reaction or anaphylaxis. If, after a few milliliters of blood is transfused, a patient becomes dyspneic and shows generalized flushing and chest pain (with or without vomiting and diarrhea), he could be having an anaphylactic reaction. Stop the blood and change the tubing. Start a slow infusion of 0.9% sodium chloride solution. Then ask another nurse to stay with the patient and administer oxygen while you call the doctor. Monitor the patient's vital signs, and keep the head of the bed elevated if the vital signs allow it. Make sure you tell the patient what's happening. Expect epinephrine and corticosteroid administration and intubation as emergency treatments.
• Send the blood bag and its tubing to the blood bank, collect a urine specimen, and call the laboratory to request a repeat crossmatching if the patient shows signs worse than a rash or slight fever. Remember, only laboratory tests can determine whether a severe reaction is hemolytic, pyrogenic, severely allergic, or anaphylactic.
• Watch elderly and cardiac patients for signs of circulatory overload. If these patients are given too much fluid, or if the blood is transfused too rapidly, they may develop congestive heart failure. Slow the transfusion to a keep-vein-open rate, raise the head of the bed, and administer oxygen. Then notify the doctor.

Don'ts
• Avoid adding any medications to the blood bag.
• Never give blood or blood products without checking the order against the blood bag label. This is the only way you can discover if the request form has been stamped with the wrong name. Most life-threatening reactions result when this step is omitted.
• Don't piggyback blood into the port of an existing line. Most solutions—including dextrose in water—are incompatible with blood, so administer blood only with 0.9% sodium chloride solution.
• When you can't give the blood as planned, don't put blood bags in the unit refrigerator. The refrigerator's temperature isn't controlled, and the blood might be damaged. Return the blood to the blood bank and get it when you're ready to hang it.
• Don't stop the transfusion if your patient develops an itchy rash or hives. Most likely, these signs indicate an allergic reaction. If the patient isn't dyspneic, just reduce the transfusion rate and call the doctor.
• Don't hesitate to stop the transfusion if your patient shows vital sign changes, is dyspneic or restless, or if he develops chills, hematuria, or pain in the flank, chest, or back. Your patient could go into shock, so don't remove the I.V. line. Instead, keep it open with a slow infusion of 0.9% sodium chloride solution while you call the doctor and the laboratory.
• Never transfuse blood that's been unrefrigerated for more than 4 hours. The risk of sepsis or bacterial contamination would be too high.

Remove the cap from the spike on the normal saline solution line. Insert the spike into the container.

Next, remove the cap from the blood line spike. Pull back the two tabs at the top of the blood bag to expose the port. Insert the blood line spike into the blood bag port.

Hang the entire Y-type set on the I.V. pole. With the clamp on the blood line closed, open the saline line clamp. Squeeze the drip chamber until it is half full. Then open the main tubing clamp and flush the entire line with saline solution. Close both clamps.

When the patient's vein can't accommodate the viscosity of the RBCs, you may need to dilute them with a small amount of saline solution. To dilute packed RBCs, hang the blood bag lower than the saline. Keep both Y-ports open. Allow a backflow of 50 to 75 ml of saline into the blood bag; then clamp the tubings. Gently rock the blood bag to distribute the normal saline.

Because infusing blood through a needle can damage the RBCs, remove the protective cap from the end of the administration tubing and flush the entire line with saline solution. Attach the tubing to the venipuncture device. Then close both clamps.

Next, open the blood line clamp. Squeeze the drip chamber on the Y-type set until the blood completely covers the filter. Open the Y-type set's main clamp and start the infusion slowly. No more than 30 ml should be transfused during the first 15 minutes.

Stay with the patient for at least the first 15 minutes of the transfusion because this is when reaction symptoms usually occur. After 15 minutes, take the patient's vital signs. If they're stable, increase the infusion rate so that the unit is infused in 2 to 4 hours, depending on the patient's condition.

Continue monitoring the patient throughout the infusion, according to the policy of your health care facility. When the blood bag is empty, close the blood line clamp. Open the saline solution clamp to flush the tubing. Then close the remaining clamps.

After the transfusion is complete, flush the filter and tubing with the saline solution. If the patient is to receive I.V. fluids, put on gloves, remove the blood tubing, and attach the primary tubing.

Return the empty blood bag to the blood bank, and discard the tubing and filter in a protective bag. Record the patient's vital signs.

Complications

Many transfusion-related complications, including transfusion reactions, are immediate, but others can be delayed up to 96 hours. Although a transfusion reaction typically results from incompatibility, contaminated blood, or too rapid an infusion, other complications stem from mechanical malfunction or other problems with the transfusion equipment. (See *Correcting transfusion problems*.)

Transfusion reactions can occur after single transfusions, or massive or multiple transfusions. Unlike a transfusion reaction, an infectious disease transmitted during a transfusion may go undetected until days, weeks, or even months later, when it produces signs and symptoms.

Single-transfusion reactions

Reactions to a single transfusion include air embolism, hemolytic reaction, febrile reaction, allergic reaction, blood contamination, circulatory overload, and plasma protein incompatibility.

Hemolytic reaction. Caused by an ABO or Rh incompatibility or by improper storage of the blood unit, a hemolytic reaction may cause such signs and symptoms as shaking, chills, fever, nausea, vomiting, chest pain, dyspnea, hypotension, oliguria, hemoglobinuria, flank pain, and abnormal bleeding.

If you note any of these signs and symptoms, stop the transfusion immediately. Keep the vein open with a secondary line of 0.9% sodium chloride solution. Treat the patient's shock by giving oxygen, fluids, and epinephrine, as ordered. Maintain his renal circulation by giving mannitol (Osmitrol) or furosemide (Lasix), and collect blood and urine samples for the laboratory. In a hemolytic reaction, the blood will show hemolysis, and the urine will contain hemoglobin. Record fluid intake and output, and watch for signs of diuresis or oliguria.

One way to prevent a hemolytic reaction is to make sure the blood you're administering is compatible with the patient's blood type. Always double-check the patient's identification before starting the transfusion, and begin the transfusion slowly. Stay with the patient for at least the first 15 minutes of the transfusion.

Febrile reaction. A common reaction, although not usually a serious one, a febrile reaction results from the presence of bacterial lipopolysaccharides. The patient's anti-human leukocyte antigen antibodies react with the transfused lymphocytes or platelet cell mem-

Correcting transfusion problems

A patient who receives excellent care can still encounter problems during a transfusion. Here's how to proceed when common transfusion problems occur.

If the transfusion stops
• Check the distance between the I.V. container and the insertion site. Make sure it's at least 3' (1 m) above the site.
• Make sure the flow clamp is open.
• Make sure the blood completely covers the filter. If it doesn't, squeeze the drip chamber until it does, as shown below.

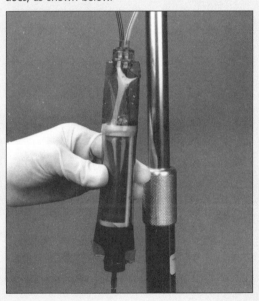

• Rock the bag back and forth gently to agitate blood cells that may have settled to the bottom.
• Squeeze the tubing and flashbulb to get the fluid moving again.
• Untape the dressing over the insertion site, and make sure the needle or catheter is still correctly placed in the vein. Reposition if necessary.
• Close the primary line's flow clamp. Lower the blood bag and open the 0.9% sodium chloride solution line. Dilute the blood with 50 to 100 ml of this solution to facilitate blood flow.

If a hematoma develops at the needle site
• Stop the transfusion immediately.
• Remove the needle or catheter, and cap the tubing with a new needle and guard.
• Notify the doctor. Expect an order to apply ice intermittently to the site for 24 hours and warm compresses after that.
• Promote reabsorption of the hematoma by gently exercising the involved limb.
• Document your observations and actions.

If the blood bag empties before the next one arrives
• Hang a container of 0.9% sodium chloride solution, if you haven't already, and administer it slowly until the new blood arrives.
• If you used a Y-type set, close the blood line clamp, open the 0.9% sodium chloride solution line clamp, and let it run slowly until the new blood arrives. Make sure to decrease the flow rate or clamp the line before attaching the new unit of blood.

---

branes. He may experience signs ranging from mild chills and fever to the more serious signs and symptoms of a hemolytic reaction.

For mild cases, administer antipyretics and antihistamines, as ordered. Treat severe cases as you'd treat a hemolytic reaction.

You can help prevent this reaction by keeping the patient covered and warm. Using a leukocyte-removal filter during the transfusion may prevent febrile reaction, as may administering saline-washed RBCs or frozen saline–

washed packed cells. You may administer antipyretics with the blood, but never add antihistamines to the blood bag.

Allergic reaction. Like a febrile reaction, an allergic reaction is common but shouldn't become serious. An allergic reaction results from an atopic substance in the blood. The patient may experience pruritus, urticaria, facial swelling, chills, fever, nausea, and vomiting. If you note any of these signs and symptoms, notify the doctor and give parenteral antihistamines. For more serious cases, give epinephrine or corticosteroids, as needed.

To prevent an allergic reaction, find out if the patient has ever had such a reaction to a transfusion. If so, he has a two in three chance of having another one.

Blood contamination. Although blood contamination is rare, it's a serious complication. Caused by cold-growing, gram-negative bacteria, such as *Pseudomonas,* cloiform, or *Achromobacter,* blood contamination may cause chills, fever, vomiting, abdominal cramping, diarrhea, shock, and signs of renal failure. Notify the doctor at the first indication of blood contamination. He may order a broad-spectrum antibiotic and corticosteroids.

To prevent blood contamination, examine the blood for gas, clots, or a dark purple color. Make sure that blood storage is strictly controlled, and use aseptic technique during administration. Change the blood tubing and filter every 4 hours, and transfuse each unit of blood over 2 to 4 hours.

Circulatory overload. Common and fairly easy to treat, circulatory overload occurs when too large a transfusion is given and the patient cannot handle the extra fluid over a short period. The patient may have engorged neck veins, constricting chest pain with breathing difficulties, moist crackles and, eventually, acute edema.

If these signs and symptoms occur, stop the transfusion and notify the doctor immediately. He may prescribe a diuretic. Once the transfusion is stopped, give D_5W — not 0.9% sodium chloride solution — to keep the vein open.

To prevent circulatory overload, the doctor may order packed RBCs rather than whole blood. He also may order a diuretic before or during the transfusion. You should keep the patient warm and in a sitting position. With high-risk patients, transfuse the blood at a reduced rate.

Plasma protein incompatibility. Caused by immunoglobulin A (IgA) incompatibility, a

plasma protein incompatibility reaction is rare but serious. The patient may experience flushing, abdominal pain, diarrhea, chills, fever, dyspnea, and hypotension. Usually he goes into shock, so the doctor may order oxygen, fluids, and epinephrine. Sometimes, corticosteroids are given. To prevent plasma protein incompatibility, transfuse only IgA-deficient blood or washed RBCs.

Multiple-transfusion reactions
Multiple-transfusion reactions include hemosiderosis, bleeding tendencies, elevated blood ammonia level, increased oxygen affinity for hemoglobin, hypothermia, hypocalcemia, and hyperkalemia.

Hemosiderosis. Caused by RBC destruction, hemosiderosis is an increase in hemosiderin (iron-containing pigment levels). The patient will have a plasma iron level greater than 200 mg/dl. Excess iron must be removed by phlebotomy. To prevent hemosiderosis, blood should be administered only when absolutely necessary.

Bleeding tendencies. Dilutional thrombocytopenia results from the low platelet count in stored blood. The patient may complain of abnormal bleeding and oozing from a cut or break in the skin surface. To treat bleeding, administer platelets and monitor the patient's platelet count. To prevent bleeding, make sure the patient receives only fresh blood (less than 7 days old) whenever possible.

Hypothermia. The result of a rapid transfusion of large amounts of cold blood, hypothermia decreases myocardial temperature. The patient may experience shaking, chills, and hypotension. If his core temperature falls below 86° F (30° C), the patient may experience ventricular fibrillation and cardiac arrest. To treat hypothermia, stop the transfusion and warm the patient with blankets. You should also obtain an electrocardiogram (ECG) to assess for any heart irregularities. To prevent hypothermia in a patient receiving multiple transfusions, use a blood warmer to warm the blood to 95° to 98.6° F (35° to 37° C) before transfusing it.

Hypocalcemia. Multiple transfusions can lead to hypocalcemia. Citrate toxicity occurs when citrate-treated blood is infused rapidly. Citrate binds with calcium, causing a calcium deficiency. Normal citrate metabolism may also be hindered by hepatic disease. The patient may experience tingling in the fingers, muscle cramps, nausea, vomiting, hypotension, cardiac arrhythmias, and seizures.

To treat hypocalcemia, slow or stop the transfusion, depending on the severity of the reaction. Expect a worse reaction in hypothermic patients and in patients with elevated potassium levels. The doctor may order a slow I.V. infusion of calcium gluconate.

To prevent hypocalcemia, transfuse the blood slowly, monitor potassium and calcium levels, and use blood less than 2 days old when administering multiple units.

Hyperkalemia. A potentially serious reaction, hyperkalemia results from an abnormally high level of potassium in stored plasma, which is caused by RBC lysis. The patient may develop intestinal colic; diarrhea; renal failure; ECG changes with tall, peaked T waves; or bradycardia leading to cardiac standstill. You may need to run an ECG and administer sodium polystyrene sulfonate (Kayexalate) orally or by enema to lower the serum potassium level. To prevent hyperkalemia, use fresh blood for multiple transfusions.

Transmittable diseases

Even though blood and blood products undergo many tests that screen for transmittable diseases, you can never be sure the blood you're transfusing is free of disease. These five diseases may be transmitted through a blood transfusion: acquired immunodeficiency syndrome (AIDS), hepatitis, malaria, syphilis, and a viral syndrome. The causes and incubation time vary for each, as do the methods of detection, treatment, and prevention.

AIDS. Caused by the presence of the human immunodeficiency virus (HIV) in the blood, AIDS has an incubation time of months to years. AIDS antibodies develop within 6 weeks to 6 months after infection. The presence of the antibodies in the blood confirms the presence of the virus. These antibodies can be detected by two tests, the enzyme-linked immunosorbent assay (ELISA) and the Western blot assay.

Although antiviral drugs may reduce a carrier's ability to infect another, no drug cures HIV infection. To prevent transmission of the virus through blood transfusion, potential donors should be educated about the disease and the need for strict compliance with the Centers for Disease Control's universal precautions.

Hepatitis. The greatest risk of hepatitis B and hepatitis C transmission is carried by pooled plasma, fibrinogen, and concentrates of factors VII and IX. Immune serum globulin, plasma protein fraction, and normal serum albumin pose no risk. Hepatitis C—formerly called non-A, non-B hepatitis—accounts for 85% of blood-borne hepatitis cases. The incubation time for this disease is 2 weeks to 6 months.

If a patient does contract hepatitis, he may exhibit these signs and symptoms: anorexia, vomiting, abdominal discomfort, enlarged liver, diarrhea, headache, fever, and jaundice. Once diagnosed with hepatitis, a patient must be isolated to avoid infecting others. He should receive gamma globulin therapy and nursing care that promotes his comfort.

To avoid hepatitis transmission, make sure the blood is tested for the hepatitis B surface antigen and the anti-hepatitis C virus before you administer it. All donor blood products should receive a radioimmunoassay for hepatitis B. Only healthy, reliable donors should be accepted. If potential donors are suspected hepatitis carriers, arrange for epidemiologic follow-up tests.

Malaria. Caused by protozoan parasites in RBCs, malaria has an incubation time of 2 weeks to 4 months. To treat malaria, administer quinine sulfate (Legatrin) or chloroquine phosphate (Aralen Phosphate). To prevent malaria transmission through a blood transfusion, avoid donors who have lived in parts of the world where the disease is endemic or those who have not taken antimalarial drugs for at least 3 years.

Syphilis. The spirochete *Treponema pallidum* causes syphilis, a disease with an incubation time of 4 to 18 weeks. The patient may have a positive serologic test and a genital chancre, which is considered proof of the disease.

To treat syphilis, administer penicillin. To prevent it, don't administer blood unless it has been tested and refrigerated for at least 2 days at 39.2° F (4° C) to kill the spirochetes.

Viral syndrome. A viral syndrome can be caused by cytomegalovirus or Epstein-Barr virus in the blood. The incubation time for these viruses is 2 to 5 weeks. The patient with a viral syndrome will develop fever, atypical lymphocytosis, and a rash. He'll also have some degree of hepatitis, with or without jaundice. Currently no treatment for a viral syndrome exists. To prevent transmission from a blood transfusion, select donors who are free of recent viral symptoms.

Nursing considerations
• You may need to use a blood or fluid warmer, a device that provides external heat to the blood or I.V. fluid before it enters the patient's vein. Blood or fluid warmers are commonly used to prevent hypothermia and patient discomfort during the transfusion of a large volume of cold blood. They're also used to prevent cardiac arrhythmias during central-line blood administration and to prevent an antigen-antibody reaction when cold agglutinins are identified in the crossmatching process. Cold agglutinins may cause clumping at temperatures below 39° F (3.9° C), leading to hemolysis.

A blood or fluid warmer may be electronic or nonelectronic. Some may require special tubing or a warming bag, but others can be used with conventional blood administration sets. Before using a blood or fluid warmer, read the manufacturer's instructions. And be sure to check the policy of your health care facility regarding their use.
• Make sure you document each step thoroughly. If your health care facility requires it, you may need to record information in a special blood administration record for legal purposes. This information includes the signatures of the two nurses who identified the blood product and the patient, the blood product administered, the patient's baseline and subsequent vital signs, the time the transfusion was started and the time it was completed, and the total volume transfused, including the blood product and the starter solution, with their individual volumes listed separately. You'll also record the patient's response to the transfusion. Include any signs or symptoms of an adverse reaction and the interventions carried out.

Patient teaching
Allay your patient's anxieties about his upcoming blood transfusion by explaining the process thoroughly before you begin. Reassure him that the blood product he'll receive has been thoroughly tested by the health care facility for impurities and transmittable diseases. Tell him that his vital signs will be taken frequently during the 2 to 4 hours of the transfusion and that he'll be watched closely. Instruct him to report any shortness of breath, chest pain, itching, or chills. If the patient can walk, encourage him to use the bathroom before you start the transfusion so that he won't be up and around while the blood product is infusing.

If you're administering a blood transfusion to a patient in his home, you'll probably need to explain the process to the patient and to a caregiver. Tell the patient that quality-control measures ensure the same safety at home as in the health care facility. (See *Administering transfusions.*)

Patient-controlled analgesia

Patient-controlled analgesia (PCA) puts the patient in charge of relieving his own pain. Steadily improving technology in this area has increased the popularity of PCA, and the method of administration is most often I.V.

An I.V. PCA pump can deliver small amounts of a narcotic at a slow, continuous rate, and it allows the patient to give himself boluses of the narcotic when pain increases. With I.V. administration, drug absorption is faster and more predictable than with I.M. administration. When patients control their own analgesia, less narcotic is used and they are sedated for less time than when they receive prescribed doses of pain reliever through another route. They tend to experience less pain and return to normal activities sooner.

Morphine is the most commonly prescribed drug for PCA, but many other drugs are also given, including hydromorphone, fentanyl, buprenorphine, meperidine, and methadone. The anesthesiologist determines the drug based on the patient's weight, age, and previous narcotics usage. He may establish a basal rate—the maximum amount the patient may receive hourly in continuous infusion. He'll also determine whether a bolus dose can be given and how often. Within these established limits, the patient can control the amount of drug he receives. You should check the pump twice a day to make sure the patient is getting enough relief and is experiencing no adverse reactions.

It is essential that patients receiving PCA therapy be mentally alert and able to understand and comply with instructions and procedures. Patients with limited respiratory reserve, a history of drug abuse, or a psychiatric disorder are ineligible for PCA.

Equipment

Many PCA pumps are available, and the technology is constantly changing. Although certain features are necessary, others simply add to the cost of the pump. Determining the type of pump to use should depend on the needs of your patients.

In evaluating a pump, first consider its cost and the cost of its operation. Does it include expensive refill cassettes or syringes? Consider cost along with the pump's complexity. How easy is it to operate, both for you and the patient? Operating the pump should be a straightforward procedure but not so simple that anyone can manipulate the program. Evaluate the pump's size and portability. An ambulatory patient should have a small, portable PCA pump. Can the pump be used on an I.V. pole

Administering transfusions

To give a transfusion in a patient's home, follow these guidelines:
• Transport the blood product in a container with the appropriate coolant for the product. The proper temperature for transporting blood is between 33.8° and 50° F (1° and 10° C); for platelets, it's between 68° and 75° F (20° and 24° C).
• Encourage the patient to void before you begin the transfusion because the procedure may take up to 2 hours.
• Set up and transfuse the product according to the policy of your health care facility.
• After the transfusion, keep the I.V. line open, and stay with the patient for at least 30 minutes to watch for delayed reaction to the transfusion.
• If no reactions occur within 30 minutes of the transfusion, remove the I.V. line and give the patient or caregiver posttransfusion instructions.
• Place all equipment, including the containers and infusion devices, in a bag labeled BIOHAZARD and then into the transport container. Return the container to the blood bank for proper disposal.
• If a transfusion reaction occurs, notify the transfusion service and the patient's doctor immediately.

and carried or worn as well?

Some pumps can provide both continuous infusion and bolus doses. Others only provide bolus doses. For many patients, bolus dosing is inferior to continuous infusion. If the patient doesn't receive a regular amount of the drug, he may suffer a rapid decline in relief following a high peak. If the bolus dose is too low, he may need up to 10 doses an hour. And if he falls asleep, he may awake in pain.

Some pumps offer a wide range of volume settings for both bolus doses and continuous infusion. They may have a panel that can display the amount delivered or, if necessary, an alarm message. You can program certain pumps to record the concentration in either

Initiating subcutaneous PCA therapy

Subcutaneous patient-controlled analgesia (PCA) therapy is often used to manage chronic pain. Therapy can be administered through a number of routes, such as the abdominal route shown below. If you're initiating PCA via this route, follow these steps:

• Insert a 27G butterfly needle or a commercial subcutaneous infusion needle into the patient's abdomen or into another area with accessible subcutaneous tissue.

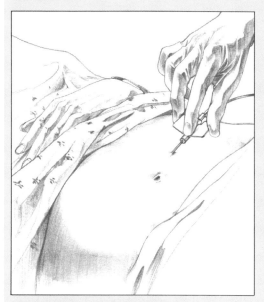

• Cover the site with a dressing.
• Calculate the hourly subcutaneous dose the same way you would an I.V. dose, considering both the hourly infusion rate and the bolus doses.
• Subcutaneous absorption of a drug depends on the patient's condition. The maximum volume per hour that a well-nourished and well-hydrated patient can usually absorb is about 2 to 2.5 ml. If your patient can't absorb that much, you may need to increase the drug's concentration. The minimum volume per hour should be about 1 ml.
• Inspect the site twice a day for signs of irritation. If it becomes irritated, change to a new site as often as necessary and apply a corticosteroid cream two or three times a day. Otherwise, change the site weekly or according to the policy of your health care facility.

milligrams (mg) or milliliters (ml), allowing greater flexibility in choosing rates. With some pumps you can vary the length of the lockout interval (how often a dose can be delivered) from 5 to 90 minutes. And some pumps can be programmed to store and retrieve information such as the total dose allowed in a specified length of time.

Drug administration

With PCA, the patient controls drug delivery by pressing a button on the pump. Before the device can be used, it must be programmed to deliver the specified doses at the correct time intervals. You can set up a pump to deliver PCA subcutaneously as well as I.V. (See *Initiating subcutaneous PCA therapy.*)

If the patient is using a pump that provides continuous infusion, he can control incidental pain (from coughing, for example) or breakthrough pain. If he's receiving continuous infusion therapy at home, the pump should allow him to stop and start the infusion.

If the patient is having steady pain that gradually increases or decreases, or pain that's worse at one time or another, he should be able to regulate the hourly infusion rate. If he has sudden but brief increases in pain, he should be able to give himself bolus doses along with the infusion. But if his pain is intermittent, he may not need continuous infusion at all.

Programming the PCA pump

You and the patient's doctor determine the initial trial bolus dose and a time interval between boluses. You'll program this information into the pump. Once these safety limits are set, the patient can push the button to receive a dose when he feels pain. You and the doctor may decide to change either the dose or the lock-out interval after you've seen how the patient responds. (See *Determining bolus doses and lock-out intervals.*)

If the patient hasn't been receiving narcotics, first give the drug until his pain is relieved (the loading dose). With morphine, for example, give 1 to 5 mg every 10 minutes until the pain subsides. Then set the pump's hourly infusion rate to equal the total number of milligrams per hour needed to control the pain. If you set the pump so that the patient can give himself bolus doses, decrease the hourly infusion rate. Check his response every 15 to 30 minutes for 1 to 2 hours.

If you can program the pump to deliver a continuous infusion plus bolus doses, remember this rule of thumb: The initial total hourly dose shouldn't exceed the cumulative bolus doses per hour needed to relieve the pain. For example, if the patient needs a total of 6 mg of morphine over 1 hour, you could begin therapy with a continuous infusion of 3 mg/ hour, allowing bolus doses of 0.5 mg every 10 minutes (six boluses/hour). If the patient needs six or more boluses, check with the doctor about increasing the hourly infusion rate.

Complications

The primary complication of PCA is respiratory depression. Other complications include anaphylaxis, nausea, vomiting, constipation, postural hypotension, and drug tolerance. Infiltration into the subcutaneous tissue and catheter occlusion may also occur, and this can cause the drug to back up into the primary I.V. tubing.

Nursing considerations

• Before giving a narcotic analgesic, review the patient's medication regimen. Concurrent use of two central nervous system (CNS) depressants may cause drowsiness, oversedation, disorientation, and anxiety.
• Use caution when programming the PCA pump. After changing the program, don't start the pump until another nurse has double-checked the new settings.
• Monitor vital signs every 2 hours for the first 8 hours after starting PCA.
• Because narcotic analgesics can cause postural hypotension, guard against accidents. Keep the side rails raised on the patient's bed. If the patient is mobile, help him out of bed and assist him in walking. Encourage him to practice coughing and deep breathing to promote ventilation and to prevent pooling of secretions, which could lead to respiratory difficulty.
• In case of anaphylaxis, treat the symptoms

Determining bolus doses and lock-out intervals

Follow these suggestions for determining bolus doses for bolus-only patient-controlled analgesia pumps and lock-out intervals in bolus-only or bolus plus continuous infusion devices.

Determining bolus doses

If the patient has only intermittent pain, simply estimate a dose and increase or decrease it until you determine the amount that relieves pain. Calculate the mg/dose and the total dose (or number of boluses) that he may receive per hour.

Determining lock-out intervals for bolus doses

• For I.V. boluses (whether bolus only or bolus plus continuous infusion), set the lock-out interval for 6 minutes or more. Typically, pain relief following an I.V. narcotic bolus takes 6 to 10 minutes.
• For subcutaneous boluses (whether bolus only or bolus plus continuous infusion), set the lock-out interval for 30 minutes or more. Typically, pain relief following a subcutaneous bolus takes 30 to 60 minutes.
• For spinal boluses (whether bolus only or bolus plus continuous infusion), set the lock-out interval for 60 minutes or more. Typically, pain relief following a spinal bolus takes 30 to 60 minutes.

and give another drug for pain relief, as ordered.
• Watch for respiratory depression during administration. If the patient's respiratory rate declines to 10 or fewer breaths per minute, call his name and touch him. Tell him to breathe deeply. If he can't be roused, or is confused or restless, notify the doctor and prepare to give oxygen. If ordered, give a narcotic antagonist such as naloxone. Respiratory depression during PCA isn't common. That's because if a patient receives too much narcotic, he'll fall asleep and be unable to press the bolus button. Make sure family or staff members don't give extra doses of the narcotic when a patient hasn't requested them.
• Evaluate the effectiveness of the drug at regular intervals. Is the patient getting relief? Does

Teaching your patient about PCA

When your patient plans to receive patient-controlled analgesia (PCA) therapy at home, make sure that he and his family fully understand the method. Explain how the pump works and precisely how he can increase or decrease his dose. Also, make sure that he and his caregivers know when to contact the doctor.

Managing doses
A narcotic analgesic relieves pain best when taken before the pain becomes intense. Stress that the patient shouldn't increase the dose or the frequency of administration. If he misses a dose, he should take it as soon as he remembers. But, if it's almost time for the next dose, tell him to skip the missed dose. Advise the patient never to double-dose.

Using caution
Advise the patient to get up slowly from his bed or a chair because the drug may cause postural hypotension. Instruct him to eat a high-fiber diet, to drink plenty of fluids, and to take a stool softener if one has been prescribed. Caution him against drinking alcohol because this may enhance central nervous system depression.

Calling the doctor
Your patient should notify his doctor if the drug loses its effectiveness. His family should report signs of an overdose: slow or irregular breathing, pinpoint pupils, or loss of consciousness. Teach family members how to maintain respiration until help arrives.

• If a patient has persistent nausea and vomiting during therapy, the doctor may change the medication. If ordered, give the patient an antiemetic such as chlorpromazine.
• To prevent constipation, give the patient a stool softener and, if necessary, a senna derivative laxative. Provide a high-fiber diet and encourage the patient to drink fluids. Regular exercise may also help. In case of urine retention, monitor the patient's intake and output.
• Always document the drug given, the amount (including boluses), the effectiveness of the treatment, and the patient's vital signs.

Patient teaching
Your patient must understand how PCA works for therapy to succeed. Although some patients receive excellent preoperative teaching, not all patients who receive PCA go through planned surgery. Often you, as the patient's nurse, are in the best position to teach him and his family about PCA. And you may have to reinforce your teaching several times, especially with an elderly or a confused patient. Keep in mind that PCA isn't for everyone. A patient won't do well with this method if he can't understand it.

When teaching your patient the techniques involved in PCA, be sure to stress that he'll be able to control his pain. Reassure him that the method is safe and effective, but that he may experience mild discomfort.

Home care patients must receive particularly good instructions. Include the patient's family in your teaching session, if possible, and instruct the family members to contact the doctor whenever they suspect a problem. (See *Teaching your patient about PCA.*)

the dosage need to be increased because of persistent or worse pain? Is the patient developing a tolerance to the drug? Although you should give the smallest effective dose over the shortest time period, narcotic analgesics shouldn't be withheld or given in ineffective doses. Psychological dependence on narcotic analgesics occurs in fewer than 1% of hospitalized patients.

Using infusion controllers and pumps

When administering an I.V. infusion, you'll probably use one of the many electronic infusion devices available. Classified as either infusion controllers or infusion pumps, these electronic control devices permit accurate, on-

How infusion devices operate

The most common electronic systems for delivering an I.V. infusion include the peristaltic system, the syringe pump, the cassette system, and the elastomeric reservoir. These four systems operate on different principles.

Peristaltic system
Infusion devices that work by peristaltic action deliver fluid using rotary cams (rotary peristaltic) or fingerlike projections (linear peristaltic). The fluid is propelled along its pathway when the rotating cams or projections press on the tubing. The action is similar to GI peristalsis.

With most peristaltic devices, a special piece of tubing attaches to a reservoir bag, which determines the range of volumes for pump delivery. One disadvantage of this method: The tubing may eventually become stretched because of the constant pressure of the moving fluid.

Syringe pump
A common choice for I.V. drug infusion, the syringe pump is less costly and more widely available than other infusion devices. A syringe pump is generally more accurate than a peristaltic pump.

With most syringe pumps, a motor-driven lead screw or gear mechanism drives the syringe plunger. The speed of the motor determines the plunger's rate of movement and thus the rate of infusion. The syringe plunger moves and delivers a measure of fluid, followed by a pause before the plunger's next motor movement.

The main disadvantage of a syringe pump is its 60-ml volume limit.

Cassette system
A pump that uses a cassette system includes an electronic infuser and a disposable administration set with a measured chamber. The disposable cassette attaches easily to the infuser.

Pumps using a cassette system need two separate sequential cycles to deliver fluid: one cycle to fill the chamber with the right amount of fluid and another cycle to infuse that volume. Many large-volume infusion pumps (such as the IMED 900 pump) use the cassette system. The Parker Micropump is frequently used with ambulatory patients.

Elastomeric reservoir
Pumps that use this system work by exerting a constant pressure on a balloonlike reservoir. Medication is forced through a flow restrictor that controls the flow rate. The internal pressure of the elastomeric reservoir is low; thus, its one disadvantage is that the accuracy of medication delivery may depend on such external factors as temperature and solution viscosity.

---

time delivery of drugs and fluids. With controllers and pumps, you can adjust flow rates immediately, and you'll make fewer hands-on infusion checks. These devices prevent rapid infusions, reduce the incidence of infiltration, and maintain catheter patency. The primary difference between controllers and pumps is this: A pump can add pressure to the infusion to overcome resistance but a controller can't.

Recent advances in infusion technology and computer technology have produced devices with very sophisticated operating and programming capabilities. Some devices allow you to program different rates for a single solution. Others permit the infusion of several solutions at different rates, meaning you'll need only one device per patient. (See *How infusion devices operate.*)

Controllers and pumps have various detectors and alarms that automatically signal or respond to the completion of an infusion, air in the line, low battery power, an occlusion, and inability to deliver at the preset rate. Depending on the problem, these devices may sound or flash an alarm, shut off, or switch to a keep-vein-open rate.

Equipment
Besides your pump or controller, you may need an I.V. pole. Also, gather a sterile I.V. administration set; sterile peristaltic tubing or cassette, if needed; alcohol sponges; and adhesive tape.

ADVANCED EQUIPMENT

I.V. infusion pumps

This chart presents four categories of the newest infusion pumps used in peripheral venous therapy.

PUMP AND MAKER	RESERVOIR	FLOW RATES	PUMPING MECHANISM	SPECIAL FEATURES
Pumps for multiple intermittent infusions				
Autosyringe AS20A (Autosyringe)	Syringe (up to 60 ml)	0.03 to 99.9 ml/hr	Lead screw	None
Bard 400 (Bard)	Syringe (60 ml)	10 to 120 ml/hr	Lead screw	None
Pumps designed for patient-controlled analgesia				
Harvard (Bard)	Syringe (60 ml)	0.1 to 99.9 ml/hr (continuous 150 ml/hr)	Lead screw	Can be connected to an external printer; delivers dose volumes of 0.1 to 9.9 ml; possible lock-out intervals of 3 to 60 min
Life Care Classic (Abbott)	Abbott syringe, vial injector	1 ml/14 sec continuous	Lead screw	Delivers dose volumes of 0.1 to 5 ml; possible lock-out intervals of 5 to 99 min; doses can be programmed in mg
Life Care Plus 4100 (Abbott)	Abbott syringe, vial injector	1 ml/14 sec continuous	Lead screw	Delivers dose volumes of 0.1 to 5 ml; possible lock-out intervals of 5 to 99 min; can be connected to an external printer; doses can be programmed in mg
BD Infuser (Becton Dickinson)	Syringe (20, 30, or 60 ml)	1 to 60 ml/hr	Lead screw	Delivers dose volumes of 0 to 10 ml; possible lock-out intervals of 5 to 99 min; doses can be programmed in mg
Pumps with multiple-rate programming capabilities				
Quest 521 Intelligent Pump (Quest [Kendall McGaw])	Bag, bottle, or syringe	1 to 999 ml/hr	Volumetric positive pressure displacement reservoir	Variable pressure settings of 100 to 400 mm Hg; programmable delivery of up to nine flow rates per time period
Micropump 2100 (Parker)	Bag (100 or 200 ml)	0.1 to 4.5 ml/hr continuous	Pulsatile piston cassette	Patient-controlled ranges of flow rate
MiniMed 504S (MiniMed)	MiniMed 3-ml syringe	1 to 72 mcl/hr	Lead screw	Programmable delivery of up to four rates per 24 hr; can be programmed in insulin units to deliver maximum basal, bolus, and temporary basal doses; immersion-proof

ADVANCED EQUIPMENT

I.V. infusion pumps *(continued)*

PUMP AND MAKER	RESERVOIR	FLOW RATES	PUMPING MECHANISM	SPECIAL FEATURES
Pumps with multiple-rate programming capabilities *(continued)*				
MiniMed 404 SP (Minimed)	MiniMed 3-ml syringe	2 to 720 mcl/hr	Lead screw	Programmable delivery of up to four rates per 24 hr; can be programmed to deliver maximum basal and bolus doses; immersion-proof
Pumps with multiple-solution programming capabilities				
Gemini PC-2 (IMED)	Bag, bottle	1 to 500 ml/hr (controller) of 1 to 999 ml/hr (pump)	Linear peristaltic	Can be operated as a pump or controller; can deliver two fluids at independent rates
Life Care 5000 Plum (Abbott)	Bag, bottle, syringe	0.1 to 999 ml/hr	Piston diaphragm	Can be operated as a pump or controller; can deliver two fluids at independent rates
Intelliject (Intellimed)	Intellimed 30-ml/syringes	0.3 to 40.5 ml/hr per channel	Rack and pinion drive	Can deliver up to four fluids at independent rates; patient-controlled analgesia capability
Omniflo 4000 (Omniflo)	Bag, bottle, syringe	1.4 to 800 ml/hr	Piston diaphragm	Can deliver up to four fluids; automatic air elimination

The type of tubing you'll use depends on the I.V. infusion device.

Controllers

With a controller, the maximum flow rate depends on how high you hang the I.V. bag above the I.V. site. Hanging an I.V. bag 36″ (91.4 cm) above a patient's head while he's lying flat will provide adequate gravity pressure for the flow. The controller then delivers a preset amount of fluid over a given period. In case of resistance to the flow caused by an occlusion in the I.V. system or increased vascular backflow, the alarm will sound, signaling that the controller can't maintain the preset I.V. rate. Because resistance can occur when the patient moves, this alarm may sound often. Some controllers have indicator lights that signal a need to check the I.V. site and correct a resistance problem before the alarm sounds.

Pumps

Pumps are often preferred to controllers because of their greater accuracy in delivering infusions and because they have fewer nuisance alarms. (See *I.V. infusion pumps.*)

An infusion pump controls the flow rate completely. If gravity pressure doesn't deliver the infusion at a preset rate, the pump adds a driving pressure to the system. The amount of pressure, measured in pounds per square inch (psi), determines how much resistance the pump can overcome, but the pump won't exceed preset limits. When it exerts maximum preset pressure, the machine's alarm sounds and the infusion stops. Newer pump models don't exceed 15 psi, which is considered a safe limit. But some pumps include an optional setting called "variable pressure," which allows you to set the pressure limit.

Other new pumps, such as the IMED Gemini PC-2 and the Baxter Multiplex series 100,

ADVANCED EQUIPMENT

Using a multiple-solution infusion pump

A multiple-solution infusion pump, such as the IMED Gemini PC-2, is a pump that lets you give several drugs or fluids simultaneously. Solutions can be infused to the same site or to two different sites.

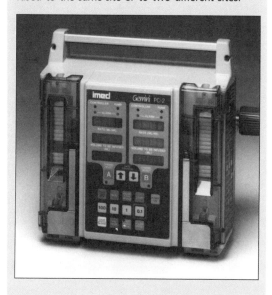

Other new pumps, such as the IMED Gemini PC-2 and the Baxter Multiplex series 100, allow you to give several drugs and fluids simultaneously. (See *Using a multiple-solution infusion pump.*)

Drug administration
To set up a controller, first attach the controller to the I.V. pole. Expose the port on the I.V. solution bag, and insert the spike on the administration tubing into the bag. Fill the drip chamber no more than halfway to avoid miscounting the drops. Rotate the chamber so that the fluid touches all sides and removes any vapor that could interfere with drop counting. Next, prime the tubing and close the clamp. Position the drop sensor above the fluid level in the drip chamber and below the drop port to ensure correct drop counting. Insert the peristaltic tubing into the controller, close the door, and open the flow clamp completely.

To set up a volumetric pump, attach the pump to the I.V. pole. Insert the administration set spike into the I.V. solution bag. According to directions, fill the drip chamber halfway or completely to prevent air bubbles from entering the tubing. Next, prime the tubing and close the clamp. Then follow the manufacturer's instructions for placement of the tubing.

Operating the controller or pump
Begin by positioning the controller or pump on the same side of the bed as the I.V. or anticipated venipuncture site to avoid crisscrossing I.V. lines over the patient. Plug in the machine.

If necessary, perform the venipuncture. Attach the tubing to the needle or catheter hub. If you're using a controller, position the drip chamber 30" (76 cm) above the infusion site to ensure gravity flow. Depending on the machine, you'll then turn it on and press the START button. Set the appropriate dials on the front panel to the desired infusion rate and volume.

Check the patency of the I.V. line and watch for infiltration. If you're using a controller, monitor the accuracy of the infusion rate. Securely tape all of the connections, and recheck the controller's drip rate because taping may alter it. The alarm switches should all be turned on.

Complications
The risks and potential problems associated with I.V. controllers and pumps are the same as those associated with peripheral venous lines. The pressure generated by pumps does not cause infiltration. However, infiltration may develop rapidly with an infusion pump because the increased pressure won't slow the infusion rate until significant edema occurs.

Nursing considerations
• Remove I.V. solutions from the refrigerator 1 hour before infusing them to help release small gas bubbles from the solutions. Small bubbles in the solution can join to form larger bubbles, which can activate the pump's air-in-line alarm.
• Check the manufacturer's recommendations

before administering opaque fluids such as blood. Some pumps are designed to dilate the chamber so the fluid touches all sides to remove any vapor that could interfere with correct drop counting.

• Frequently monitor the pump or controller and the patient to make sure the flow rate is correct. Look for infiltration and signs and symptoms of complications, such as infection and air embolism.

• Move the tubing in controllers every few hours to prevent permanent compression or damage. Change the tubing and cassette every 48 hours or according to the policy of your health care facility.

• Keep in mind that if electrical power fails, the pumps will automatically switch to battery power.

• If the pump doesn't have free-flow protection, remember to close the roller clamp before removing tubing from the pump.

Patient teaching

Teach your patient not to touch the controller or pump. Explain that it's set to a specific rate and that if it's touched, he could receive too much or too little of the drug. Encourage the patient to call you if he hears any alarms from the pump or controller.

If the patient will be using the device at home, demonstrate how it works. Also demonstrate how to maintain the system and assess the I.V. site. Discuss which complications to watch for and review which measures to take if any complications occur.

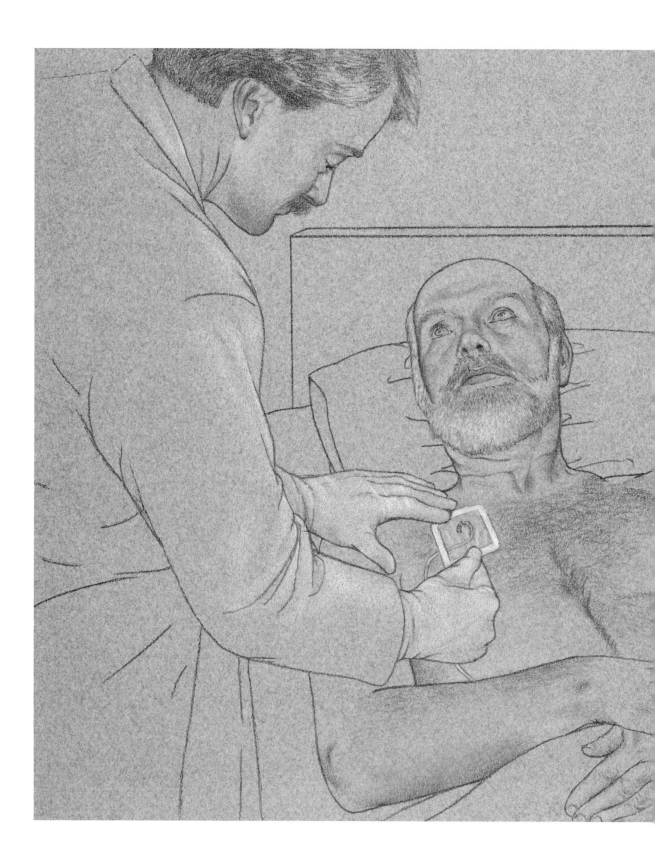

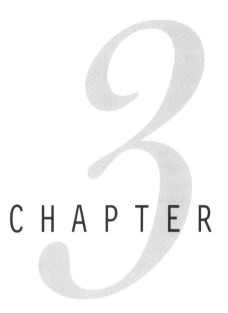

CHAPTER

3

Providing central venous therapy

Intravascular therapy provides essential fluids and medications to patients in the hospital or at home. But if a patient's veins are in poor condition, he may not be able to withstand the repeated venipunctures required for peripheral I.V. therapy. So giving drugs or fluids through the central veins may prove the best alternative. As a nurse, you can evaluate your patient's veins and, if appropriate, recommend central venous (CV) therapy.

In the past, CV therapy was available only to hospital patients—typically those in critical care units. But in recent years, changing health insurance regulations, the growing number of gravely ill patients, and technologic advances have made CV therapy more common among patients in medical-surgical units and even those at home.

Today, nurses provide care in almost every setting for patients receiving CV therapy. And with one type of CV catheter—a peripherally inserted central catheter (PICC)—you can re-

Recognizing CV catheter pathways

The illustrations here show several common pathways for central venous (CV) catheter insertion. Typically, a CV catheter is inserted into the subclavian or internal jugular vein. It may terminate in the superior vena cava or in the right atrium.

Insertion: Subclavian vein
Termination: Right atrium

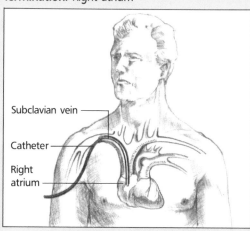

Subclavian vein
Catheter
Right atrium

Insertion: Internal jugular vein
Termination: Superior vena cava

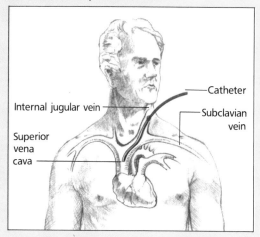

Catheter
Internal jugular vein
Subclavian vein
Superior vena cava

Insertion: Subclavian vein
Termination: Superior vena cava

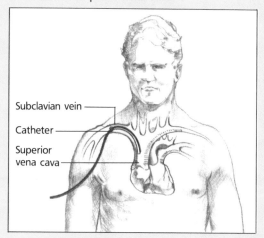

Subclavian vein
Catheter
Superior vena cava

ceive training to insert the line yourself. With these expanding opportunities, you'll need to understand each type of CV therapy so that you can recommend the best one for your patient.

A CV catheter, which can be implanted or tunneled under the skin, can be used on a long-term or short-term basis. Other types of CV lines are inserted peripherally and threaded into a central vein. Besides knowing how these devices work, you need to know how to care for a patient who has a CV line, how to care

Insertion: Basilic vein (peripheral)
Termination: Superior vena cava

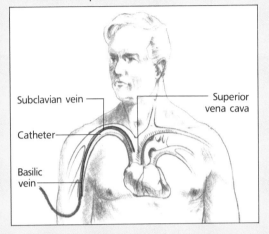

Subclavian vein

Superior
vena cava

Catheter

Basilic
vein

Insertion: Through subcutaneous tunnel to
subclavian vein (Dacron cuff helps hold catheter
in place)
Termination: Superior vena cava

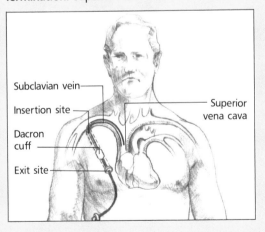

Subclavian vein

Insertion site

Superior
vena cava

Dacron
cuff

Exit site

for the line itself, and how to recognize and
manage any complications that arise.

This chapter explains how to provide effective care for a patient receiving CV therapy.
First, it presents the underlying pharmacologic
principles of CV therapy. Then it describes the

three major types of CV devices currently
used: the traditional short- or long-term CV
catheter, the vascular access port, and the PICC
catheter. It details the catheter insertion procedure and describes how to administer drugs,
change the dressing and I.V. tubing, obtain
blood samples, and remove the catheter. It
also discusses possible complications and describes related nursing considerations and patient teaching.

Pharmacologic principles

A CV line delivers drugs and other substances
directly into the superior vena cava or right
atrium. It's also used to measure CV pressure.
Typically, the line is inserted into the patient's
subclavian or internal jugular vein. In some patients, it's inserted into a peripheral vein and
threaded into a central vein. (See *Recognizing
CV catheter pathways.*) If subclavian or internal
jugular access is difficult or impossible, the line
may be inserted into the femoral vein and
threaded into the inferior vena cava.

Because a CV catheter delivers substances
into a large vessel, it's commonly used to administer drugs or fluids that may be too caustic for a peripheral vein. Drugs given through a
CV line mix directly with the patient's blood.
Besides promoting rapid absorption, such mixing produces a high drug concentration in the
blood and tissues. A large volume of blood
mixed with a drug helps when the administered substance is caustic or when several incompatible substances are given through
different lumens of the same device. In this
case, you'll need to monitor your patient for
both therapeutic and toxic drug effects.

Although CV therapy is preferable for many
patients, it's not without difficulties. Insertion
of a CV device may require surgery, thereby increasing the cost. And caregivers must use extreme caution to prevent life-threatening
complications when inserting and maintaining

the line. The CV line may also restrict the patient's activities and choice of clothing. To avoid complications, patients and their families must understand the advantages and limitations of CV therapy as well as how to care for the device.

Which drugs can be given by CV line?

Consult the policy of your health care facility to find out which drugs can and can't be given through a CV line. Many facilities, for instance, prohibit amphotericin B administration by this method because it increases the likelihood of hypokalemia, which may cause cardiac arrhythmias. Some facilities prohibit CV delivery of dopamine because this drug can also cause arrhythmias. Others, in contrast, specify that dopamine must be given *only* through a CV line because of the risk of extravasation with a peripheral line.

Despite the controversy about which drugs can and can't be administered safely through a CV line, experts generally agree on which ones should always be given this way. For instance, most facilities require CV therapy for delivering highly osmolar fluids, such as hypertonic sodium chloride solution, dextrose 50% solution (often used in total parenteral nutrition [TPN]), and certain chemotherapeutic agents.

CV lines

A CV line may be inserted in a patient who needs multiple infusions of fluid, blood or blood products, antibiotics, chemotherapy, or TPN. These infusions may be given for short or prolonged periods, using a single-lumen or multilumen catheter. A single-lumen catheter allows infusion of just one solution at a time. A multilumen catheter allows simultaneous infusion of several solutions regardless of their compatibility.

The doctor inserts the CV line directly into the patient's subclavian or internal jugular vein. Depending on the catheter type, the line ter-

minates in the superior vena cava.

Short-term CV therapy (less than 4 weeks) typically requires hospitalization. The line is used for TPN and is especially useful for patients who need multiple infusions. Usually, the doctor inserts the catheter at the patient's bedside. You may need to assist him and reassure the patient during the procedure. After insertion, you must keep the catheter patent and monitor for complications.

If your patient needs CV therapy for 4 weeks or more, the doctor will insert a catheter designed for long-term use. Candidates for long-term CV therapy include patients receiving home care or chemotherapy.

The growing number of patients receiving long-term CV therapy at home makes your role more vital than ever. By teaching your patient and his family about catheter insertion and maintenance, you can help prevent complications and keep the catheter in good condition. Your teaching should include how to change dressings and injection caps and how to recognize problems. If your patient is receiving I.V. fluids or TPN at home, you must also assist him and his family in maintaining the infusion and changing the I.V. tubing.

Equipment

Your patient's needs will determine the choice of CV catheter. Catheters used for short-term therapy are usually stiffer than those designed for long-term use. (See *Comparing common CV catheters*, pages 68 and 69.)

Short-term catheters

Short-term CV catheters provide access for drug and fluid administration and withdrawal of blood samples. The increased risk of infection and thrombus formation at the insertion site makes short-term catheters undesirable for prolonged use. However, short-term catheters have a heparin coating to help prevent clot formation. Still, when caring for a patient with a short-term catheter, you must flush it with a heparin sodium solution to ensure its patency. The Intravenous Nurses Society recommends changing these catheters every 3 to 7 days.

The first short-term catheters were made of polyvinyl chloride. Because this material is stiff, patients using these catheters had a high incidence of thrombus formation. With the introduction of polyurethane catheters, complications have decreased.

Short-term catheters may have a single lumen or multiple lumens (up to four). A multilumen catheter provides better access because of the multiple injection ports. Lumen size varies. The most commonly used catheter has a 16G distal lumen, 18G proximal lumen, and 18G medial lumen. The distal lumen is used to monitor CV pressure. The end of each lumen has a luer-lock connection for attaching I.V. tubing or applying an injection cap. Your health care facility may direct you to use one lumen for TPN.

Long-term catheters

Made of silicone rubber, catheters for long-term use are softer and more flexible than short-term catheters and thus are more comfortable for the patient. They're also more durable and biocompatible and cause fewer complications when managed properly. Their flexibility allows surgical insertion in subcutaneous tissue, although insertion is more difficult and time-consuming than with short-term catheters. A Dacron cuff placed under the skin just in front of the exit site helps secure the catheter and acts as a barrier to migrating microorganisms.

Long-term catheters may have one or more lumens, each with a luer-lock on the end. Common long-term catheters include the Hickman and Broviac catheters, which have blunt open ends. The Groshong catheter, another common catheter, comes in single- and double-lumen versions and has a closed tip. Its unique pressure-sensitive valve opens during fluid administration or blood withdrawal and closes when the infusion is discontinued. (See *How the Groshong catheter works,* page 70.) Hickman and Broviac catheters must be flushed with heparin solution to maintain their patency. The Groshong catheter can be flushed and locked off with 0.9% sodium chloride solution.

Insertion of the access device

The doctor may insert a short-term CV catheter at the patient's bedside. However, he must insert a long-term catheter in the operating room using sterile technique. In either situation, assist him by preparing the patient physically and psychologically, gathering equipment, and ensuring sterile conditions throughout the procedure.

To insert a short-term catheter, the doctor uses a percutaneous stick and advances the catheter over a guide wire. Besides gathering equipment, you'll position the patient, making him as comfortable as possible, and prepare the insertion site. During insertion, you'll hand equipment to the doctor. After insertion and before therapy starts, monitor the patient for complications.

If your patient needs a long-term catheter, prepare him by explaining where the doctor will place the catheter and teach how to care for it after insertion. Expect the doctor to order a sedative before the procedure. He inserts the catheter into a central vein using a percutaneous or cutdown technique; then he tunnels it through subcutaneous tissue to an exit site at the third or fourth intercostal space.

Gathering the equipment. Today, most hospitals have prepared disposable trays for CV line insertion. Make sure the tray includes all the necessary equipment. If you don't have a preassembled tray, gather the following items: sterile gloves, gowns, goggles, and masks for each participant; sterile drapes and a linen-saver pad; sterile towel; scissors; povidone-iodine sponges and ointment; alcohol sponges; 70% alcohol solution; hydrogen peroxide; 0.9% sodium chloride solution; antiseptic ointment; 3-ml syringe with a 25G 1" needle (if necessary); 1% or 2% injectable lidocaine (depending on the doctor's preference); syringes for blood samples; suture material; sterile gauze pads or a transparent semipermeable dressing; nonporous tape; I.V. solution (if ordered); I.V. infusion pump or controller; heparin flush solution (if the doctor hasn't ordered an I.V. solution); and CV catheter.

(Text continues on page 70.)

Comparing common CV catheters

DESCRIPTION

Short-term catheters
Single-lumen catheter
- Polyurethane or polyvinyl chloride (PVC)
- Approximately 8" (20.3 cm) long
- Lumen gauge varies

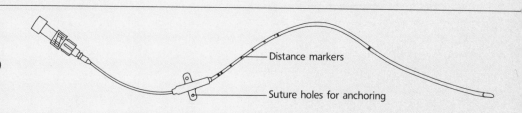

Multilumen catheter
- Polyurethane or PVC
- Double, triple, or quadruple lumens, exiting at ¾" (2-cm) intervals
- Lumen gauge varies
- Most models have color-coded lumen parts

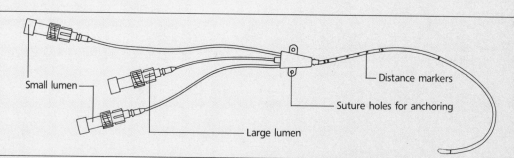

Long-term catheters
Groshong catheter
- Silicone rubber
- Approximately 35" (89 cm) long
- Closed end with pressure-sensitive, two-way valve
- Polyester fiber (Dacron) cuff
- Single lumen or multilumen

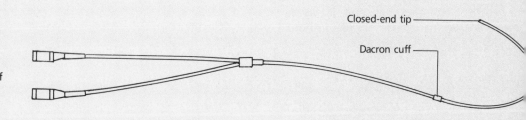

Triple-lumen Hickman catheter
- Silicone rubber
- Approximately 35" long
- Open ended with clamp
- Dacron cuff
- Single lumen or multilumen

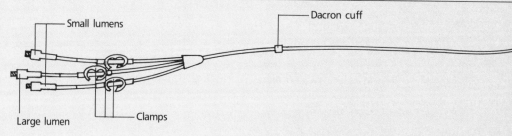

Broviac catheter
- Identical to Hickman but has smaller diameter

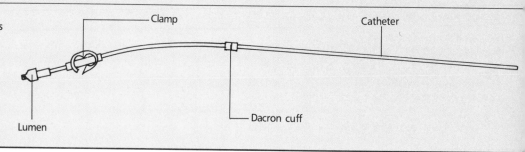

INDICATIONS	NURSING CONSIDERATIONS
• Short-term CV access • Emergency access • Single-purpose therapy: I.V. therapy, antibiotics, total parenteral nutrition (TPN), blood transfusions, chemotherapy • CV pressure (CVP) monitoring • Blood sampling for diagnostic testing	• Use sterile technique when caring for insertion site. • Assess frequently for signs of infection and clot formation. • If necessary, use air elimination filter to minimize the risk of air embolism. • Obtain a chest X-ray to verify catheter placement after insertion.
• Short-term CV access • Emergency access • Patient with multiple CV infusion needs • Patient with limited venous access sites who needs simultaneous multiple infusions that may not be compatible • CVP monitoring • Blood sampling for diagnostic testing	• Realize that nursing considerations for short-term catheters apply. • Know the gauge and purpose of each lumen. • Use the same lumen for the same task. • Remember to label the lumen used for each task. • Heparinize ports not in use to prevent clotting, according to the policy of the health care facility.
• Long-term CV access • Heparin allergy • Infusion of I.V. fluids, antibiotics, TPN, blood, or chemotherapy • Blood sampling for diagnostic testing	• Dress two surgical sites immediately after insertion. • Use gauze dressing until drainage stops, then use transparent semipermeable dressing. • Handle catheter gently because silicone tears easily. • Have catheter repair kit readily available. • Check external portion of catheter for kinks or fluid leakage. • Flush with enough saline solution to clear length of catheter (especially after blood sampling or blood administration). • Encourage patient to participate in care and use of device as soon as he is able.
• Long-term CV access • Home I.V. therapy • Infusion of I.V. fluids, antibiotics, TPN, blood, and chemotherapy • Blood sampling for diagnostic testing	• Handle catheter gently and check frequently for kinks, leakage, or tears. • Clamp catheter any time it is open or becomes disconnected (use clamps without teeth). • Heparinize unused ports, according to the policy of the health care facility. • Encourage patient to participate in care and use of device as soon as he is able.
• Long-term CV access • Patients with small central vessels, especially children and elderly patients • Infusion of fluids, antibiotics, TPN, blood, or chemotherapy • Blood sampling for diagnostic testing	• Handle catheter gently and check frequently for kinks, leakage, or tears. • Clamp catheter any time it's open or becomes disconnected (use clamps without teeth); clamp eliminates need for Valsalva's maneuver. • Heparinize unused ports, according to facility policy. • Encourage patient to participate in care and use of device as soon as he is able.

How the Groshong catheter works

Developed in 1978, the Groshong central venous (CV) catheter is positioned and inserted the same way as other CV catheters, with its tip placed in the superior vena cava. However, because the Groshong catheter has a pressure-sensitive valve, it works differently than other catheters. As these illustrations show, the valve, located near the proximal tip of each lumen, resembles a horizontal slit. The valve remains closed when the lumen isn't in use, but it opens inward during blood aspiration and opens outward during fluid or blood administration.

Valve closed (lumen not in use)

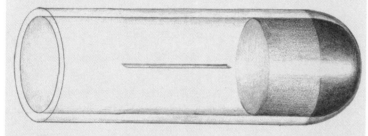

Valve opens inward during blood aspiration

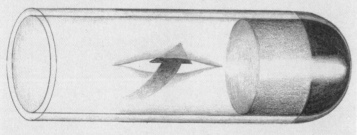

Valve opens outward during fluid or blood infusion

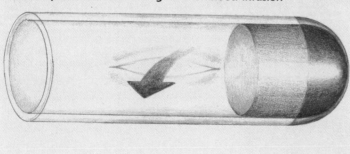

Preparing the patient. Make sure the chosen venipuncture site is hairless. If necessary, snip hair close to the skin in an area about 5" (13 cm) around the site; then rinse the skin with 0.9% sodium chloride solution. (Avoid shaving the area because this can cause skin irritation.)

Next, explain the procedure. Tell the patient that although he may have a drape covering his face, the staff will be present to take care of his needs. (If his face is draped, you can ease his anxiety by uncovering his eyes.) Make sure the patient, his spouse or partner, or other family member has signed a consent form. Be sure to check the patient's history for hypersensitivity to local anesthetics.

Put on sterile gloves, a mask, a gown, and goggles. Clean the insertion site with the povidone-iodine sponges and let it air-dry for at least 2 minutes. Repeat this procedure twice. Make sure the patient keeps his head turned away from the insertion site to make the site more accessible and to prevent contamination from airborne pathogens.

Inserting the catheter. Place a linen-saver pad under the patient's head and right shoulder. Expose the right side of his chest. If his condition permits, place him in Trendelenburg's position, which causes the vein to dilate and fill, reducing the risk of air embolism. To further increase vein dilation, place a rolled-up towel or blanket lengthwise between the patient's shoulder blades.

Surround the site with sterile drapes. Wipe the top of the lidocaine vial with an alcohol sponge; then invert the bottle for the doctor.

The doctor usually inserts the catheter on the patient's right side because the central veins there provide a more direct pathway to the superior vena cava. After inserting the 25G 1" needle and withdrawing the solution, he then injects the local anesthetic into the insertion site. If you haven't done so already, prepare the I.V. solution while the doctor anesthetizes the site. Also prepare the infusion pump or controller.

The doctor inserts the needle into the vein. He then inserts a guide wire through the needle and removes the needle, leaving the guide wire in place. He then slips the catheter over the guide wire and sutures it in place.

If the doctor wants to draw blood samples, he does this after catheter insertion, before connecting the I.V. solution. He may use either a syringe or Vacutainer to obtain the samples. Hand the doctor a sterile 5- to 10-ml syringe (depending on the tests ordered). A Vacutainer can be applied to the end of the catheter.

When inserting a multilumen catheter, the doctor draws blood back through each lumen to prevent air embolism. Connect the I.V. solution to the appropriate lumen or lumens. (The lumens that aren't connected to I.V. lines should have injection caps applied.) Flush these capped lumens with 0.9% sodium chloride solution, followed by heparin flush solution. Start the infusion at a rate of 20 ml/hour until catheter placement is verified. Then select the ordered administration rate. To prevent disconnection, tape over any non-leur-lock connections.

Using 0.9% sodium chloride solution, clean around the site to remove any dried blood. Your health care facility may also direct you to clean around the site with alcohol sponges. Then clean the site with povidone-iodine sponges. If required by your facility's policy, place a small drop of antiseptic ointment at the site; then cover the site with a dry, sterile gauze dressing or apply a transparent semipermeable dressing. Apply nonporous tape. Label the dressing with the date, time, and your initials.

Place the patient in high Fowler's position to permit a chest X-ray, which confirms catheter placement. If the X-ray shows improper placement (which can cause pneumothorax or cardiac tamponade), the doctor may try to reposition the catheter or replace it with a new one. If the X-ray verifies correct catheter placement, start infusing I.V. fluids at the prescribed rate, as ordered.

Drug administration

I.V. solutions may be administered by continuous or intermittent infusion through the CV line. A bolus dose can be given through an injection cap on the catheter.

Administering a continuous infusion

When giving an I.V. solution by continuous infusion (usually longer than 30 minutes), first prepare the solution and tubing. To ensure accurate delivery of the solution, use a volumetric control device.

Prepare the patient by explaining the procedure. Then put on clean gloves. If you plan to attach I.V. tubing to a capped lumen, you should first flush the lumen with 0.9% sodium chloride solution to ensure compatibility.

Clamp the catheter, but only where indicated. If the catheter doesn't have its own clamp or designated clamp location, choose a smooth-edged clamp or apply tape to the catheter and clamp over the tape. Don't use a clamp with teeth because this may damage the catheter. If a clamp isn't available, have the patient perform Valsalva's maneuver to help prevent air embolism. As he bears down and takes a deep breath, remove the cap and plug in the I.V. tubing. (See *Teaching Valsalva's maneuver,* page 72.) Set the ordered flow rate on the I.V. controller or pump. Tape over any non-luer-lock connections to prevent disconnection.

Flushing the catheter. You must always flush the CV catheter after drug or fluid administration. If the patient has a CV catheter in place but isn't currently receiving a drug or fluid, you'll need to flush the catheter to keep it patent.

Gather alcohol sponges, 3 to 5 ml of sterile 0.9% sodium chloride solution in a syringe, heparin flush solution, and clean gloves.

Explain the procedure to the patient. Then put on gloves and clean the injection cap with the alcohol sponge. Next, insert the syringe with sterile 0.9% sodium chloride solution and gently flush the catheter. Clean the injection cap again, insert the heparin solution in a syringe, and flush the catheter a second time. As you withdraw the syringe with the flush solu-

Teaching Valsalva's maneuver

Inserting or removing a central venous catheter may reduce the patient's intrathoracic pressure, leading to air embolism. To help avoid this complication, have the patient perform Valsalva's maneuver (forced exhalation against a closed airway) during catheter insertion and removal. This maneuver initially increases intrathoracic pressure from its normal level of −3 to −4 mm Hg to 60 mm Hg or higher. It also slows the pulse, decreases blood return to the heart, and increases venous pressure.

Instruct the patient to take a deep breath and hold it, and then to bear down for 10 seconds. Next, tell him to exhale and breathe quietly. If he can't perform the maneuver or if he has a condition that precludes its use (such as bradycardia, recent eye surgery, myocardial infarction, respiratory distress, or increased intracranial pressure), try increasing intrathoracic pressure another way. For instance, remove the catheter while he holds his breath after a deep inspiration, while he exhales, or while delivering positive pressure via a hand-held resuscitation bag.

tion, continue to put pressure on the plunger to prevent blood from entering the catheter.

For a short-term catheter, flush a heparin solution of 10 to 100 units/3 to 5 ml (depending on your facility's guidelines) through the catheter every 12 hours, or according to the manufacturer's recommendations. For a long-term catheter, flush with a heparin solution of 100 units/5 ml every 12 to 24 hours or longer, depending on the catheter. Remember to flush the catheter after each drug or fluid administration.

If your patient has a Groshong catheter, you won't need heparin flush solution. Because of this catheter's pressure-sensitive valve, you should flush with 5 ml of sterile 0.9% sodium chloride solution every 7 days. If the patient is receiving a highly viscous fluid, such as TPN, or if blood samples have been drawn through the catheter, you should flush with 20 ml of this

sodium chloride solution to prevent crystallization of the catheter tip.

Administering an intermittent infusion

Antibiotics and other drugs may be given intermittently through a CV line (typically for 40 to 60 minutes). You'll either inject a drug into an existing I.V. line that feeds into the CV line or administer it through an injection cap.

To give a drug through an injection cap, gather the prescribed medication, I.V. tubing, a short needle (1" or smaller), two 3- to 5-ml syringes filled with sterile 0.9% sodium chloride solution, heparin solution, and alcohol sponges.

Attach a needle or appropriate needleless system to the end of the I.V. tubing, according to your facility's policy. Then explain the procedure to the patient.

Put on clean gloves, and clean the top of the injection cap with an alcohol sponge. If you're unsure of compatibility, flush the catheter through the injection cap with 3 to 5 ml of sterile sodium chloride solution. Plug the needle into the injection cap and start the infusion at the desired rate. Tape over the non-leur-lock connections to prevent disconnection.

When the infusion is complete, close the roller clamp on the I.V. tubing. Unplug the needle and discard it, but don't recap it because this could cause a needle-stick injury. Clean the top of the injection cap with alcohol and flush it with 3 to 5 ml of sterile 0.9% sodium chloride solution. Clean the cap again and flush with heparin solution, according to your facility's policy. (If the patient has a Groshong catheter, don't use heparin solution.)

Administering a bolus dose

To give a bolus dose through a CV line, gather a syringe with the prescribed drug, alcohol sponges, two 3- to 5-ml syringes with 0.9% sterile sodium chloride solution, and heparin solution.

Explain the procedure to the patient. Then put on clean gloves. Clean the injection cap with an alcohol sponge and flush the cap with sterile 0.9% sodium chloride solution. Insert the needle of the syringe containing the drug; then slowly inject the drug according to the manufacturer's directions or your facility's policy. Withdraw the needle and discard it (but don't recap it).

Clean the injection cap again with an alcohol sponge; then inject the cap with 3 to 5 ml of the sterile sodium chloride solution. Clean the cap a third time; then inject it with heparin solution, according to your facility's policy.

Changing the dressing

You should change the dressing on a CV line every 48 to 72 hours or whenever it becomes soiled or nonocclusive. You'll need sterile gloves, alcohol sponges, povidone-iodine swabs, antiseptic or povidone-iodine ointment, sterile transparent semipermeable dressing, sterile gauze pads, and adhesive tape. Always use sterile technique to prevent contamination and, again, be sure to follow your facility's policy.

To remove the old dressing, put on clean gloves. Then pull the edges of the dressing toward the exit site for a long-term catheter or toward the insertion site for a short-term catheter. Be careful not to dislodge the catheter. Remove and discard the gloves and the dressing.

Put on sterile gloves and clean the skin around the site with alcohol sponges, hydrogen peroxide, or chlorhexidine. Start at the center of the site and move outward, using a circular motion. Repeat twice, using a fresh sponge each time. Allow the skin to dry; then repeat the procedure using povidone-iodine swabs.

After the solution has dried, apply a small amount of antiseptic or povidone-iodine ointment to the site, if facility policy allows. Then secure the catheter to the skin and cover the site with a transparent semipermeable or sterile gauze dressing. (If you're using gauze, tape the dressing securely.) Label the dressing with the date, time, and your initials. (See *Changing a CV dressing*, page 74.)

Changing I.V. tubing and solution

You should change your patient's I.V. tubing and solution every 24 hours, or as often as your facility requires. After preparing the new tubing and solution, explain the procedure to the patient. Then put on clean gloves.

Stop the current infusion and clamp the catheter, using either the clamp attached to the catheter or the designated clamp location on the catheter. Be sure not to use a clamp with teeth. If a clamp isn't available, have the patient perform Valsalva's maneuver if he can.

Disconnect the old I.V. tubing and apply the new tubing. Set the infusion pump to the prescribed rate and discard the old solution and tubing.

Changing the injection cap

You must regularly change the injection cap on a CV catheter used for intermittent infusion — every 3 to 7 days in most facilities.

First explain the procedure to the patient. Then put on clean gloves. Clean the old injection cap with alcohol at its connection to the catheter. Clamp the catheter at the proper location, or have the patient perform Valsalva's maneuver. Remove the old cap and connect the new cap, using aseptic technique.

Removing the catheter

Depending on your facility's policy, you may remove your patient's CV catheter if necessary. In most facilities, a nurse may remove a short-term catheter but a doctor must remove a long-term catheter.

To remove the catheter, gather sterile gloves, suture-removal material, a gauze pad, tape, povidone-iodine sponges, alcohol sponges, and antiseptic ointment. If the doctor has ordered cultures, you'll also need a specimen container for the catheter tip.

Place the patient in the supine or modified Trendelenburg's position. Make sure he can perform Valsalva's maneuver. Then remove the old dressing.

Wearing sterile gloves, clean the site with alcohol sponges, then with povidone-iodine sponges. Inspect the site for drainage or in-

Changing a CV dressing

If the dressing on the patient's central venous (CV) line becomes soiled or nonocclusive, you'll need to change it. You should also change it routinely every 48 to 72 hours, depending on the policy of your health care facility. Be sure to use sterile technique to prevent contamination. Here are the basic steps to follow.

Remove the old dressing and clean the skin around the site. Then secure the CV catheter to the patient's skin and cover with one or two Steri-Strips.

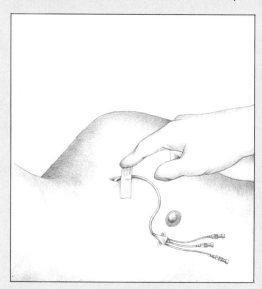

Cover the entire site with a transparent semipermeable dressing.

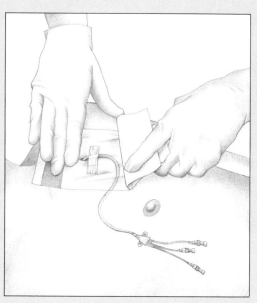

flammation. If you see drainage, obtain a specimen for culture and notify the doctor.

Remove the sutures securing the catheter, taking care not to cut the catheter. Have the patient perform Valsalva's maneuver to reduce the risk of air embolism, then withdraw the catheter from the vein in one slow, even motion. Immediately apply antiseptic ointment to the insertion site; then place a gauze dressing over it. Apply manual pressure to the site for 1 minute.

Next, inspect the catheter. Alert the doctor immediately if it looks ragged or damaged because this could indicate a catheter embolus.

After 1 hour, remove the dressing and inspect the site. Then apply more antiseptic oint-

ment and a gauze dressing, taping all sides. Leave the dressing in place for 24 to 72 hours.

Obtaining a culture

If your patient develops sepsis, the doctor may order a culture. The catheter tip can yield valuable information about the infection source. To prepare the tip for a culture, cut it off with sterile scissors, letting it drop directly into a sterile specimen container.

Obtaining a blood sample

To obtain a blood sample through a CV catheter (such as when the patient has poor peripheral veins), use a Vacutainer to collect and discard the filling volume of blood or fluid in the catheter.

If a solution is infusing, stop it and place an injection cap on the catheter lumen. (Always use the distal port to ensure the most accurate results.) Wait approximately 1 minute before drawing blood from the catheter.

Put on sterile gloves; then clean the top of the injection cap with an alcohol sponge or a povidone-iodine sponge. Place a 5-ml, lavender-top evacuated tube into the Vacutainer; then insert the needle on the Vacutainer into the injection cap. The first milliliter of I.V. solution may be clear until blood flows through the catheter. Usually, 5 ml is enough to remove any I.V. solution.

Remove the tube and withdraw the blood sample. Discard the first tube of blood. Label the remaining tubes and take them to the laboratory. (In some facilities, the first 5 ml of blood isn't discarded if the patient is scheduled for multiple blood studies. Instead, it's infused into the patient after the sample is withdrawn.)

Flush the catheter with 0.9% sodium chloride solution and resume the infusion. If you're not going to use the lumen immediately, you must flush the catheter with heparin solution (unless the patient has a Groshong catheter).

If you can't get a blood sample from the catheter, suspect that the catheter tip is lodged against the vessel wall. To correct this, ask the patient to raise his arms over his head, turn on his side, cough, or perform Valsalva's maneuver. You can also try flushing the catheter with 0.9% sodium chloride solution before your next attempt to withdraw blood.

Instead of obtaining blood through the CV catheter, you can use a syringe to withdraw up to 10 ml of blood; then inject it into the appropriate tube. Or you can remove the injection cap and apply the syringe directly to the end of the catheter lumen. You may do this when starting an infusion or just after catheter insertion, when changing the injection cap.

If you suspect inaccurate laboratory results (this is most common with serum potassium and glucose tests), try withdrawing blood from a peripheral venipuncture. Also, be aware that results may be more accurate if you discard more blood or fluid that's in the catheter or flush the catheter with 10 ml of 0.9% sodium chloride solution before withdrawing blood.

Complications
Complications can occur at any time during CV therapy. Traumatic complications, such as pneumothorax, typically occur during catheter insertion but may go unnoticed until afterward. Systemic complications, such as sepsis, typically occur later. Other complications may include air embolism, local infection, cardiac tamponade, thrombus formation, and phlebitis. (See *Dealing with CV therapy problems,* pages 76 and 77.)

Nursing considerations
• After catheter insertion, document the entire procedure, including catheter type and size, insertion site location, X-ray confirmation of catheter placement, the distance of catheter insertion (in centimeters), and the patient's tolerance of the procedure. Also document any blood studies ordered.
• During continuous infusion, monitor your patient's fluid status. When the infusion ends, change the injection cap and flush the catheter with 0.9% sodium chloride solution and heparin solution, according to facility policy. (If your patient has a Groshong catheter, however, don't use a heparin solution.)
• If your patient is receiving antibiotics every 4 hours, monitor him for bleeding because he may be receiving more than the therapeutic level of heparin.
• After administering an intermittent infusion or bolus dose, document the procedure and the patient's response. Monitor the patient for adverse drug reactions.
• Document all dressing changes, including the condition of the catheter insertion site and the patient's reaction to the procedure.

(Text continues on page 78.)

Dealing with CV therapy problems

COMPLICATION	SIGNS AND SYMPTOMS	POSSIBLE CAUSES
Pneumothorax, hemothorax, chylothorax, hydrothorax	• Chest pain • Dyspnea • Cyanosis • Decreased breath sounds • With hemothorax, reduced hemoglobin from blood pooling • Abnormal chest X-ray	• Lung puncture by catheter during insertion or exchange over guide wire • Puncture of large blood vessel with bleeding inside or outside of lung • Puncture of lymph nodes with leakage of lymph fluid • Infusion of solution into chest area through infiltrated catheter
Air embolism	• Respiratory distress • Unequal breath sounds • Weak pulse • Elevated CV pressure • Decreased blood pressure • Churning murmur over precordium • Loss of consciousness	• Intake of air into CV system during catheter insertion or tubing change • Inadvertent catheter opening, cutting, or breakage
Thrombosis	• Edema at puncture site • Erythema • Ipsilateral swelling of arm, neck, and face • Pain along vein • Fever, malaise • Tachycardia	• Sluggish flow rate • Catheter material (some materials, such as polyvinyl chloride, are more thrombogenic) • Patient's hematopoietic status • Preexisting limb edema • Infusion of irritating solutions • Repeated or long-term use of same vein • Preexisting cardiovascular disease
Local infection	• Redness, warmth, tenderness, and swelling at catheter insertion or exit site • Purulent exudate • Local rash or pustules • Fever, chills, malaise	• Failure to maintain aseptic technique during insertion or site care • Failure to comply with dressing change protocol • Wet or soiled dressing remaining on site • Immunosuppression • Irritated suture line
Systemic infection	• Unexplained fever, chills • Leukocytosis • Nausea, vomiting • Malaise • Elevated urine glucose level	• Contaminated catheter or infusate • Failure to maintain aseptic technique during solution hookup • Frequent catheter opening or long-term use of single I.V. access • Immunosuppression
Cardiac tamponade	• Pulsus paradoxus • Jugular vein distention • Narrowed pulse pressure • Muffled heart sounds • Diaphoresis • Dyspnea	• Perforation of heart wall by catheter

NURSING INTERVENTIONS	PREVENTION
• Notify doctor. • Remove catheter or assist with removal. • Administer oxygen, as ordered. • Prepare for and assist with chest tube insertion. • Document your actions.	• Place the patient in Trendelenburg's position with rolled towel between shoulder blades to dilate and expose vein as much as possible during insertion. • Assess for early signs of fluid infiltration (swelling in shoulder, neck, chest, and arm). • Ensure patient immobilization through adequate preparation for procedure and restraint during it; active patients may need to be sedated or taken to operating room for CV line insertion.
• Clamp catheter immediately. • Turn patient onto left side with head down so air can enter right atrium and disperse via pulmonary artery; have him maintain this position for 20 to 30 minutes. • Administer oxygen, as ordered. • Notify doctor. • Document your actions.	• Purge all air from tubing before hookup. • Have patient perform Valsalva's maneuver during catheter insertion and tubing changes. • Use air-elimination filters proximal to patient. • Use infusion control device with air detection capability. • Use locking tubing, tape connections, or locking devices for all connections.
• Notify doctor. • Remove catheter, if ordered. • Infuse anticoagulant doses of heparin, if ordered. • Verify thrombosis with diagnostic test results. • Apply warm, wet compresses locally. • Don't use limb on affected side for venipuncture. • Document your actions.	• Maintain flow through catheter at steady rate with infusion pump, or flush at regular intervals. • Use catheter made of less thrombogenic material or one coated to discourage thrombosis (if permitted). • Dilute irritating solutions. • Use 0.22-micron filter on line.
• Monitor patient's temperature frequently. • Obtain culture from site. • Redress aseptically. • Use antibiotic ointment locally, as ordered. • Treat systemically with antibiotic or antifungal agents, depending on culture results and doctor's orders. • Remove catheter, as ordered. • Document your actions.	• Maintain strict aseptic technique. • Adhere to dressing change protocols. • Teach patient about swimming and bathing restrictions, if necessary. • Change dressing immediately if it becomes wet. • Change dressing more frequently if catheter is located in femoral area or near tracheostomy.
• Draw central and peripheral line blood cultures; if results show the same organism, catheter is primary source of sepsis and should be removed. • If cultures don't match but are positive, catheter may be removed or infection may be treated through catheter. • Administer antibiotics, as ordered. • Culture tip of device, if removed. • Assess for other infection sources. • Monitor patient's vital signs closely. • Document your actions.	• Examine fluid container for cloudiness, leaks, and turbidity before infusing. • Monitor urine glucose level in patients receiving total parenteral nutrition; if greater than 2, suspect early sepsis. • Use strict aseptic technique for hookup and fluid discontinuation. • Use 0.22-micron filter. • Change catheter frequently, if necessary, to decrease infection risk. • Disturb catheter as little as possible and maintain closed system. • Teach staff and patient about need for aseptic technique.
• Give oxygen, if ordered. • Prepare patient for emergency surgery, if ordered. • Monitor patient continuously. • Keep emergency equipment available.	• Ensure patient immobilization for insertion procedure. • Assess for signs and symptoms of cardiac tamponade. • Monitor chest X-rays to assess catheter position.

• When changing the I.V. tubing and solution, label the new I.V. bag and tubing with the date and time.

• If you change the injection cap or remove the catheter, document the procedure and the patient's response. Be sure to include the date and time that the injection cap was changed or the catheter was removed. Note the condition of the catheter at removal.

Patient teaching

Preparing your patient for CV therapy is an essential nursing responsibility. It's especially important if your patient will be discharged with a long-term CV catheter in place. You'll need to work with him and his spouse, family member, or caregiver to make sure they understand all aspects of care.

Before discharge, teach the patient or caregiver how to change dressings and injection caps, flush the catheter, and infuse drugs. Verify their learning by having them demonstrate these skills. Discuss any required changes in daily routine. Also make sure the patient or caregiver can recognize signs and symptoms of complications and knows what to do if they occur.

Make sure the patient and caregiver are familiar with both clean technique and sterile technique. Usually, when a patient is home in familiar surroundings, the infection risk decreases and clean technique can be substituted for sterile technique when changing dressings, I.V. tubing, and injection caps. However, if you have any doubt about your patient's personal hygiene practices or sanitary conditions in his home, encourage him to use sterile technique.

Vascular access ports

Surgically inserted under local anesthesia, vascular access ports (VAPs) are typically used in patients who need intermittent long-term I.V.

therapy but can't use an external CV catheter. The VAP, the most common implantable CV device, allows for bolus and intermittent doses, blood sampling, and continuous infusion. It poses a lower risk of infection than an external device because it has no exit site to serve as an entry for microorganisms. (See *Vascular access port*.)

Too expensive for short-term use, the VAP is normally implanted for 3 months to several years. It's not used for daily or continuous infusion because it's harder to access than an external catheter. Also, the needle, which is injected through subcutaneous tissue, must remain in place, which makes it easier to dislodge.

Candidates for VAPs include patients with poor peripheral veins; patients who need long-term periodic infusion of such drugs as antibiotics or chemotherapy; patients requiring parenteral nutrition, blood, or I.V. fluids; and patients who need regular blood testing.

Because VAPs protrude only slightly beneath the skin and don't restrict activity, many patients accept them more easily than external CV devices. VAPs may also be easier to maintain than external devices (unless the patient needs daily I.V. drugs or fluids).

A VAP usually isn't inserted in an obese patient because extra subcutaneous tissue presents problems with placement, port access, and healing. It also shouldn't be inserted at the site of radiation therapy or a previous mastectomy.

Equipment

A VAP consists of a silicone catheter attached to a reservoir made of titanium, plastic, or stainless steel. With a capacity volume of 0.2 to 0.5 ml, the reservoir is covered with a self-sealing, silicone rubber septum designed to withstand up to 2,000 punctures. The septum, which resembles the head of a stethoscope, measures 7 to 10 mm in diameter. The port's base measures ¾" to 2½" (2 to 5 cm) in diameter. (Smaller VAPs are usually used for children and small adults.)

Vascular access port

The large illustration below provides a cutaway view of drug injection through a vascular access port (VAP). The inset shows the entire VAP device.

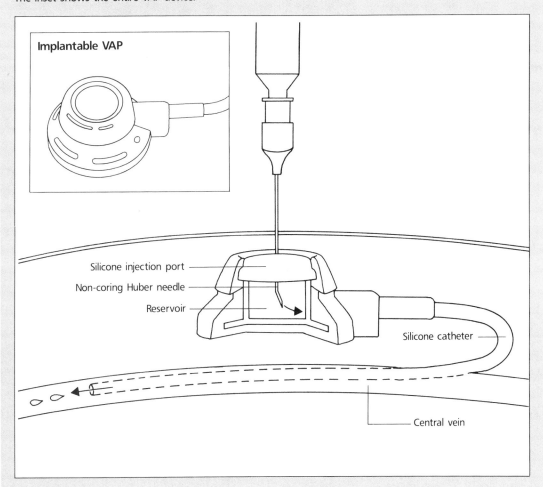

Implantable VAP

Silicone injection port

Non-coring Huber needle

Reservoir

Silicone catheter

Central vein

VAPs come in two basic designs: top entry (such as Med-i-port, Port-A-Cath, and Infus-A-Port) and side entry (such as S.E.A. Port). The Infus-A-Port P.A.S. port, a small device with a 16-mm base, is designed for peripheral venous access. Single- or double-lumen ports are available for different therapeutic needs.

VAPs are also classified as high- or low-profile depending on their height—usually ½" to 1" (1.3 to 2.5 cm). Low-profile VAPs are typically more stable, whereas high-profile VAPs allow easier access.

The VAP reservoir is attached to a radiopaque silicone catheter that is 20" to 30" (50.8 to 76.2 cm) long. Catheter placement can be verified by fluoroscopy or X-ray. A Hickman or Groshong catheter may also be used. Other VAPs are available as one unit, preconnected, or as a two-part system that's connected after placement.

To implant a VAP, the doctor uses a noncoring needle with a deflected and angled point. This needle design prevents coring or rubber removal during insertion and removal from the septum. The needle may be straight or bent at a 90-degree angle. Generally, the doctor uses a straight needle when implanting a side port and a bent needle when implanting a top-entry port. A straight needle can also be used to administer a bolus drug dose or draw blood from a top-entry port.

Needle length varies from 1/2" to 1 1/2" (1.3 to 3.8 cm). Half-inch needles usually are adequate for low-profile VAPs and the Infus-A-Port P.A.S. Needle width varies from 22G (for flushes only) to 19G (for administration of blood). A 20G needle, the largest size recommended for the Infus-A-Port P.A.S., can be used for almost any procedure performed with a VAP.

The needle may be plain or winged, with a stainless steel or plastic hub. The winged version is more stable and easier to grasp. Needles are available with or without a preconnected extension tube.

Using an over-the-needle catheter (such as the Surecath) gives the patient more freedom of movement. With this model, a 19G flexible catheter is left in place when the solid introducer spike is removed. The catheter conforms to the patient's chest contour, making dislodgment less likely.

VAP insertion
Usually, the doctor inserts and removes an implantable CV device in the operating room, using local anesthesia. The procedure is usually performed on an outpatient basis. Some VAPs can be inserted in the doctor's office. Nursing responsibilities include preparing the patient, assisting during insertion, and providing follow-up care and teaching.

Before the procedure
The doctor will recommend the device most suitable for the patient. Obtain the patient's allergy history because an allergic patient could develop problems with the port components. Also find out if he's likely to undergo magnetic resonance imaging in the near future. If he is, he should have a plastic or titanium port because a stainless steel port may cause image distortion.

If the patient has had a VAP device before, he may check to make sure you're using the right needle. So be sure to tell him you're using a non-coring needle. Warn him that he'll feel the needle prick during insertion. Mention that he may feel discomfort initially, but reassure him that the site will become less sensitive over time.

Make sure the patient has signed a consent form before VAP insertion. Answer all of his questions frankly and make sure he understands any other long-term CV therapy options available to him.

During the procedure
Have your patient assume Trendelenburg's position. Let him know you'll be present throughout the procedure. As necessary, provide periodic explanations or reassurance during insertion. Be prepared to hand the doctor the equipment he requests. To prepare the catheter, he may ask for a 3-ml flush of heparinized 0.9% sodium chloride solution (100 units/ml), although flushing is sometimes done only after the reservoir is connected to the catheter. (Keep in mind, however, that a Groshong catheter is flushed with 0.9% sodium chloride solution only.)

Insertion techniques are similar for both one-part and two-part VAPs. The doctor makes two incisions: one for the pocket that will hold the reservoir port and another for catheter placement in the vein. After insertion, he confirms placement by fluoroscopy or chest X-ray. He also confirms the port's stability, patency, and flow. Then he sutures the incisions shut.

To insert a two-part VAP, the doctor surgically places the distal end of the catheter into the vessel (usually the subclavian vein), with the catheter tip at the junction of the superior vena cava and right atrium. (Doctors no longer insert catheter tips in the right atrium because that may increase the risk of cardiac arrhythmias.) After he inserts the distal end of the catheter, he tunnels the proximal end to the port site using a trocar.

The ideal port site for a VAP is a subcutaneous pocket located medially over a bony prominence. The right infraclavicular fossa is most often chosen. The doctor sutures the port's base to the fascia. With a two-part VAP, the locking sleeve attaches the port to the catheter. (A drawback of this type of VAP is that the catheter may become disconnected from the reservoir if subjected to excessive pressure.)

After the procedure

Immediately after insertion, examine the port's pocket incision carefully. Note any signs of hematoma, excess swelling, exudate, thrombosis, port rotation, or port extrusion. Assess both incisions for redness, swelling, or drainage related to infection. Expect some tenderness and swelling around the insertion site for about 72 hours after the procedure. No special care is required after the incisions heal (usually in 5 to 7 days).

Drug administration

Once the doctor inserts the port, you can use it immediately unless he asks you to wait or unless the site is extremely painful, tender, or swollen. When ready to proceed, you'll access the port and either give a bolus injection or initiate a continuous infusion. Be sure to follow universal safety precautions whenever necessary.

Giving a bolus injection

Gather povidone-iodine swabs, a needle and syringe containing 3 to 5 ml of heparin solution (100 units/ml), a 10-ml syringe (with needle) containing sterile 0.9% sodium chloride

solution, a non-coring needle, 6″ (15 cm) I.V. extension tubing, the prescribed drug, and sterile gloves and mask.

Wash your hands. Then palpate the port, assessing its depth and size.

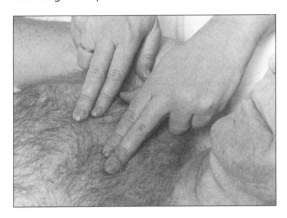

If you have trouble palpating a deeply inserted port, try using a 1½″ needle when gaining access. You'll need a longer needle to access a deeply implanted port. If the patient is anxious about needle insertion, try applying an ice pack for 1 or 2 minutes to numb the port area. You can also use a topical anesthetic, such as 0.1 to 0.15 ml of 2% lidocaine solution. If the port has been in place for a long time, a chest X-ray can confirm the port's location.

Prepare the site by cleaning it with povidone-iodine swabs, according to facility policy. Put on sterile gloves and mask. Stabilize the reservoir between your thumb and forefinger. Hold the non-coring needle like a dart, and position it at a 90-degree angle over the septum.

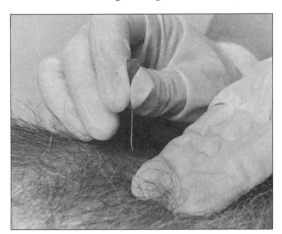

Push the needle straight through the skin and septum until it hits the needle stop at the back of the septum. (Don't insert the needle at an angle because this may damage the septum.) Now, attach the extension tubing to the needle hub.

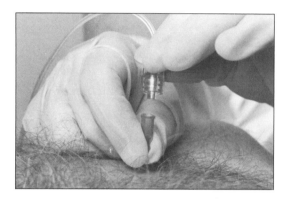

Note: As an alternative, you can attach a stopcock to the needle hub. However, extension tubing maintains a closed system for drug administration and other uses while minimizing needle manipulation.

Check needle placement by aspirating for blood return. If you don't see blood return, have the patient cough, turn, raise his arm, or take a deep breath. If these actions don't induce blood return, take out the needle and repeat the access procedure at a different site. (Repeated sticks in the same area may cause skin erosion over the septum and possibly infection.)

Steadily inject 5 ml of 0.9% sodium chloride flush solution.

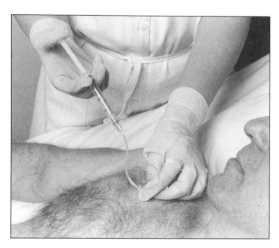

If you can't inject the solution, the needle tip is probably not positioned correctly. Make sure you've advanced the needle tip to the needle stop and try to inject the solution again. If you fail again, remove the needle and start over.

After injecting the flush solution, remove the syringe.

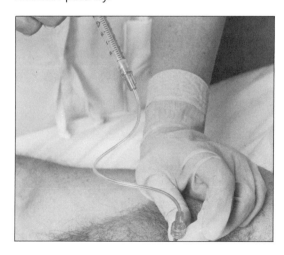

Then inject the prescribed drug into the extension tubing port. Flush the tubing again with 5 ml of 0.9% sodium chloride solution. *Important:* To prevent problems caused by drug incompatibility, flush the device with the sodium chloride solution before and after each drug injection and before each heparin flush.

Flush the tubing with 3 to 5 ml of heparin flush solution, according to facility policy. *Note:* During regular use, the port doesn't need more heparin flushing. However, when not in use, it should be flushed monthly to maintain patency.

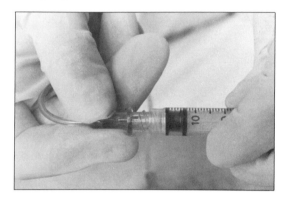

To remove the needle, stabilize the reservoir between your thumb and forefinger. Then withdraw the needle, taking care not to twist or angle it.

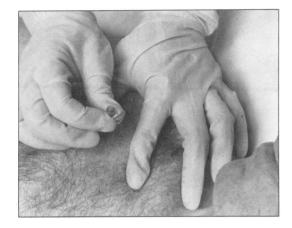

After needle withdrawal, you may see a slight serosanguineous discharge at the insertion site.

Giving a continuous infusion
To give a continuous infusion, use extension tubing with a luer-lock and clamp and a right-angle non-coring needle.

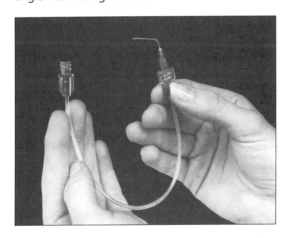

Remove all air from the extension tubing by priming it with an attached syringe of normal saline solution. Clean the insertion site and prime the I.V. tubing.

Using sterile technique, insert the needle. To prevent rotation, stabilize it at its hub.

After insertion, the needle's upper portion should lie just above the skin surface. If it lies more than 0.5 cm above the surface, support it with a folded 2″ × 2″ gauze pad. Connect the I.V. administration set and secure the connection with sterile tape, if necessary. Unclamp the I.V. administration set and start the infusion.

Use sterile adhesive Steri-Strips to secure first the needle hub, then the extension tubing. Apply povidone-iodine ointment to the insertion site. Then apply a transparent semipermeable dressing.

Monitor the site carefully for infiltration. If the patient complains of stinging, burning, or pain at the site, discontinue the infusion and intervene appropriately.

When the solution container is empty, obtain a new I.V. solution container, as ordered.

If your patient is receiving a continuous or prolonged infusion, you'll need to change the dressing and needle every 3 to 5 days. In addition, you'll need to change the tubing and solution, just as you would for a long-term CV infusion.

Obtaining a blood sample
To obtain a blood sample, access the port and verify placement the same way as when giving a drug or fluid. If a solution is infusing, stop it 2 to 3 minutes before drawing blood.

Flush the port with 10 ml of 0.9% sodium chloride solution to verify patency. Then, using either a syringe or an evacuated tube system, withdraw approximately 5 ml of blood and discard it. Next, withdraw the amount of blood needed for the sample. If you need blood for a coagulation study, you should draw that sample last. (Blood for a baseline coagulation study should be withdrawn when the port is first inserted because the heparin solution that is used to maintain patency may interfere with test results.)

After obtaining the blood sample, flush the port vigorously with 20 ml of the sodium chloride solution. Then restart the infusion, flush with heparin solution and cap, or deaccess the port.

Removing the needle from the port

To remove the needle from the port, put on sterile gloves. Discontinue any infusion. Using the thumb and forefinger of your nondominant hand, stabilize the port by pressing down on either side of it while removing the needle with your dominant hand. Keep exerting pressure until the needle is completely out.

Most patients prefer to have a small adhesive bandage applied, although little or no bleeding will occur. Dispose of the needle as you would any other sharp object.

Complications

A patient with a VAP faces risks similar to those associated with a traditional CV catheter. Make sure you can recognize signs and symptoms of these complications and know how to intervene appropriately. (See *Managing problems caused by a vascular access port.*)

Thrombosis

Thrombosis results from inadequate flushing of the system, too-frequent blood sampling, or blood transfusion. To detect thrombosis, examine your patient's hand, neck, and shoulder on the side of the port. Suspect thrombosis if he has edema and tenderness on that side. Treatment usually includes fibrinolytic therapy.

Erythema

Erythema, or skin breakdown, can occur from excessive patient movement while the needle is in place or from repeated use of the same site to access the port. Localized infection may develop, causing redness and drainage at the site. Erythema also can lead to systemic infection, which causes fever, lethargy, and other flulike symptoms. Expect the doctor to prescribe antibiotics and possibly port removal. If the port is the suspected infection source, he may want you to obtain blood cultures from both the port and a site in the opposite arm. An organism found in the port sample but not in the other sample confirms the port as the infection source. (However, some doctors believe the port can still be used as long as the patient receives antibiotics.)

Blocked catheter

The most common problem associated with VAPs, a blocked catheter can result from various problems, including kinked tubing, pump malfunction, improper needle or catheter position, port rotation, or port dislodgment. Kinked tubing should be straightened, a malfunctioning pump must be replaced, and improper needle placement should be corrected by removing and replacing the needle. If the port rotates or becomes dislodged, the doctor must intervene.

If you suspect that the catheter is lodged against the vessel wall, have the patient change position, reaccess the port, or gently irrigate and flush the catheter with 0.9% sodium chloride solution. If these measures fail, suspect clotting of the catheter and notify the doctor. He may order instillation of a fibrinolytic or declotting agent, such as urokinase or streptokinase.

Before using a declotting agent, check your patient's blood platelet count and the results of any coagulation studies. Then access the port, instill the prescribed agent, and attempt to declot the catheter using a gentle push-pull action. You can repeat the procedure three times within 4 hours if the patient's platelet count exceeds 20,000/mm^3. But if his count is less than 20,000/mm^3, limit the procedure to once in a 4-hour period.

Burning sensation

If your patient complains of a burning sensation around the port site, suspect that the needle has become dislodged from the port, causing infiltration or extravasation. Edema may develop under the arm or in the neck area.

Stop the infusion. If you suspect infiltration, notify the doctor. However, be aware that treatment usually consists only of reaccessing the port and verifying placement. If you suspect extravasation, don't remove the needle. Follow the policy of your health care facility for treating extravasation and notify the doctor. Be prepared to give the prescribed antidote.

Managing problems caused by a vascular access port

PROBLEM	POSSIBLE CAUSE	INTERVENTIONS
Erythema	• Patient movement • Infected incision or port pocket • Poor postoperative healing	• Assess daily for redness and drainage. Notify doctor. Administer antibiotics, as ordered.
Inability to flush or withdraw from system	• Kinked I.V. tubing • Pump malfunction • Catheter lodged against vessel wall • Incorrect needle placement • Fibrin sheath formation • Occlusion (clots) • Kinked catheter, port rotation	• Check tubing. • Check equipment. • Reposition patient by moving upper torso and arms. • Reposition needle and advance tip to bottom of reservoir. Verify correct positioning by blood aspiration. • Flush with 3 ml of sterile 0.9% sodium chloride solution and repeat, if necessary. Increase frequency of flushing to prevent sheath formation. • Use a declotting or fibrinolytic agent, such as urokinase, as ordered. • Contact doctor.
Burning sensation	• Needle dislodgment into subcutaneous tissue	• Don't remove needle. Stop infusion and notify doctor immediately.

"Twiddler's syndrome"

If your patient plays with the port area, the VAP may rotate or the catheter may migrate. (Catheter migration also can occur for no apparent reason.) To correct these problems, loop and tape the catheter securely, use a transparent semipermeable dressing, and teach the patient not to pull on or manipulate the device.

"Pinch-off syndrome"

In this syndrome, the catheter becomes pinched between muscles in the patient's upper chest. When this occurs, you're able to infuse fluid but unable to get a blood return. More of a nuisance than a complication, this syndrome can also occur when a fibrin sheath forms within the catheter. In this case, you're able to infuse fluid but unable to draw blood. The problem requires surgical correction.

Nursing considerations

• Once a port is accessed, you'll need to examine it at least every 8 hours. If the patient is receiving a vesicant drug, monitor the site hourly.

• Don't inject or infuse any drug until you verify needle placement. If you have trouble getting a blood return, notify the doctor. If this has been a working port, the catheter may have migrated out of the vessel. Some ports don't show a blood return; for instance, when the catheter is lodged against the vessel wall or when a fibrin sheath covers the catheter tip. If you can't get a blood return, a dye study can determine needle placement. This study should be repeated periodically.

• For a continuous infusion, be sure to attach a filter. Also use an I.V. pump with an automatic shut-off of 25 psi to prevent the catheter's disconnection from the reservoir. If you're not using a luer-lock connection, tape all connections securely to prevent air embolism.

• After each use, or at least every 4 weeks, flush the port with 5 ml of 0.9% sodium chloride solution (100 units/ml). Follow with heparinized sodium chloride solution to prevent clot formation and ensure the catheter's patency. To help prevent reaccessing problems, flush the port even if the needle is being changed. (If no extension is used, 3 ml of heparin flush solution is sufficient. However, your facility may have a different recommendation.)

• Maintain pressure on the syringe until the extension is clamped or, if the clamp doesn't have an extension, until the needle is removed from the port. (Remember to use only 0.9% sodium chloride solution to flush a Groshong catheter.)

• Never use anything smaller than a 10-ml syringe with a VAP. A syringe with a smaller lumen may put more pressure on the port. A 20G non-coring needle is appropriate for almost any injection or infusion with a VAP.

• If your patient has a double-lumen port, access and dress each port separately. Label the medial and lateral ports correctly.

• Be aware that a needle can remain in place up to 7 days, although in most facilities it's changed every 3 to 5 days. You can change the dressing during needle changes, or when necessary.

• Document every step you take when accessing and deaccessing the port. Also document each drug or fluid infusion on the medication administration record. Record needle size, number of dressing changes, patient teaching, and any complications.

• Label the dressing over the port with the date of insertion and access, your initials (if you accessed the port), and needle size used.

Patient teaching

To teach your patient about the VAP he's using, first find out how much he already knows about CV therapy. Let his level of knowledge, curiosity, and sophistication guide your teaching. If possible, provide models, pamphlets, books, or tapes supplied by the VAP manufacturer.

Inform your patient that his VAP won't restrict his activities and requires little maintenance except when the port is in use.

Mention how often the catheter and port need flushing. Tell him that if treatment is suspended for more than 4 weeks, he should

make an appointment for flushing, or you'll need to teach him how to do it himself.

Teach your patient the signs of local infection (redness, tenderness, and drainage at the site) and systemic infection (fever and malaise). Inform him that infiltration causes burning at the site and edema of the neck or underarm area on the affected side.

Instruct your patient to wear a medical identification bracelet or carry a card that informs all health care providers that he has a VAP. If he undergoes an invasive procedure, he may need prophylactic antibiotics.

If your patient is using the VAP at home for periodic infusions, make sure he knows how to access it himself. Before discharge, have him practice the procedure. Emphasize that he should feel the needle hitting the reservoir bottom or needle stop first. Teach him how to confirm needle placement with a blood return.

PICC line

For a patient who needs CV therapy for 5 days to several months or who requires repeated venous access, a PICC line may be the best option. The doctor may order a PICC line if your patient has suffered trauma or burns resulting in chest injury or if he has respiratory compromise resulting from chronic obstructive pulmonary disease, a mediastinal mass, cystic fibrosis, or pneumothorax. With any of these conditions, a PICC line helps avoid complications that may occur with a CV line.

A PICC line is used increasingly for patients receiving home care. The device is easier to insert than other CV devices and provides safe, reliable access for drugs and blood sampling. A single catheter may be used for the entire course of therapy (approximately 1 to 140 days), with greater convenience and at reduced cost.

Infusions commonly given by PICC include TPN, chemotherapy, antibiotics, narcotics, analgesics, and blood products. PICC therapy works best when introduced early in treatment and shouldn't be considered a last resort for patients with sclerosed or repeatedly punctured veins.

The patient receiving PICC therapy must have a peripheral vein large enough to accept a 14G or 16G introducer needle and a 3.8G to 4.8G catheter. The doctor or nurse inserts a PICC via the basilic, median antecubital basilic, cubital, or cephalic vein. He then threads it to the superior vena cava or subclavian vein or to a noncentral site, such as the axillary vein.

PICCs cost from $11 to $60. Insertion may cost from $50 to $300, compared with approximately $500 for insertion of short-term CV catheters and $1,200 for insertion of long-term CV catheters and implantable CV devices.

Equipment

Made of silicone or polyurethane, a PICC is soft and flexible, with increased biocompatibility. It may range from 16G to 23G (1.8 to 5 cm) in diameter and from 16" to 24" (40 to 60 cm) in length. A PICC is available in single- and double-lumen versions, with or without guide wires. A guide wire stiffens the catheter, easing its advancement through the vein, but it can damage the vessel if used improperly.

Insertion of a PICC

If your state nurse practice act permits, you may insert a PICC if you show sufficient knowledge of vascular access devices. To prove your competency in PICC insertion, it is recommended that you complete an 8-hour workshop and demonstrate three successful catheter insertions. You may have to redemonstrate competency every year.

First gather the necessary supplies. If you're administering PICC therapy in the patient's home, bring everything with you. You'll need a catheter insertion kit, three alcohol swabs, three povidone-iodine swabs, a 3-ml vial of heparin (100 units/ml), a latex injection port with short extension tubing, sterile and nonsterile measuring tape, a vial of 0.9% sodium chloride solution, sterile gauze pads, linen-saver pad, sterile drapes, tourniquet, and a sterile transparent semipermeable dressing. Gather sterile gloves (two pairs), gown, mask, and goggles to maintain sterility and universal precautions.

Describe the insertion procedure to your patient and answer her questions.

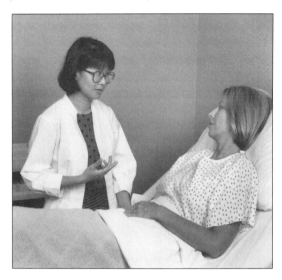

Select the insertion site and place the tourniquet on the patient's arm. Assess the antecubital fossa.

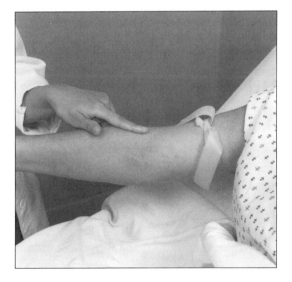

The most common veins used are the median antecubital basilic, cubital, basilic, and cephalic veins. The two basilic veins are preferred because they're straighter than the cephalic vein and they widen gradually as they become axillary veins. If you choose the cephalic vein, you may have some trouble advancing the catheter past the deltoid muscle.

Remove the tourniquet. Now, determine catheter tip placement, or the spot at which the catheter tip will rest after insertion. For subclavian vein placement, use nonsterile measuring tape to measure the distance from the insertion site to the shoulder and from the shoulder to the sternal notch.

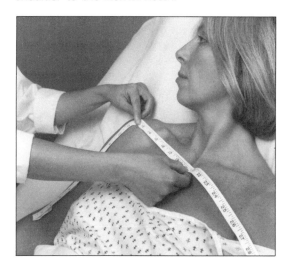

For catheter tip placement in the superior vena cava, measure the distance from the insertion site to the shoulder and from the shoulder to the sternal notch. Then add 3″ (7.6 cm).

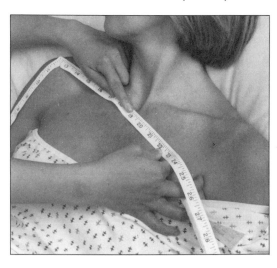

Have the patient lie supine with her arm at a 90-degree angle to her body. Place a linen-saver pad under her arm.

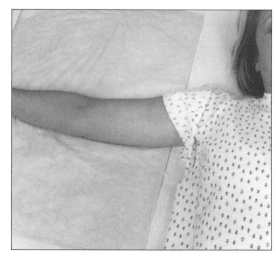

Open the PICC tray and drop the rest of the sterile items onto the sterile field. Put on the sterile gown, mask, goggles, and gloves.

Using the sterile measuring tape, cut the distal end of the catheter to the premeasured length. Cut the tip straight across to prevent the catheter from lying flush against the intima of the vein and possibly obstructing the infusion flow.

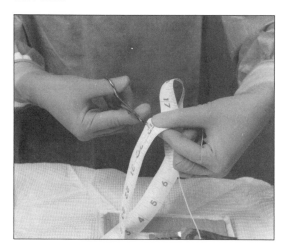

Using sterile technique, withdraw 5 ml of the sodium chloride solution and flush the extension tubing and the latex cap.

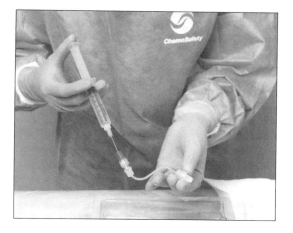

Remove the needle from the syringe. Attach the syringe to the hub of the catheter and flush.

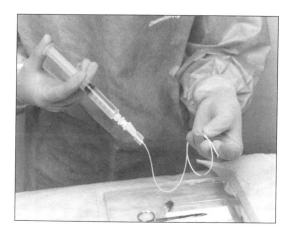

Prepare the insertion site by rubbing three alcohol swabs over it. Use a circular motion, working outward from the site about 6" (15 cm). Repeat, using three povidone-iodine swabs, as shown at the top of the next column. Pat the area dry with a sterile 4" × 4" gauze pad. Be sure not to touch the intended insertion site.

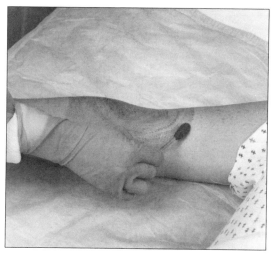

Take your gloves off. Then apply the tourniquet about 4" (10 cm) above the antecubital fossa.

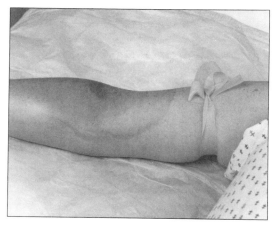

Put on a new pair of sterile gloves. Then place a sterile drape under the patient's arm and another on top of her arm. Drop a sterile 4" × 4" gauze pad over the tourniquet.

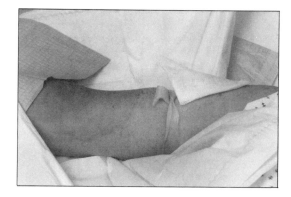

Stabilize the patient's vein. Insert the catheter introducer at a 10-degree angle, directly into the vein.

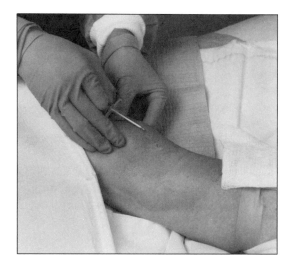

After successful vein entry, you should see a blood return in the flashback chamber. Without changing the needle's position, gently advance the plastic introducer sheath until you're sure the tip is well within the vein.

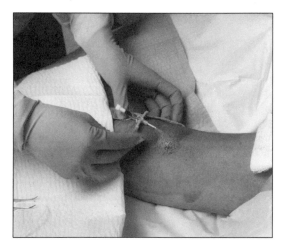

Carefully withdraw the needle while holding the introducer still. To minimize blood loss, try applying finger pressure on the vein just beyond the distal end of the introducer sheath.

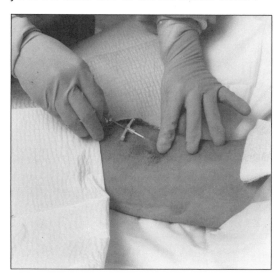

Using sterile forceps, insert the catheter into the introducer sheath and advance it into the vein. Remove the tourniquet, using the 4" × 4" gauze pad.

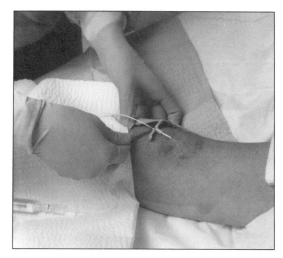

When you've advanced the catheter to the shoulder, ask the patient to turn her head toward the affected arm and place her chin on her chest. This will occlude the jugular vein and ease the catheter's advancement into the subclavian vein.

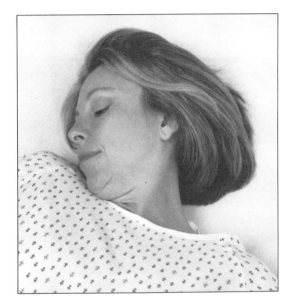

Advance the catheter until about 4″ (10 cm) remain. Then pull the introducer sheath out of the vein and away from the introducer site.

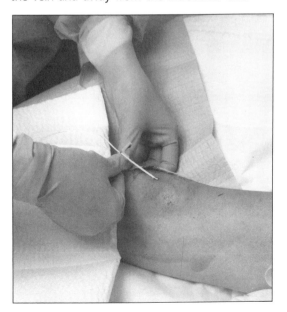

Grasp the blue tabs of the introducer sheath and flex them toward its distal end to split the sheath.

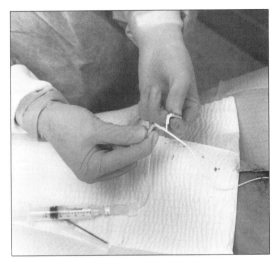

Pull the blue tabs apart and away from the catheter until the sheath is completely split. Discard the sheath.

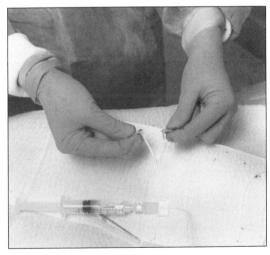

Continue to advance the catheter until about 2″ (5 cm) remain externally. Flush with 0.9% sodium chloride solution.

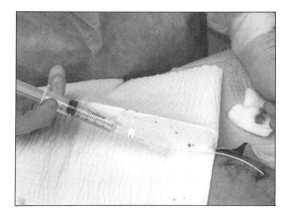

With the patient's arm below heart level, remove the syringe. Connect the capped extension set to the hub of the catheter.

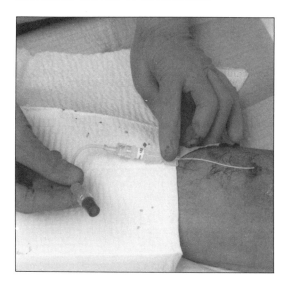

Apply a sterile 2″ × 2″ gauze pad directly over the site and a sterile transparent semipermeable dressing over that. Leave this dressing in place for 24 hours.

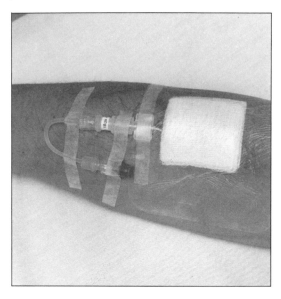

After the initial 24 hours, apply a new sterile transparent semipermeable dressing. The gauze pad is no longer necessary. You can place Steri-Strips over the catheter wings. Flush with heparin.

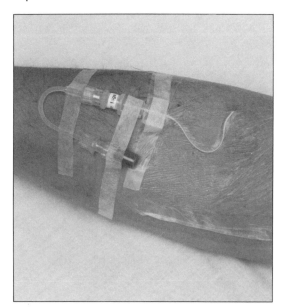

Drug administration

As with any CV line, be sure to check for a blood return and flush with 0.9% sodium chloride solution before administering a drug through a PICC line.

First clamp the 7″ extension tubing and connect the empty syringe to the tubing. Release the clamp and aspirate slowly to verify blood return. Flush with 3 ml of sodium chloride solution. Then administer the drug.

After giving the drug, flush again with 3 ml of the sodium chloride solution. (And remember to flush with the same solution between infusions of incompatible drugs or fluids.)

Changing the dressing

You should change the dressing every 4 days for an inpatient and every 5 to 7 days for a home care patient. If possible, choose a transparent semipermeable dressing, which has a high moisture-vapor transmission rate. Use aseptic technique.

First, wash your hands and assemble the necessary supplies. Position the patient with his arm extended away from his body, at a 45- to 90-degree angle. Put on a sterile mask.

Open the package of sterile gloves and use the inside of the package as a sterile field. Then open the transparent semipermeable dressing and drop it onto the field. Remove the old dressing by holding your left thumb on the catheter and stretching the dressing parallel to the skin. Repeat this last step with your right thumb holding the catheter. Free the remaining section of the dressing from the catheter by peeling toward the insertion site from the distal end to the proximal end to prevent catheter dislodgment.

Put on the sterile gloves. Clean the area thoroughly with three alcohol swabs, starting at the insertion site and working outward from the site. Repeat this step three times with povidone-iodine swabs and pat dry.

Apply the dressing carefully. Secure the tubing to the edge of the dressing over the tape with ¼″ adhesive tape.

Complications

PICC therapy causes fewer and less severe complications than conventionally placed CV lines. Pneumothorax is extremely rare because the insertion site is peripheral. Catheter-related sepsis is also rare.

Phlebitis, perhaps the most common complication, may occur during the first 48 to 72 hours after PICC insertion. It's more common in left-sided insertions and when a large-gauge catheter is used. If the patient develops phlebitis, apply warm, moist compresses to his upper arm. You may also elevate the area and encourage mild exercise. If phlebitis continues or worsens, remove the catheter, as ordered.

You should expect minimal bleeding from the insertion site for 24 hours after insertion; bleeding that persists, however, warrants additional evaluation.

Air embolism, always a potential risk of venipuncture, poses less danger in PICC therapy than with traditional CV lines because the line is inserted below heart level.

Some patients complain of pain at the catheter's insertion site, usually from chemical properties of the infused drug or fluid. Slowing the infusion rate and applying warm compresses should relieve pain.

Catheter tip migration may occur with vigorous flushing. Patients receiving chemotherapy are most vulnerable to this complication because of frequent nausea and vomiting and subsequent changes in intrathoracic pressure. If the catheter fails to show a blood return, arrange for a chest X-ray to determine the exact position of the catheter tip.

Catheter occlusion, a relatively common complication, may warrant urokinase administration. As ordered, give urokinase according to the manufacturer's recommendations to restore catheter patency. (See *Coping with PICC line problems,* page 94.)

Nursing considerations

• Be aware that the doctor or nurse probably will place the PICC in the superior vena cava if the patient will receive therapy in the hospital.

Coping with PICC line problems

PROBLEM	POSSIBLE CAUSES	INTERVENTIONS
Occlusion	• Thrombus • Improper flushing • Decreased flow rate • Precipitate formation from infusion of incompatible substances • Catheter improperly positioned in vein; catheter tip against vessel wall	• Reposition patient and check for flow. • Attempt to aspirate the clot. Don't force clot. • Notify the doctor. • Possibly, infuse thrombolytic agents such as streptokinase or urokinase. • Possibly, remove catheter (may be repositioned in vein with verification by X-ray). • Document interventions.
Damaged or broken catheter	• Pinholes, leaks, or tears in catheter	• Examine catheter for drainage after flushing. • Follow recommended clamping procedure. • Remove catheter if ordered. • To prevent, avoid using sharp objects near catheter and avoid injection of needles larger than 1" through the injection cap.
Fluid won't infuse	• Closed clamp • Displaced or kinked catheter • Thrombus	• Check infusion system and clamps. • Change the patient's position. • Have the patient cough, breathe deeply, or perform Valsalva's maneuver. • Remove the dressing and examine the external portion of the catheter. • If a kink isn't apparent, obtain an X-ray order. • Try to withdraw blood. • Try a gentle flush with saline solution.
Unable to draw blood	• Closed clamp • Displaced or kinked catheter • Thrombus • Catheter movement against vessel wall with negative pressure	• Check the infusion system and clamps. • Change the patient's position. • Have the patient cough, breathe deeply, or perform Valsalva's maneuver. • Remove dressing and examine external portion of catheter. • Obtain an X-ray order.
Disconnected catheter	• Patient movement • Not securely connected to tubing	• Apply catheter clamp, if available. • Place sterile syringe or catheter plug in catheter hub. • Change extension set. Don't reconnect contaminated tubing. • Clean catheter hub with alcohol or povidone-iodine. Don't soak hub. • Connect clean I.V. tubing or a heparin lock plug to the site. • Restart the infusion.

• For a hospital patient receiving intermittent PICC therapy, flush the catheter with 6 ml of 0.9% sodium chloride solution and 6 ml of heparin (10 units/ml) after each use. For catheters that are not being used, a weekly flush of 2 ml (1,000 units/ml) of heparin will maintain patency.

• You can use a declotting agent, such as urokinase, to clear a clotted PICC line, but make sure you read the manufacturer's recommendations first.
• Remember to add an extension set to all PICC lines so that you can start and stop an I.V. away from the insertion site. An extension

set will also make using a PICC line easier for the patient who will be administering infusions himself.

• If a patient will be receiving blood or blood products through the PICC line, you should use at least an 18G catheter.

• Assess the catheter insertion site through the transparent semipermeable dressing every 24 hours. Look at the catheter and check for any bleeding, redness, drainage, and swelling. Ask your patient if he's having any pain associated with therapy. Although bleeding is common for the first 24 hours after insertion, excessive bleeding after that period of time must be evaluated.

• Document the entire procedure, including any problems with catheter placement. Also document the size and type of catheter as well as the insertion location.

Patient teaching

Describe the PICC insertion procedure to the patient in advance, and discuss dressing changes and the flushing procedure. Make sure he knows how to recognize the signs and symptoms of complications and when to report them.

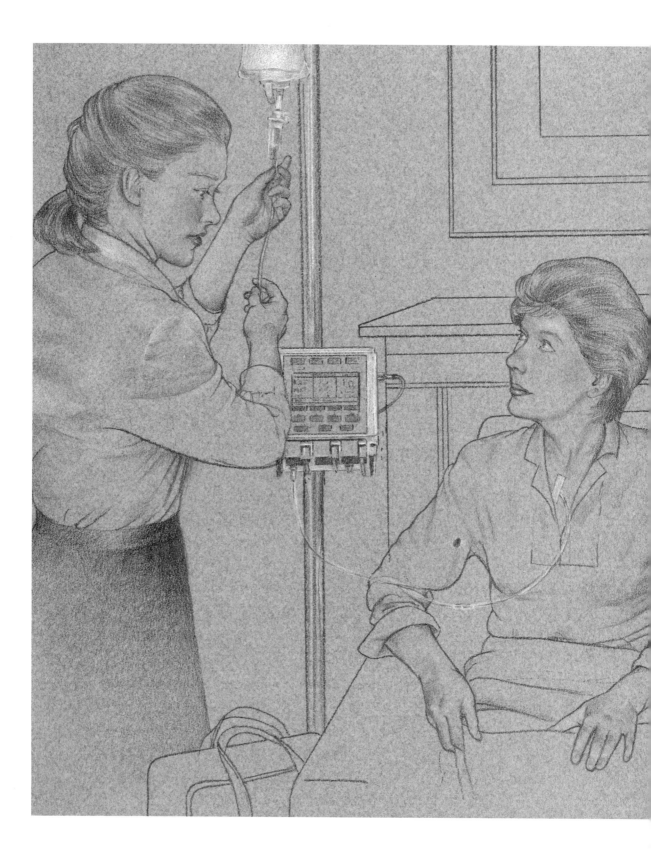

Providing parenteral nutrition

When a patient can't meet his nutritional needs by oral or enteral feedings, he may require I.V. nutritional support, or parenteral nutrition. The patient's diagnosis, history, and prognosis determine the need for parenteral nutrition. Generally, this treatment is prescribed for any patient who can't absorb nutrients through the GI tract for more than 10 days. More specific indications for parenteral nutrition include:

• debilitating illness lasting longer than 2 weeks
• weight loss of 10% or more of pre-illness weight
• serum albumin level below 3.5 g/dl
• excessive nitrogen loss from wound infection, fistulas, or abscesses
• renal or hepatic failure
• nonfunctioning GI tract for 5 to 7 days when the patient is severely catabolic.

Common illnesses that can trigger the need for parenteral nutrition include inflammatory bowel disease, radiation enteritis, severe diarrhea, intractable vomiting, and moderate to se-vere pancreatitis. A massive small-bowel resection, a bone marrow transplant, high-dose chemotherapy or radiation therapy, or major surgery can also hinder a patient's ability to absorb nutrients and necessitate parenteral nutrition.

Infants with congenital or acquired disorders may need parenteral nutrition to promote their growth and development. Specific disorders that could require parenteral nutrition include tracheoesophageal fistula, gastroschisis, duodenal atresia, cystic fibrosis, meconium ileus, diaphragmatic hernia, volvulus, malrotation of the gut, and annular pancreas.

But parenteral nutrition isn't right for all patients. It has limited value for well-nourished patients whose GI tracts will resume normal function within 10 days. It also shouldn't be given if the patient has a normally functioning GI tract. It may be inappropriate for a patient with a poor prognosis or if the risks of parenteral nutrition outweigh the benefits. Also, depending upon state law and health care facility policy, parenteral nutrition can be refused by the patient or by his legal guardian.

Besides helping to identify patients who need parenteral nutrition, you'll also monitor the effects of therapy. This chapter will help you gain the skills to do so. It starts by reviewing the pharmacologic principles of parenteral nutrition, including the solution's composition and distribution within the body. Next, parenteral solution and lipid emulsion—the two basic components of total parenteral nutrition—are introduced. You'll find the same categories of information for both: the equipment you'll need, the administration procedure, possible complications, and special nursing considerations. You'll also find patient-teaching concerns.

Pharmacologic principles

The prescribed parenteral solution depends on the patient's condition and metabolic needs, and on whether it's to be given through a peripheral line or a central venous (CV) line. The solution usually contains protein, carbohydrates, electrolytes, vitamins, and trace minerals. Lipid emulsion provides the necessary fat. (See *Comparing I.V. and parenteral solutions.*)

Protein content
The parenteral solution typically provides 42 g of protein per liter of amino acid solution. To reach this level of concentration, 500 ml of 8.5% amino acid solution (such as FreAmine, Travasol, or Aminosyn) are mixed with 500 ml of dextrose 50% in water. This ratio may be changed according to the patient's metabolic needs, but most patients require 2 to 3 liters of parenteral nutrition daily to meet their protein requirement.

Carbohydrate content
Dextrose 50% in water supplies the parenteral solution with its carbohydrate content. Five hundred milliliters of dextrose solution per liter of parenteral nutrition provides 250 g of glucose, but some patients may need a more concentrated source of energy. If so, the doctor may order a 70% dextrose solution, which provides 350 g of glucose per 500 ml.

Fat content
Fats, or lipids, provide a major source of nonprotein calories. Typically, lipids provide 25% to 35% of the total calories delivered by parenteral nutrition. In some instances, this percentage may be higher, but fats should never exceed 60% of the total calories.

Four different lipid emulsions may be used. These include Intralip, Travamulsion, and Soyacal (all soybean oil) as well as Liposyn II (safflower and soybean oils).

Lipids are supplied in 250-ml or 500-ml bottles at concentrations of 10% to 20%. The 10% concentration provides 1.1 kcal/ml, whereas the 20% solution supplies 2.2 kcal/ml. You'll usually give lipid emulsions separately from other parenteral nutrition solutions. While some solutions mix lipids with the protein-carbohydrate solution, these ingredients may not be compatible with each other and the solution may not be stable. Also, these mixtures tend to clog I.V. filters.

Comparing I.V. and parenteral solutions

TYPE AND COMPONENTS	USES	SPECIAL CONSIDERATIONS
Standard I.V. solution Composed of dextrose, water, and electrolytes. Doesn't contain vitamins unless ordered. Dextrose 5% in water contains 170 calories/liter; 0.9% sodium chloride solution contains no calories.	Given for less than 1 week as a nutritional source. Maintains hydration. Also facilitates and maintains normal metabolic function.	Nutritionally incomplete. Standard I.V. solutions contain insufficient calories to maintain adequate nutritional status.
Total parenteral nutrition (TPN) Composed of dextrose 15% to 25% in water (1 liter of dextrose 25% contains 850 nonprotein calories) and crystalline amino acids 2.5% to 8.5%. Contains electrolytes, minerals, vitamins, and trace elements. Lipid emulsion 10% or 20% is given as a separate solution.	Given for 2 weeks or longer. Can provide 2,000 to 4,000 calories/ day. Helps restore nitrogen balance and replaces electrolytes, minerals, vitamins, and trace elements. Also promotes tissue synthesis, wound healing, and normal metabolic function; allows the bowel to rest and heal; reduces activity in the gallbladder, pancreas, and small intestine; and improves the patient's tolerance for surgery.	Must be administered through a central venous (CV) line. The *basic solution* is nutritionally complete, highly hypertonic, and may cause metabolic complications (such as glucose intolerance, electrolyte imbalances, and acid/base disturbances). The *lipid emulsion* may be ineffective in severely stressed patients, such as those with burns. It may interfere with immune mechanisms and, in patients suffering respiratory compromise, it reduces carbon dioxide buildup.
Total nutrient admixture Also called 3-in-1 solution; combines lipid emulsion with other parenteral nutrition components. A 3-liter bag contains a one-day supply of nutrients.	Given for 2 weeks or longer. Typically administered to patients who are relatively stable because solution components can only be adjusted once daily. Other uses are the same as those for TPN.	Because the bag is hung only once a day, the risk of contamination decreases. Allows for increased patient mobility and is easier to use in a home setting. The solution and tubing require changing every 24 hours. Use is limited because not all types and amounts of components are compatible. The solution precludes the use of certain infusion pumps (because many can't accurately deliver large volumes), as well as standard I.V. tubing filters (because 0.22-micron filters block lipid molecules).
Peripheral parenteral nutrition Composed of dextrose 5% to 10% in water, crystalline amino acids 2.5% to 5%, electrolytes, minerals, vitamins, and trace elements. Lipid emulsion 10% or 20% is given as a separate solution. Heparin or hydrocortisone is administered as ordered.	Given for 2 weeks or less. Can provide up to 2,000 calories/day. Used to maintain nutritional status in patients who can tolerate relatively high fluid volumes, who will resume oral feedings after a few days, and who are susceptible to CV catheter infections.	The *parenteral solution* is nutritionally complete for short-term use. Because the site must be rotated every 72 hours, the patient must have accessible veins. Although the solution is less hypertonic than TPN given through a CV line, it can't exceed 900 mOsm/liter. May cause phlebitis, and increases risk of metabolic complications. Contraindicated in nutritionally depleted patients and volume-restricted patients. Does not cause weight gain. The *lipid emulsion* is as effective a calorie source as dextrose. If infused with the nutrient solution, the patient's risk for phlebitis decreases.
Protein-sparing therapy Contains crystalline amino acids (in the same amount as in TPN), electrolytes, vitamins, minerals, and trace elements.	Given for 2 weeks or less. Used to augment oral or tube feedings. May preserve body protein in a stable patient.	Nutritionally complete solution requires little mixing. May be started and stopped at any time during the patient's stay. Other I.V. fluids, medications, and blood by-products may be administered through the same line. Carries a lower risk of phlebitis but is expensive and has limited benefits.

Electrolyte content

For efficient tissue synthesis, the body requires the proper amounts of certain electrolytes. The electrolytes usually contained in parenteral nutrition solution include:
• sodium: 60 mEq or more (adults) or 3 to 5 mEq/kg/day (infants and children)
• potassium: 60 mEq or more (adults) or 3 mEq/kg/day (infants and children)
• magnesium: 12 to 20 mEq/kg/day or more (adults) or 0.3 to 0.5 mEq/kg/day (infants and children)
• calcium: 10 to 25 mEq/kg/day (adults) or 12 mEq/kg/day (infants and children)
• phosphorus: 450 mg/day (adults) or 15 to 30 mEq/kg/day (infants and children).

Vitamin content

All patients require a certain number and amount of vitamins. Vitamin D aids in bone metabolism and helps maintain serum calcium levels, whereas vitamin B complex helps in the final absorption of carbohydrates and protein. Also, trace elements (such as zinc, copper, chromium, and manganese) stimulate wound healing, aid in the metabolism of nutrients, and act as catalysts in enzyme systems.

The vitamin content of a parenteral nutrition solution varies according to the patient's needs. For example, a burn patient demands an increased amount of ascorbic acid, whereas a patient with an infection requires other vitamins. Because pharmacists prepare parenteral nutrition solution for each individual patient, these varying vitamin requirements can be easily satisfied.

Parenteral solution

Parenteral nutrition may be given through a peripheral or a central line. Depending on the solution, parenteral nutrition may be used to boost the patient's caloric intake, to supply full caloric needs, or to surpass the patient's caloric requirements.

Total parenteral nutrition (TPN) refers to any nutrient solution, including lipids, given through a central line. Peripheral parenteral nu-

trition (PPN), which is given through a peripheral line, has the advantage of being able to supply full caloric needs while avoiding the risks that accompany a CV line. However, to keep from sclerosing the vein through which it's administered, the dextrose in PPN solution must be limited to 10%. Therefore, the success of PPN depends on the patient's tolerance for the large volume of fluid necessary to supply his nutritional needs.

Many times you'll need to increase the glucose content beyond the level a peripheral vein can handle. For example, most TPN solution is six times more concentrated than blood. As a result, it must be delivered into a vein with a high rate of blood flow to dilute the solution.

The most common delivery route for TPN is through a central venous catheter (such as a Hickman or a Broviac) into the superior vena cava. The catheter may also be placed through an infraclavicular approach or, less commonly, the supraclavicular, internal jugular, or antecubital fossa approach. (See *Indications for using a peripheral or central vein*.)

Regardless of the delivery route, your care of the patient and the catheter site will be the same.

Equipment

Gather the following equipment: a bag or bottle of prescribed parenteral nutrition solution, sterile I.V. tubing with attached extension tubing, a 0.22-micron filter (or a 1.2-micron filter if the solution contains lipids or albumin), a reflux valve, time tape, alcohol sponges, and an electronic infusion pump. You'll also need a test kit for urine glucose and ketones (or a glucose enzymatic test strip if the patient is receiving cephalosporins, methyldopa, aspirin, or large doses of ascorbic acid), a scale, and an intake and output record.

Drug administration

Before giving parenteral nutrition, you'll need to make sure the solution, the patient, and the equipment are ready. Remove the bag or bottle of solution from the refrigerator at least 1 hour before use to avoid the pain, hypothermia, venous spasm, and venous constriction that can accompany delivery of a chilled solu-

Indications for using a peripheral or central vein

PERIPHERAL VEIN	CENTRAL VEIN
• Interrupted enteral intake, but patient can resume enteral feedings in 5 to 7 days • Mild-to-moderate malnutrition • Normal or mildly elevated metabolic rate • Absence of fluid restrictions • Supplement to enteral feedings needed	• Inability to tolerate enteral intake for more than 7 days. • Moderate-to-severe malnutrition that can't be corrected with enteral feedings • Moderately or severely elevated metabolic rates • Restricted fluid intake • Poor or inaccessible peripheral veins • Readily accessible central vein

tion. Check the solution against the doctor's order for correct patient name, expiration date, and formula components. Also observe the container for cracks and the solution for cloudiness, turbidity, or particles. If any of these are present, return the solution to the pharmacy. If you'll be administering a total nutrient admixture solution, look for a brown layer on the solution, which can indicate that the lipid emulsion has "cracked" or separated from the solution. If you see a brown layer, return the solution to the pharmacy.

When you're ready to administer the solution, explain the procedure to the patient. Check the name on the solution container against the name on the patient's wristband. Then put on gloves and, if specified by your the policy at your health care facility, a mask. Throughout the procedure, use strict aseptic technique.

Preparing the tubing
In sequence, connect the pump tubing, the micron filter with attached extension tubing (if the tubing doesn't contain an in-line filter), and the reflux valve. Be sure to insert the filter so that it will be as close to the catheter site as possible. If the tubing doesn't have luer-lock connections, tape all connections to prevent accidental separation, which could lead to air embolism, exsanguination, and sepsis. Next, squeeze the I.V. drip chamber and, holding the drip chamber upright, insert the tubing spike into the I.V. bag or bottle. Then release the drip chamber. Squeezing the drip chamber be-

fore spiking an I.V. *bottle* prevents accidental dripping of the parenteral nutrition solution. An I.V. bag, however, shouldn't drip.

Prime the tubing, gently tapping it to dislodge air bubbles trapped in the Y-ports. If indicated, attach a time tape to the parenteral nutrition container for accurate measurement of fluid intake. Record the date and time you hung the fluid, and initial the parenteral nutrition solution container. Next, attach the setup to the infusion pump and prepare it according to the manufacturer's instructions.

With the patient in the supine position, flush the sterile I.V. tubing with heparin or 0.9% sodium chloride solution, according to the policy at your health care facility. Then wipe the connection between the catheter hub and the existing line with an alcohol sponge and allow it to dry.

Connecting the line
If you'll be attaching the parenteral nutrition solution to a CV line, clamp the CV line before disconnecting it to prevent air from entering the catheter. If a clamp isn't available, ask the patient to perform the Valsalva maneuver just as you change the tubing, if possible. Or, if the patient is being mechanically ventilated, change the I.V. tubing immediately after the machine delivers a breath at peak inspiration. Both of these measures increase intrathoracic pressure and prevent air embolism. (See *Administering parenteral nutrition through a CV line*, page 102.)

Administering parenteral nutrition through a CV line

This illustration shows the infusion of a parenteral solution through a CV line. Because of its gentle arch, the left subclavian vein is commonly used for CV infusion. Make sure that no air enters the catheter because of the vein's proximity to the heart.

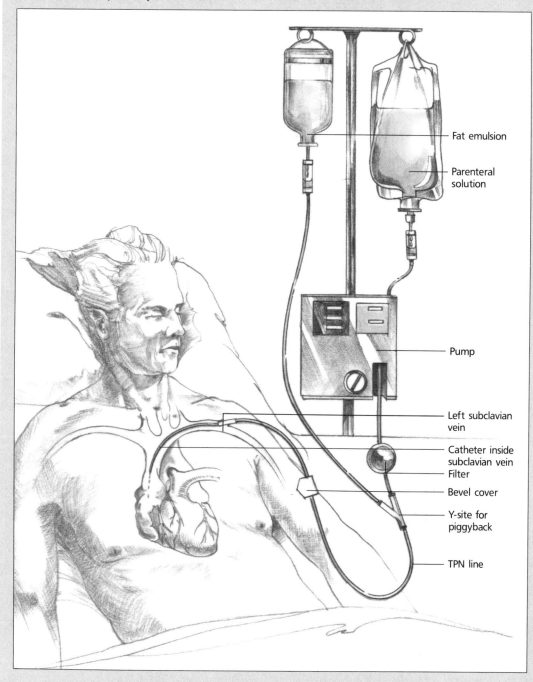

Fat emulsion

Parenteral solution

Pump

Left subclavian vein

Catheter inside subclavian vein

Filter

Bevel cover

Y-site for piggyback

TPN line

Then, using aseptic technique, remove the old I.V. tubing from either the peripheral or central line and attach the new I.V. line. Once you've connected the new tubing, remove the clamp, if applicable. Set the infusion pump at the ordered flow rate and start the infusion. Check to make sure the catheter junction is secure. Tag the tubing, indicating the date and time of change.

Starting the infusion

Because parenteral nutrition solution often contains large amounts of glucose, you may need to start the infusion slowly to allow the patient's pancreatic beta cells time to increase their output of insulin. Depending on the patient's tolerance, parenteral nutrition is usually initiated at a rate of 40 to 50 ml/hour and is advanced 25 ml/hour every 6 hours until the desired rate of infusion is achieved. However, when the concentration of glucose is low, as occurs in most peripheral parenteral nutrition formulas, you can initiate the rate necessary to infuse the complete 24-hour volume. In this instance, you can also discontinue the solution without tapering.

You may allow a parenteral nutrition solution to hang for 24 to 72 hours, or according to the policy at your health care facility. However, if the patient has a 3-in-1 solution (a solution that contains lipids in addition to carbohydrates and protein), you'll need to hang a new solution container every 24 hours.

Changing solutions

Prepare the new solution and I.V. tubing as described earlier. Put on sterile gloves. Remove the protective caps from the solution containers and wipe the tops of the containers with alcohol sponges. Turn off the infusion pump and close the flow clamps. Using strict aseptic technique, remove the spike from the solution container that's hanging and insert it into the new container. Hang the new container and tubing alongside the old. Turn on the infusion pump, set the flow rate, and open the flow clamp completely.

If you'll be attaching the solution to a peripheral line, examine the skin above the insertion site for signs of phlebitis, such as redness

and warmth, and assess for pain. If such signs exist, remove the existing I.V. line and start a line in a different vein. Also, insert a new line if the present I.V. catheter has been in place for 72 hours or more, to reduce the risk of phlebitis and infiltration.

Next, turn off the infusion pump and close the flow clamp on the old tubing. Disconnect the tubing from the needle or catheter hub, and connect the new tubing. Open the flow clamp on the new container to a keep-vein-open rate to prevent clot formation in the needle or catheter while you insert the tubing into the infusion pump.

Remove the old tubing from the infusion pump, and insert the new tubing according to the manufacturer's instructions. Then turn on the infusion pump, set it to the desired flow rate, and open the flow clamp completely. Remove the old equipment and dispose of it properly.

Complications

Catheter-related sepsis is the most serious complication of parenteral nutrition. Although rare, a malpositioned subclavian or jugular vein catheter may lead to thrombosis or sepsis.

An air embolism, a potentially fatal complication, can occur during I.V. tubing changes if the tubing is inadvertently disconnected. An embolism may also result from undetected hairline cracks in the tubing. Extravasation of parenteral nutrition solution can cause necrosis, with sequential sloughing of the epidermis and dermis. (See *Correcting common problems with parenteral nutrition,* page 104.)

Nursing considerations

• Always infuse a parenteral nutrition solution at a constant rate without interruption to avoid fluctuations in blood glucose. If the infusion slows, consult the doctor before changing the infusion rate.
• Monitor the patient's vital signs every 4 hours, or more often if necessary. Be alert for an increased temperature, which may be an early sign of catheter-related sepsis.
• Check the patient's urine for glucose and ketones every 4 to 6 hours. Some patients may require supplementary insulin throughout par-

COMPLICATIONS

Correcting common problems with parenteral nutrition

COMPLICATIONS	SIGNS AND SYMPTOMS	INTERVENTIONS
Metabolic problems		
Hepatic dysfunction	Elevated serum aspartate aminotransferase (formerly serum glutamic oxaloacetic transaminase), alkaline phosphatase, and bilirubin levels	Reduce total caloric intake and dextrose intake, making up lost calories by administration of lipid emulsion. Change to cyclical infusion. Use specific hepatic formulations only if the patient has encephalopathy.
Hypercapnia	Heightened oxygen consumption, increased carbon dioxide production, measured respiratory quotient of 1 or greater	Reduce total caloric and dextrose intake, and balance dextrose and fat calories.
Hyperglycemia	Fatigue, restlessness, confusion, anxiety, weakness, polyuria, dehydration, elevated serum glucose levels and, in severe hyperglycemia, delirium or coma	Restrict dextrose intake by decreasing either the rate of infusion or the dextrose concentration. Compensate for calorie loss with administration of lipid emulsion. Begin insulin therapy.
Hyperosmolarity	Confusion, lethargy, seizures, hyperosmolar nonketotic syndrome, hyperglycemia, dehydration, and glycosuria	Discontinue dextrose infusion. Administer insulin and 0.45% sodium chloride solution with 10 to 20 mEq/liter of potassium to rehydrate the patient.
Hypocalcemia	Polyuria, dehydration, and elevated blood and urine glucose levels	Increase calcium supplements.
Hypoglycemia	Sweating, shaking, and irritability after the infusion has stopped	Increase dextrose intake or decrease exogenous insulin intake.
Hypokalemia	Muscle weakness, paralysis, paresthesia, and arrhythmias	Increase potassium supplements.
Hypomagnesemia	Tingling around the mouth, paresthesia in fingers, mental changes, and hyperreflexia	Increase magnesium supplementation.
Hypophosphatemia	Irritability, weakness, paresthesia, coma, and respiratory arrest	Increase phosphate supplements.
Hypozincemia	Dermatitis, alopecia, apathy, depression, taste changes, confusion, poor wound healing, and diarrhea	Increase zinc supplements.
Metabolic acidosis	Elevated serum chloride level, reduced serum bicarbonate level	Increase acetate and decrease chloride in parenteral nutrition solution.
Metabolic alkalosis	Diminished serum chloride level, elevated serum bicarbonate level	Decrease acetate and increase chloride in parenteral nutrition solution.

enteral nutrition feeding, which the pharmacist may add directly to the solution.

• Because most patients receiving PPN are in a protein-wasted state, the therapy causes marked changes in fluid and electrolyte status and in levels of glucose, amino acids, minerals, and vitamins. Therefore, record daily fluid intake and output accurately. Specify the volume and type of each fluid, and calculate the daily caloric intake.

• Monitor the results of routine laboratory tests

COMPLICATIONS	SIGNS AND SYMPTOMS	INTERVENTIONS
Mechanical problems		
Clotted I.V. catheter	Interrupted flow rate, resistance to flushing and blood withdrawal	Attempt to aspirate the clot. If unsuccessful, instill urokinase to clear catheter lumen, as ordered.
Cracked or broken tubing	Fluid leaking from the tubing	Apply a padded hemostat above the break to prevent air from entering the line.
Dislodged catheter	Catheter out of the vein	Apply pressure to the site with a sterile gauze pad.
Too-rapid infusion	Nausea, headache, and lethargy	Adjust the infusion rate and, if applicable, check the infusion pump.
Other problems		
Air embolism	Apprehension, chest pain, tachycardia, hypotension, cyanosis, seizures, loss of consciousness, and cardiac arrest	Clamp the catheter. Place the patient in a steep, left lateral Trendelenburg position. Administer oxygen, as ordered. If cardiac arrest occurs, begin cardiopulmonary resuscitation. When the catheter is removed, cover the insertion site with a dressing for 24 to 48 hours.
Extravasation	Swelling and pain around the insertion site	Stop the infusion. Assess the patient for cardiopulmonary abnormalities; a chest X-ray may be required.
Phlebitis	Pain, tenderness, redness, and warmth	Apply gentle heat to the area, and elevate the insertion site, if possible.
Pneumothorax and hydrothorax	Dyspnea, chest pain, cyanosis, and decreased breath sounds	Assist with chest tube insertion and apply suction, as ordered.
Septicemia	Red and swollen catheter site, chills, fever, and leukocytosis	Remove the catheter and culture the tip. Obtain a blood culture if the patient has a fever. Give appropriate antibiotics.
Thrombosis	Erythema and edema at the insertion site; ipsilateral swelling of the arm, neck, face, and upper chest; pain at the insertion site and along the vein; malaise; fever; tachycardia	Remove the catheter promptly. If not contraindicated, systemic thrombolytic therapy may be used. Apply warm compresses to the insertion site and elevate the affected extremity. Venous flow studies may be done.

and report any abnormal findings to the doctor to allow for appropriate changes in the parenteral nutrition solution. Typical laboratory tests include serum electrolytes, calcium, blood urea nitrogen, creatinine, and blood glucose at least three times weekly; serum magnesium and phosphorus twice weekly; liver function studies, complete blood count and differential, serum albumin, and transferrin weekly; and urinary nitrogen balance and creatinine-height index studies weekly. A zinc serum level is obtained at the start of parenteral nutrition ther-

apy. Other studies the doctor may order include serum prealbumin, total lymphocyte count, aminogram, fatty acid–phospholipid fraction, skin testing, and expired gas analysis.
• Physically assess the patient daily. If ordered, measure arm circumference and skinfold thickness over the triceps. Weigh the patient at the same time each morning after he voids; he should be weighed in similar clothing, and on the same scale. Suspect fluid imbalance if the patient gains more than 1.1 lb (0.5 kg) daily.
• Change the dressing over the catheter according to the policy at your health care facility or whenever the dressing becomes wet, soiled, or nonocclusive. Always use strict aseptic technique. When performing dressing changes, watch for signs of phlebitis or catheter retraction from the vein. Measure the catheter length from the insertion site to the hub for verification.
• Change the tubing and filters every 24 to 72 hours, or according to the policy at your health care facility.
• Closely monitor the catheter site for any sign of swelling, which may indicate infiltration. Extravasation of parenteral nutrition solution can lead to tissue necrosis.
• Always document the times of the dressing, filter, and solution changes; the condition of the catheter insertion site; your observations of the patient's condition; and any complications and resulting treatments.
• Use caution when using the parenteral nutrition line for other functions. If using a single-lumen CV catheter, don't use the line to infuse blood or blood products, to give a bolus injection, to administer simultaneous I.V. solutions, to measure CV pressure, or to draw blood for laboratory tests. Never add medication to a parenteral nutrition solution container. Also, don't use a three-way stopcock, if possible, because add-on devices increase the risk of infection. In addition, don't administer parenteral nutrition solution through a pulmonary artery catheter because of the high risk of phlebitis. After infusion, flush the catheter with heparin or 0.9% sodium chloride solution, according to the policy at your health care facility.

• Provide regular mouth care.
• Provide emotional support. Keep in mind that patients commonly associate eating with positive feelings and become disturbed when they can't eat.

Patient teaching

You'll need to teach the patient the potential adverse effects and complications of parenteral nutrition. Encourage him to inspect his mouth regularly for signs of parotitis, glossitis, or oral lesions. Tell the patient he may have fewer bowel movements while receiving parenteral nutrition therapy.

Encourage the patient to remain physically active. Explain that being physically active will help his body use the nutrients more fully.

Patients who require prolonged or indefinite parenteral nutrition may be able to receive the therapy at home. Home parenteral nutrition reduces the need for long hospitalizations and allows the patient to resume many of his normal activities. Meet with a home care patient before discharge to make sure he knows how to perform the administration procedure and how to handle complications. (See *Teaching patients about parenteral nutrition.*)

Lipid emulsion

Typically given as a separate solution, lipid emulsion is a source of calories and essential fatty acids. A deficiency in essential fatty acids can hinder wound healing, adversely affect production of red blood cells, and impair prostaglandin synthesis.

Although lipids are usually given in conjunction with parenteral nutrition solution, lipid emulsion may also be given by itself. You may administer the emulsion through either a peripheral or a central line.

Give lipid emulsion cautiously to patients who have liver disease, pulmonary disease, anemia, or coagulation disorders, or who are at risk for developing a fat embolism. Its use is contraindicated in patients who have a condi-

Teaching patients about parenteral nutrition

Sometimes patients can receive parenteral nutrition at home. Common indications for home parenteral nutrition include the need for bowel rest because of a GI fistula or pancreatitis, or impaired GI function from chronic radiation enteritis, Crohn's disease, intestinal obstruction, inflammatory bowel disease, short-bowel syndrome, or scleroderma.

Eligibility for home therapy

You may be asked to assess a patient's suitability for home therapy. To do so, consider the patient's motivation, his mental aptitude, and his job or other daily activities. Assess his relationships with family or other household members: Can they assist him with parenteral nutrition therapy? Also consider the accessibility of hospitals, home nursing services, and other health care support systems. If a patient's psychological state or home environment interferes with his safety, he shouldn't receive parenteral nutrition at home. Home parenteral nutrition is also contraindicated if the patient's primary disease is untreatable or if other medical problems require in-patient care.

What to teach the patient

If your patient is scheduled to receive parenteral nutrition at home, you'll need to provide careful teaching before discharge. (Include a family member or caregiver if possible.) Conduct your teaching sessions in a quiet area where you and the patient will be undisturbed.

Teach the patient to change the catheter site dressing as ordered (usually every 2 to 3 days) or whenever it becomes soiled or nonocclusive. Also emphasize the importance of changing the I.V. tub-

ing as scheduled.

Instruct the patient to take only sponge baths, and to wash gently around the catheter site. Tell him he may be allowed to remove his dressing and bathe or shower after the implanted catheter has been in place for 1 month or longer.

Tell the patient to protect his catheter against contact with granular or lint-producing surfaces. Explain that airborne particles and surface contaminants could cause a local tissue reaction.

Work with the patient to devise a suitable parenteral nutrition schedule, considering both his nutritional needs and his life-style. Suggest that he wear a medical identification bracelet or subscribe to a medical alert service. Reassure him that a nurse from the home health care team will always be available in case of an emergency.

Because the financial burden of long-term or permanent home parenteral nutrition can be devastating, even if the patient has health insurance, make a social services referral. Tell the elderly patient that Medicare may assume the cost of supplies and medications if he meets eligibility requirements.

Realize that many patients receiving home parenteral nutrition experience depression related to a change in body image, a loss of ability to eat normally, a change in family structure, financial strain, and a change in activity level. Encourage the patient and his family to verbalize their concerns and to join a support group of other persons receiving home parenteral nutrition. Also encourage the patient to resume his normal activities as soon as possible.

---

tion that disrupts normal fat metabolism (such as pathologic hyperlipidemia, lipid nephrosis, and acute pancreatitis).

Equipment

To administer lipid emulsion, you'll need an I.V. administration set with a vented spike, an access pin with a reflux valve, tape, time tape, and alcohol sponges.

If you can't get an I.V. administration set with a vented spike, you can use a separate adapter. Also, if you'll be administering the lipid emulsion as part of a 3-in-1 solution, obtain a filter that is 1.2 microns or greater because lipids will clog a smaller filter.

Drug administration

Inspect the lipid emulsion for opacity and for consistency of color and texture. If the emulsion looks frothy, oily, or contains particles, or if you think its stability or sterility is questionable, return the bottle to the pharmacy. To prevent aggregation of fat globules, don't shake the lipid container excessively. Protect the emulsion from freezing, and never add anything to the lipid emulsion. Make sure you have the correct lipid emulsion and verify the doctor's order and the patient's name.

Connecting the tubing

First, connect the I.V. tubing to the access pin. Access pins with reflux valves take the place of needles when connecting piggyback tubing to primary tubing.

Close the flow clamp on the I.V. tubing. If the tubing doesn't contain luer-lock connections, tape all connections securely to prevent accidental separation, which can lead to air embolism, exsanguination, or sepsis.

Using aseptic technique, remove the protective cap from the lipid emulsion bottle, and wipe the rubber stopper with an alcohol sponge. Hold the bottle upright and, using strict aseptic technique, insert the vented spike through the inner circle of the rubber stopper. Invert the bottle, and squeeze the drip chamber until it fills to the level indicated in the tubing package instructions. Open the flow clamp and prime the tubing. Gently tap the tubing to dislodge air bubbles trapped in the Y-ports. If necessary, attach a time tape to the lipid emulsion container to allow accurate measurement of fluid intake. Label the tubing, noting the date and time the tubing was hung.

Starting the infusion

If this is the patient's first lipid infusion, administer a test dose at the rate of 1 ml/minute for 30 minutes. Monitor the patient's vital signs and watch for signs and symptoms of an adverse reaction, such as an elevated temperature; flushing, sweating or chills; a pressure sensation over the eyes; nausea; vomiting; headache; chest and back pain; tachycardia; dyspnea; and cyanosis. An allergic reaction is usually due either to the source of lipids or to eggs, which occur in the emulsion as egg phospholipids, an emulsifying agent.

If the patient has no adverse reactions to the test dose, begin the infusion at the prescribed rate. Use an infusion pump if you'll be infusing the lipids at less than 20 ml/hour. The maximum infusion rate is 125 ml/hour for a 10% lipid emulsion and 60 ml/hour for a 20% lipid emulsion.

Complications

Immediate or early adverse reactions to lipid emulsion therapy, which occur in fewer than 1% of patients, include fever, dyspnea, cyanosis, nausea and vomiting, headache, flushing, diaphoresis, lethargy, syncope, chest and back pain, slight pressure over the eyes, irritation at the infusion site, hyperlipidemia, hypercoagulability, and thrombocytopenia. Thrombocytopenia has been reported in infants receiving a 20% I.V. lipid emulsion.

Delayed but uncommon complications associated with prolonged administration of lipid emulsion include hepatomegaly, splenomegaly, jaundice secondary to central lobular cholestasis, and blood dyscrasias (such as thrombocytopenia, leukopenia, and transient increases in liver function studies). Dry or scaly skin, thinning hair, abnormal liver function studies, and thrombocytopenia may indicate a deficiency of essential fatty acids. For unknown reasons, some patients develop brown pigmentation in the reticuloendothelial system.

In premature or low-birth-weight infants, PPN with lipid emulsion may cause lipids to accumulate in the infants' lungs.

Report any adverse reactions to the patient's doctor, so that he can change the parenteral nutrition regimen as needed.

Nursing considerations

• Always maintain strict aseptic technique while preparing and handling equipment.
• Observe the patient's reaction to the lipid emulsion. Most patients report a feeling of satiety, but some complain of an unpleasant metallic taste.

• Change the I.V. tubing and the lipid emulsion container every 24 hours.
• Monitor the patient for hair or skin changes.
• Closely monitor the patient's lipid tolerance rate. Cloudy plasma in a centrifuged sample of citrated blood indicates that the lipids haven't been cleared from the patient's bloodstream.
• Lipid emulsion may clear from the blood at an accelerated rate in patients with full-thickness burns, multiple traumatic injuries, or a metabolic imbalance. This is because catecholamines, adrenocortical hormones, thyroxine, and growth hormone enhance lipolysis and embolization of fatty acids.
• Obtain weekly laboratory tests, as ordered. Usual tests include liver function studies, prothrombin time, platelet count, and serum triglycerides. Whenever possible, draw triglyceride levels at least 6 hours after the completion of the lipid emulsion infusion to avoid falsely elevated results.
• Lipid emulsion is an excellent medium for bacterial growth. Therefore, never rehang a partially empty bottle of emulsion.

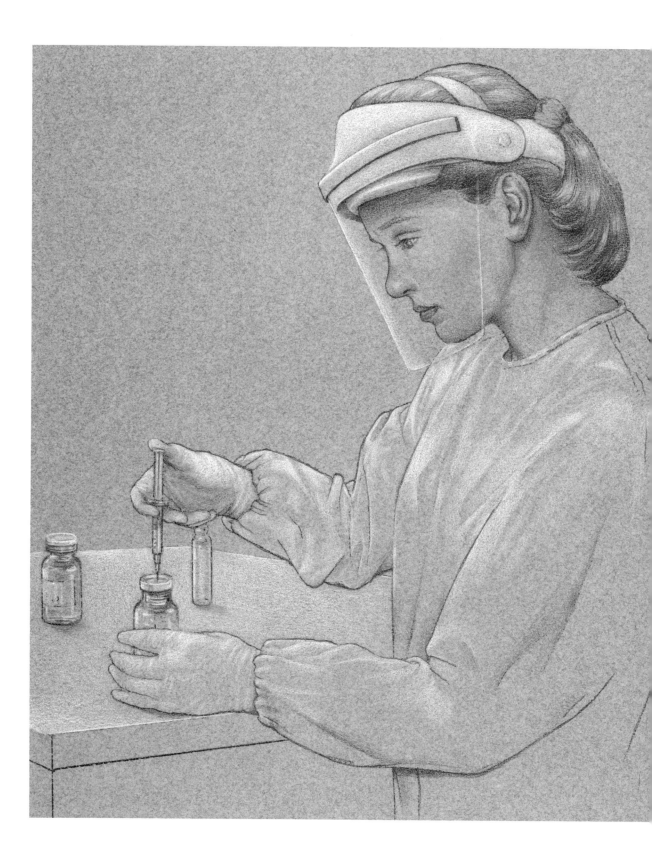

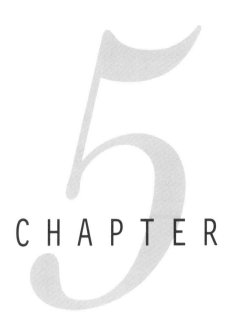

CHAPTER 5

Giving chemotherapy

No longer a treatment of last resort, chemotherapy has joined surgery and radiation therapy as mainstays for treating cancer. In fact, thanks to the development of certain chemotherapeutic drugs, many childhood and adult cancers are now curable.

Rapidly growing cancers, such as acute leukemia and lymphomas, respond best to chemotherapy. Slower-growing cancers, which have fewer cells undergoing division at any given moment, prove less responsive to chemotherapy. Such cancers include GI and pulmonary tumors.

Today, doctors may order any of 30 different chemotherapeutic drugs. These drugs may be given alone or in various combinations to cure cancer, prevent metastasis, or relieve symptoms. For example, a patient with acute leukemia may receive chemotherapy as a curative treatment, whereas a patient with ovarian cancer may receive it postoperatively to guard against undetectable metastasis. A patient with an advanced cancer may receive chemotherapy to reduce the size of a tumor, which, in turn, may relieve pain and other symptoms. A patient may also receive chemotherapy preoperatively to reduce the size of a tumor and improve the odds for surgical success.

Chemotherapeutic drugs attack all rapidly dividing cells, both normal and malignant. Therein lies the challenge of chemotherapy: to provide a drug dose large enough to kill the greatest number of cancer cells, but small enough to avoid extensively damaging normal tissue or causing toxicity.

In many cases, the challenge can be met by prescribing smaller doses of different chemotherapeutic drugs. Given in combination, the drugs potentiate each other, and the tumor responds as it would to a larger dose of a single drug. At the same time, combination chemotherapy is less likely to cause toxicity. Also, because different drugs work at different stages of the cell cycle or employ different mechanisms to kill cancer cells, using several drugs decreases the likelihood of tumor resistance.

The patient's overall condition, his allergies or sensitivities, and the cancer's stage all determine drug selection. However, doctors know that cancer cells respond best to the first dose of chemotherapy. For this reason, they strive to select the potentially most effective drugs for the first round of chemotherapy.

This chapter, you'll learn how to prepare and administer chemotherapeutic drugs. You'll find sections on equipment; preparation and administration of drugs; complications; and nursing considerations, including patient teaching and home care. However, before these sections, a discussion of pharmacologic principles reviews how chemotherapeutic drugs act on the cell cycle and how they're classified.

Pharmacologic principles

To understand how chemotherapeutic drugs work and why they produce adverse effects, you'll need to understand cellular kinetics — the study of the growth patterns of normal and malignant cells.

Cell cycle

Both normal and malignant cells pass through similar life phases. The first phase of the cell cycle is the G_1 (GAP1) *phase*. During this phase, active ribonucleic acid (RNA) and protein syntheses take place. After that, the cell moves into the S (synthesis) *phase*, during which it manufactures deoxyribonucleic acid (DNA). During this phase, which constitutes one-third to one-half of the total cell cycle, cells are particularly sensitive to many chemotherapeutic drugs.

During the G_2 (GAP2) *phase*, the cell continues to manufacture DNA and begins to assemble the mitotic spindle apparatus and to synthesize more RNA and protein. Then, the cell divides, or enters the M (mitosis) *phase*. Some experts feel that after the cell divides, it may enter a long resting state, the G_0 *phase*.

Some drugs are designed to disrupt a specific biochemical process. As a result, they're effective only during a specific phase of the cell cycle. These are called *cycle-specific* drugs. Other drugs, called *cycle-nonspecific,* have a prolonged action independent of the cell cycle. (See *How chemotherapeutic drugs disrupt the cell cycle.*)

Treating cancer

Because a tumor consists of cells at varying phases of the cell cycle, chemotherapy typically employs more than one drug. This way, each drug can either target a different site or take action during a different phase of the cell cycle. During a single administration of a chemotherapeutic drug, a fixed percentage of cells die — both normal and malignant cells. Afterward, the remaining cells — again, both normal and malignant — reproduce. Cells that were in the resting phase when the chemotherapy was administered may return to the reproduction phase.

To eradicate a tumor, then, a patient needs repeated drug doses. At the same time, the drug doses need to be spaced at certain intervals so that normal cells can regenerate. Most patients require at least three treatments before they show any beneficial response. Even then, it can be difficult to accurately evaluate

How chemotherapeutic drugs disrupt the cell cycle

Chemotherapeutic drugs may be either cycle-specific or cycle-nonspecific. Cycle-specific drugs, such as methotrexate, act at one or more cell-cycle phases. Cycle-nonspecific drugs, such as busulfan, can act on both replicating and resting cells. (Drugs listed in this diagram are only examples of cycle-specific agents.)

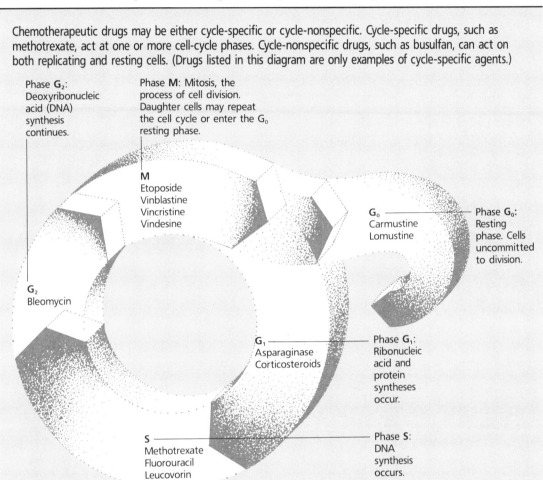

Phase G_2: Deoxyribonucleic acid (DNA) synthesis continues.

Phase M: Mitosis, the process of cell division. Daughter cells may repeat the cell cycle or enter the G_0 resting phase.

M
Etoposide
Vinblastine
Vincristine
Vindesine

G_0
Carmustine
Lomustine

Phase G_0: Resting phase. Cells uncommitted to division.

G_2
Bleomycin

G_1
Asparaginase
Corticosteroids

Phase G_1: Ribonucleic acid and protein syntheses occur.

S
Methotrexate
Fluorouracil
Leucovorin

Phase S: DNA synthesis occurs.

how effective the chemotherapy has been because undetectable cancer cells may still be present. That's why doctors continue to administer chemotherapy for a period after the cancer seems to have been eradicated.

How well a tumor responds to chemotherapy depends on the percentage of cells killed, the rate of regrowth, and the development of resistant cells. It also depends on the size of the tumor. As a general rule, small tumors tend to respond to drugs that affect DNA synthesis, especially cycle-specific drugs, because these tumors have a higher percentage of actively dividing cells than do large tumors. Large

tumors respond better to cycle-nonspecific drugs. Once the large tumor shrinks, the doctor may switch to a cycle-specific drug.

Classifying chemotherapeutic drugs
Of the drugs currently being used, each can be placed into one of the following eight classes.

Alkylating agents
One of the largest classifications of chemotherapeutic drugs, alkylating agents bind directly and irreversibly to important compounds (such

as DNA) to disrupt cell division. An example of an alkylating agent is nitrogen mustard.

Antimetabolites
These drugs inhibit nucleic acid synthesis, which is necessary for the production of DNA and protein, by interfering with the action of crucial enzymes. Methotrexate and fluorouracil are examples.

Antibiotic chemotherapeutic drugs
Like many antibacterial drugs, most antibiotic chemotherapeutic drugs evolved from various species of fungi. By inserting themselves into DNA strands, they break the chromosome chain and inhibit RNA synthesis. The most commonly used member of this class, doxorubicin effectively treats many types of cancer.

Plant alkaloids
Derived from naturally occurring plant materials, plant alkaloids prevent mitotic spindle formation. In turn, this stops cell duplication and separation. Examples of plant alkaloids include vincristine (which is derived from the periwinkle plant) and etoposide (which comes from the mayapple, or American mandrake).

Hormones and hormone inhibitors
Although their mechanisms of action are unclear, these drugs help treat a number of cancers. Examples include estrogen, progesterone, and tamoxifen (an estrogen antagonist).

Enzymes
Certain tumor cells require an amino acid called asparagine to synthesize protein. The enzyme L-asparaginase blocks asparagine, which causes the cells to die. Unfortunately, the only cancer that this enzyme has treated successfully is acute lymphocytic leukemia.

Biological response modifiers
The newest class of chemotherapeutic drugs, biological response modifiers are produced naturally by the immune system. When administered to a patient, they enhance the body's ability to destroy cancer cells by altering the way cells grow and mature as well as by boosting the immune system.

Miscellaneous drugs
Several other drugs fight cancer through various actions but most, such as cisplatin, bind directly to DNA and prevent DNA synthesis.

New frontiers in chemotherapy
The search for new ways to treat cancer is ongoing. In fact, the National Cancer Institute (NCI) has screened more than 250,000 substances for potential antineoplastic action, and it continues to screen about 15,000 new compounds each year. Unfortunately, though, for every 40,000 substances tested in animals, only about 10 show actions that warrant testing in humans. And, of those 10, only one substance will eventually prove effective.

Despite years of such screening, the Food and Drug Administration has approved only 34 drugs to treat cancer in humans. However, the NCI is investigating more than 60 new drugs. Among these are biological response modifiers and their subgroup, cytokines, which include interferon, interleukin-2, and tumor necrosis factor. Interferon (which itself is subdivided into three major species known as alfa, beta, and gamma) inhibits viral replication. It may also directly inhibit tumor proliferation. Hematologic cancers, including malignant lymphomas, cutaneous T-cell lymphoma, and chronic myelogenous and hairy-cell leukemia, are the most responsive to interferon.

Lymphokines, another type of cytokine, fight cancer by stimulating the production of T cells, activating the lytic mechanisms of killer cells, promoting the immigration of lymphoid cells from the bloodstream, and stimulating the release of other lymphokines, such as tumor necrosis factor and interferon gamma. Examples of lymphokines include interleukin-1 and interleukin-2. Interleukin-2 has been effective in treating renal cell cancer and malignant melanoma. Unfortunately, though, most patients taking the drug experience toxic reactions, including chills and fever, nausea, vomiting, diarrhea, cutaneous erythema, weight gain, anemia, hypotension, tachycardia, and hepatic and renal dysfunction.

Scientists are also developing a method of treating cancer that uses liposomes to carry an antineoplastic drug directly to a cancerous tumor. Besides exerting a maximum effect on the malignant cells, this treatment minimizes the risk of toxicity.

Liposomes consist of a series of phospholipid bilayers in the shape of a ring. Although these layers may be composed of numerous synthetic or naturally occurring polar lipids, the most common substance is phospholipids. Between each ring is a space that contains an aqueous solution. Drugs can be placed in the lipid layer or, if they're water-soluble, in the aqueous spaces. (See *Learning about phospholipid liposomes.*)

What makes liposomes so effective for treating cancer is that scientists can design them to travel to a specific body area. Knowing this, scientists can create a liposome that's susceptible to pH gradients. Once injected in the body, the liposome can gravitate to the tumor and release its medication. Furthermore, modified phospholipids added to the surface of the liposome can bind to specific tumor cells, making targeting even more specific. (See *Using common chemotherapeutic drugs,* pages 116 to 119.)

Preparing chemotherapeutic drugs

When preparing chemotherapeutic drugs, take extra care, both for the patient's safety and for your own. While patients who receive chemotherapeutic drugs risk teratogenic, mutagenic, or carcinogenic effects, the people who prepare and handle the drugs have a risk as well. Although the risk from handling these drugs hasn't been fully determined, chemotherapeutic drugs can increase the handler's risk of reproductive abnormalities. These drugs also pose certain environmental dangers. To make matters worse, the best method for handling them hasn't been determined.

The Occupational Safety and Health Administration (OSHA) has set down guidelines for handling chemotherapeutic drugs. Although these guidelines are simply recommendations, adhering to them will help ensure both your

Learning about phospholipid liposomes

This illustration shows the concentric phospholipid rings that form the liposome. These rings are separated by a series of concentric aqueous layers. A water-soluble drug, shown as green squares, can be stored in the aqueous spaces. A lipid-soluble drug, shown as black circles, can be stored in the lipid layers. When delivered to a specific body site, the liposome gravitates to the targeted cell and releases its medication.

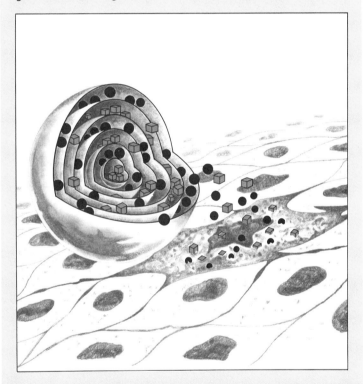

safety and the safety of your environment.

The OSHA guidelines outline two basic requirements. The first is that all health care workers who handle chemotherapeutic drugs must be educated and trained. A key element of such training involves learning how to reduce your exposure when handling the drugs. The second requirement states that the drugs should be prepared within a Class II biological safety cabinet.

(Text continues on page 119.)

Using common chemotherapeutic drugs

DRUG	INDICATIONS AND DOSAGE	MECHANISM OF ACTION	NURSING CONSIDERATIONS
carboplatin	Used for palliative treatment of recurrent ovarian cancer, even in patients previously treated with cisplatin. *Usual adult dosage:* 360 mg/m² I.V. once every 4 weeks. However, dosage depends on renal function; a creatinine clearance of less than 60 ml/minute requires a dosage adjustment.	A cycle-nonspecific alkylating agent that produces cross-linking of deoxyribonucleic acid (DNA) strands. Eliminated primarily by the kidneys. In patients with normal renal function, 71% of a dose is excreted within 24 hours. Not protein-bound. Ineffective when administered orally. Elimination of carboplatin is biphasic; initial half-life is 1.1 to 2 hours, and terminal half-life is 2½ to 6 hours.	• Do not use I.V. infusion sets and needles containing aluminum. • Determine serum electrolyte and creatinine levels, complete blood count (CBC) and platelet count, and creatinine clearance levels before the first infusion and before each course of therapy. • Administer an antiemetic before carboplatin therapy because carboplatin produces severe emesis. • Because of the possibility of infant toxicity, mothers who are breast-feeding should discontinue this practice. • Advise woman of childbearing age to avoid becoming pregnant during therapy. • Have epinephrine, corticosteroids, and antihistamines available when administering carboplatin because anaphylaxis-like reactions may occur within minutes of administration.
cisplatin	Metastatic testicular cancer; lung, head, neck, bladder, or metastatic ovarian cancer. *Usual adult dosages:* For metastatic testicular tumors, 20 mg/m² I.V. daily for 5 days when administered with other drugs. For metastatic ovarian tumors, 50 mg/m² every 3 weeks when used with doxorubicin; 100 mg/m² I.V. every 4 weeks when used as a single agent. For advanced bladder cancer, 50 to 70 mg/m² I.V. once every 3 to 4 weeks.	Cross-links strands of cellular DNA and interferes with ribonucleic acid (RNA) transcription, causing an imbalance of growth that leads to cell death. Drug is cell-cycle-nonspecific. When administered I.V., cisplatin spreads throughout the body, with the highest concentrations in the liver, large and small intestines, and kidneys. Has poor penetration into the central nervous system (CNS). The initial half-life is 25 to 49 minutes, and the terminal half-life is 58 to 78 hours. More than 90% of the drug is bound to plasma proteins. It is partially excreted in the urine.	• Cisplatin is contraindicated in patients with renal impairment, hearing impairment, myelosuppression, or known hypersensitivity to the drug or other platinum-containing compounds. • Use extreme caution when administering to pregnant patients. • Determine serum magnesium, potassium, calcium, and creatinine levels, blood urea nitrogen levels, and creatinine clearance before first infusion and before each course. • Maintain urine output of 100 to 200 ml/hour for 18 to 24 hours after therapy. Hydrate patient well before, during, and after treatment. • Administer antiemetics before, during, and for 24 hours after treatment. • To prevent or minimize uric acid nephropathy from elevated serum uric acid levels, provide adequate hydration, alkalinize the patient's urine, and administer allopurinol, as ordered. • Advise women of childbearing age to avoid becoming pregnant during therapy.
cyclophosphamide (nitrogen mustard family)	Chronic lymphocytic leukemia; neuroblastoma; breast, ovarian, or lung cancer; multiple myeloma; Burkitt's lymphoma; and retinoblastoma. *Usual adult dosages:* When used as the only agent, 40 to 50 mg/kg I.V. in divided doses every 7 to 10 days. Lower doses are usually given when combined with other drugs. Orally, the usual dose is 1 to 5 mg/kg P.O. daily.	Cross-links strands of cellular DNA and interferes with RNA transcription, causing an imbalance of growth that leads to cell death. The drug is cell-cycle-nonspecific. It is completely absorbed from the GI tract and injection site. Its half-life after I.V. administration is 4 to 6 hours. Of the total dose, 10% to 56% is protein-bound. It's metabolized in the liver and excreted in urine as active metabolites, with less than 25% of the drug remaining unchanged. The drug crosses the placenta and will appear in breast milk.	• Administer with caution to patients with leukopenia, thrombocytopenia, tumor cell infiltration of bone marrow, or impaired hepatic or renal function. • Encourage the patient to drink plenty of fluids before, during, and for 72 hours after treatment to avoid hemorrhagic cystitis. If this occurs, discontinue the drug immediately. • Infuse the drug slowly to prevent facial flushing. • Monitor CBC, kidney and liver function, and uric acid levels. • To prevent or minimize hyperuricemia, provide good hydration, alkalinize the urine, and administer allopurinol, as ordered. • Inform the patient that reversible alopecia is common.

Using common chemotherapeutic drugs *(continued)*

DRUG	INDICATIONS AND DOSAGE	MECHANISM OF ACTION	NURSING CONSIDERATIONS
daunorubicin	Acute nonlymphoblastic leukemia; childhood tumors, such as Ewing's tumor, rhabdomyosarcoma, Wilms' tumor, and neuroblastoma. *Usual adult dosage:* 30 to 45 mg/m² I.V. for 1 to 3 days.	Interferes with DNA-dependent RNA synthesis by intercalation. After I.V. administration, 25% of the drug concentrates in the liver, while the rest concentrates in cardiac, renal, and pulmonary tissue. The plasma half-life is 18 hours. The drug is metabolized in the liver; 25% is eliminated in active form in the urine and 40% is excreted in bile.	• Daunorubicin is contraindicated in patients who are pregnant or who have drug-induced bone marrow suppression (unless the benefit of daunorubicin treatment warrants the risk). • To prevent or minimize uric acid nephropathy, keep the patient well hydrated, alkalinize his urine, and administer allopurinol, as ordered. • Be aware that using a scalp tourniquet to prevent or minimize alopecia increases the risk of micrometastatic scalp lesions.
doxorubicin	Used in combination regimens against acute leukemias as well as Hodgkin's disease and malignant lymphomas. Used in breast, lung, ovarian, bladder, and thyroid carcinomas. Also, osteogenic sarcoma, Ewing's tumor, and Wilms' tumor. *Usual adult dosage:* 60 to 70 mg/m² I.V. every 3 weeks. Lifetime maximum dose is 550 mg/m². Lower doses are necessary in patients who receive radiotherapy to the mediastinum or other cardiotoxic agents such as cyclophosphamide.	Interferes with DNA-dependent RNA synthesis by intercalation. Can be given as bladder instillations. Distributed rapidly and widely to the heart, kidneys, lungs, liver, and spleen. Metabolized in the liver, producing a major metabolite with antineoplastic activity and several inactive metabolites. Of the total drug administered, 40% to 50% is excreted in bile or feces within 7 days, with half of the drug in an unchanged state.	• Cardiac problems usually preclude doxorubicin use. The lifetime dose should be decreased to 400 mg/m² for patients receiving mediastinal radiation therapy. • Patients with hepatic dysfunction should receive a reduced dosage based on their serum bilirubin level. • Watch for increased toxic effects (mucositis, leukopenia, and thrombocytopenia). • Regularly monitor electrocardiogram (ECG) or echocardiogram in patients who have received 300 mg/m² or more of the drug. Also monitor CBC and liver function tests for signs of toxicity. • Be alert for early signs of congestive heart failure (CHF) because this drug-induced condition often fails to respond to therapy. However, if CHF occurs, give cardiac glycosides, diuretics, and peripheral vasodilators, as ordered. • Inform the patient that his urine may be red for 1 to 2 days and that reversible alopecia may occur.
etoposide	Testicular cancer. *Usual adult dosage:* 50 to 100 mg/m² I.V. daily for 5 days, or 100 mg/m² I.V. daily on days 1, 3, and 5, repeated every 3 to 4 weeks. Small-cell lung cancer. *Usual adult dosage:* 35 mg/m² I.V. daily for 4 days up to 50 mg/m² I.V. daily for 5 days, repeated every 3 to 4 weeks.	A semisynthetic derivative of podophyllotoxin that arrests cell mitosis. Less than 10% of the drug will penetrate into cerebrospinal fluid (CSF). About 94% of drug is plasma protein-bound, and probably metabolized in the liver. It has a biphasic half-life; the initial phase is 3 hours and the terminal phase is 15 hours. About 44% to 60% of the drug is excreted in urine within 48 to 72 hours.	• Etoposide is contraindicated in pregnant or breastfeeding patients and in those who have a known hypersensitivity to the drug. • Give antiemetics to control nausea and vomiting. • To treat anaphylaxis, give pressor agents, adrenocorticosteroids, antihistamines, and volume expanders, as ordered. • Monitor CBC weekly.

(continued)

Using common chemotherapeutic drugs (continued)

DRUG	INDICATIONS AND DOSAGE	MECHANISM OF ACTION	NURSING CONSIDERATIONS
fluorouracil	Carcinomas of the GI tract and breast. *Usual adult dosage:* 12 mg/kg I.V. daily, up to 800 mg daily for 4 successive days; if no toxicity, give 6 mg/kg/day on the 6th, 8th, 10th, and 12th days. Basal cell carcinomas. *Usual adult dosage:* Cover lesions twice daily.	Inhibits DNA synthesis. Minimal absorption with topical application on intact skin. Six hours after I.V. administration, 7% to 20% of the parent drug is excreted unchanged in the urine. Remaining drug is metabolized in the liver, with 90% being excreted as expired carbon dioxide and the remainder clearing as inactive metabolites in the urine over the next 3 to 4 hours.	• Fluorouracil is contraindicated in patients who have a known hypersensitivity to the drug or any of its components. • Monitor CBC and liver and kidney function. • White blood cell nadir usually occurs from the 9th to 14th day after treatment, possibly up to the 25th day. Recovery occurs by the 30th day. • Treat anorexia and nausea with antiemetics. • Advise women not to be become pregnant while on fluorouracil. • Advise mothers of infants not to breast-feed during therapy.
interferon	Hairy-cell leukemia. *Usual adult dosage:* 3 million IU S.C. or I.M. daily for 16 to 24 weeks, followed by 3 million IU S.C. or I.M. three times a week. AIDS-related Kaposi's sarcoma. *Usual adult dosage:* 36 million IU I.M. or S.C. daily for 10 to 12 weeks, followed by 36 million IU I.M. or S.C. three times a week.	Interferon alph-2a is a sterile protein product made by recombinant DNA techniques. Its mechanism of action is unknown but appears to involve direct antiproliferative action against tumor cells or viral cells to inhibit replication. Alfa-interferons achieve peak concentration 4 hours after I.M. administration or 7 hours after S.C. administration. The kidneys filter and degrade the drug. Hepatic metabolism and biliary excretion are negligible.	• Interferon is contraindicated in patients who are breast-feeding or who have a known hypersensitivity to the drug. • Administer the drug with caution to patients who are pregnant, who have recently had a myocardial infarction, or who have a history of recurrent arrhythmias.
methotrexate	Maintenance of remission in acute lymphoblastic leukemia. *Usual adult dosage:* 20 to 30 mg/m² P.O. or I.M. twice weekly or 2.5 mg/kg I.V. every 14 days. Choriocarcinoma. *Usual adult dosage:* 15 mg/m² P.O. or I.M. daily for 5 days at 1- to 2-week intervals. Meningeal leukemia. *Usual adult dosage:* 12 mg/m² intrathecally at 2- to 5-day intervals. Osteogenic sarcoma. *Usual adult dosage:* 12 to 15 g/m² I.V. with leucovorin.	Prevents reduction of folic acid to tetrahydrofolate by binding to dihydrofolate reductase. Rapidly absorbed from GI tract, reaching a peak serum level 1 to 2 hours after oral administration and 30 to 60 minutes after I.V. administration. Half-life is 2 to 4 hours after I.M. or oral administration; 3 to 10 hours for a low dose, 8 to 15 hours for a high dose. Approximately 50% of the drug is bound to serum proteins, and it is widely distributed through the tissue. Kidneys clear up to 90% of the drug in unchanged form; a small amount is excreted in feces.	• Methotrexate is contraindicated in patients who are pregnant or who have blood dyscrasias. • Use extreme caution when administering to pediatric or elderly patients or to any patient who has an infection, a peptic ulcer, or ulcerative colitis. • Instruct patients to avoid beverages or medications containing alcohol. Only practitioners who know the leucovorin rescue process should administer high-dose methotrexate. • To minimize adverse hematologic and GI effects in high-dose methotrexate therapy, use leucovorin calcium, as ordered. • Measure the patient's serum creatinine level before each course of therapy when treating osteogenic sarcoma, and monitor serum creatinine levels daily during high-dose methotrexate treatment. • Advise male patients that they should use contraceptives during sex while they are taking the drug and for three months after therapy ends. • Advise women not to breast-feed because of the potential for serious adverse effects on infants. • To prevent uric acid nephropathy, administer large volumes of fluids, alkalinize the patient's urine, or use allopurinol, as ordered.

Using common chemotherapeutic drugs *(continued)*

DRUG	INDICATIONS AND DOSAGE	MECHANISM OF ACTION	NURSING CONSIDERATIONS
plicamycin	Disseminated testicular cancer; hypercalcemia, when resulting from bone metastasis. *Usual adult dosage:* For testicular cancer, 25 to 30 mcg/kg I.V daily for 8 to 10 days; for hypercalcemia, 25 mcg/ kg I.V. daily for 3 to 4 days, repeated weekly as necessary, or a single weekly dose of 25 mcg/kg.	Forms a complex with DNA, thus inhibiting RNA synthesis; inhibits osteocytic activity, blocking calcium and phosphorus reabsorption from bone. Considered 100% bioavailable. It does not enter CSF. Up to 40% of a plicamycin dose is excreted in the urine within 15 hours. Crosses the blood-brain barrier, where concentrations are low but persist longer than elsewhere. Highest concentrations of the drug can be found in Kupffer's cells of the liver, in renal tubular cells, and along formed bone surfaces.	• Plicamycin may produce bleeding diathesis, including epistaxis, hematemesis, hemoptysis, ecchymoses, and prolonged clotting and bleeding times. This adverse effect may be dose-related. The drug may also produce hypotension and nephrotoxicity. Use with caution in electrolyte imbalance, especially hypocalcemia, hypokalemia, and hypophosphatemia, to avoid exacerbation. • Administer antiemetics before and during treatment. • Correct dehydration, volume depletion, or an electrolyte imbalance before plicamycin therapy. • Obtain platelet counts, prothombin times, and bleeding times during therapy and for several days after the last dose.
procarbazine	Hodgkin's disease, small-cell lung cancer, malignant lymphoma, myeloma, melanoma, and CNS tumors. *Usual adult dosage:* 2 to 4 mg/kg P.O. daily for 1 week, then increased to 4 to 6 mg/ kg P.O. daily; for maintenance therapy, 1 to 2 mg/kg P.O. daily.	Inhibits DNA, RNA, and protein synthesis. Readily absorbed from the GI tract, after which it is widely distributed. Half-life is 1 hour. The drug is metabolized in the liver and excreted in urine as the unchanged drug and as metabolites.	• Administer procarbazine cautiously to patients with impaired renal or hepatic function. • Instruct patients not to drink alcohol while taking procarbazine. • Procarbazine potentiates insulin and oral antidiabetic drugs, so the doctor may have to adjust antidiabetic drug doses. • Advise the patient to avoid prolonged exposure to sunlight.
tamoxifen	Metastatic breast cancer that is estrogen receptor-positive, especially in postmenopausal women; adjunct to surgery in postmenopausal women whose axillary lymph nodes harbor cancer cells. *Usual adult dosage:* 10 to 20 mg P.O. b.i.d.	Acts as an estrogen antagonist. Absorbed well, but its distribution has not been studied thoroughly. The drug is metabolized in the liver to various metabolites that display antiestrogenic and antitumor effects. Tamoxifen and its metabolites are excreted slowly in the feces. Less than 30% of a dose is excreted as other metabolites or the parent compound.	• Tamoxifen is contraindicated in patients who are pregnant or breast-feeding or who have a known hypersensitivity to the drug. • Administer the drug with caution to patients who have leukopenia or thrombocytopenia. • Inform the patient that hot flashes, nausea, and occasional vomiting are the most common adverse reactions to tamoxifen; teach the patient how to manage them at home. • Assure the patient and family that tumor flare is an expected adverse reaction that will subside. Because of increased pain from tumor flare, the patient may require more analgesics.

Equipment

To prepare chemotherapeutic drugs, you'll need to gather the drug or drugs prescribed, the patient's medication record and chart, I.V. solution, diluent (if necessary), a compatibility reference source, medication labels, a Class II biological safety cabinet, a disposable towel, an 18G needle, a hydrophobic filter or dispensing pin, syringes and needles of various sizes, I.V. tubing with luer-lock fittings, and an I.V. controller pump (if available).

To protect yourself and your environment, make sure you have a long-sleeved gown, latex surgical gloves, a face shield or goggles, eyewash, a plastic absorbent pad, alcohol sponges.

sterile gauze pads, show covers, and an impervious container with the label "Caution: Biohazard" for the disposal of any unused drug or equipment.

You should also keep a chemotherapeutic spill kit readily available. To create a kit, you'll need a water-resistant, nonpermeable, long-sleeved gown with cuffs and back closure; shoe covers; two pairs of gloves (for double gloving); goggles; a mask; a disposable dustpan and a plastic scraper (for collecting broken glass); plastic-backed or absorbable towels; a container of desiccant powder or granules (to absorb wet contents); two disposable sponges; a punctureproof, leakproof container labeled "Biohazard waste"; and a container of 70% alcohol for cleaning the spill area.

Directions for preparation

Prepare the prescribed drugs in accordance with current product instructions, paying attention to compatibility, stability, and reconstitution technique. To avoid unnecessary or excessive drug exposure, follow these precautions. First, wash your hands before and after drug preparation and administration. Also, prepare the drugs in a Class II biological safety cabinet. Wear protective garments (such as a long-sleeved gown, gloves, and a face shield or goggles) as indicated by the policy of your health care facility. Don't wear the garments outside the preparation area. Also, don't eat, drink, smoke, or apply cosmetics in the drug preparation area.

Before you prepare the drug (and after you finish), clean the internal surfaces of the cabinet with 70% alcohol and a disposable towel. Discard the towel into a leakproof chemical waste container. Then cover the work surface with a clean plastic absorbent pad to minimize contamination by droplets or spills. Change the pad at the end of each shift or whenever a spill occurs. You should consider all of the equipment used in drug preparation, as well as any unused drug, as hazardous waste and dispose of them according to the policy at your health care facility. Place all chemotherapeutic waste products in leakproof, sealable, plastic bags or another appropriate container. Make sure the container is appropriately labeled.

Complications

Some scientific literature suggests that chemotherapeutic drugs are mutagenic. In addition, chronic exposure to chemotherapeutic drugs may damage the liver or chromosomes. Direct exposure to these drugs may burn and damage the skin.

Nursing considerations

• Take precautions to reduce your exposure to chemotherapeutic drugs. Realize that systemic absorption can occur through ingestion of contaminated materials, contact with the skin, or inhalation. In fact, you can inhale a drug without even realizing it, such as while opening a vial, clipping a needle, expelling air from a syringe, or from producing a splash effect when discarding excess drug. You can also absorb a drug from handling contaminated feces or body fluids.

• For maximum protection, mix all chemotherapeutic drugs in an approved Class II biological safety cabinet. Also, prime all I.V. bags containing chemotherapeutic drugs under the hood. Leave the hood blower on 24 hours a day, 7 days a week.

• If a hood isn't available, prepare drugs in a quiet, well-ventilated work space, away from heating or cooling vents and away from other personnel. Vent vials with a hydrophobic filter, or use negative pressure techniques. Also, use a needle with a hydrophobic filter to remove the solution from vials. To break ampules, wrap a sterile gauze pad or alcohol sponge around the neck of the ampule to decrease chances of droplet contamination.

• Make sure the biological safety cabinet is examined every 6 months, or any time the cabinet is moved, by a company specifically prepared for this work. If the cabinet passes certification, the certifying company will affix a sticker to the cabinet attesting to its approval.

• Use only syringes and I.V. sets that have luer-lock fittings. Label all chemotherapeutic drugs with a chemotherapy hazard label.

• Don't clip needles, break syringes, or remove the needles from the syringes used in drug preparation. Use a gauze pad when removing chemotherapy syringes and needles from I.V. bags of chemotherapeutic drugs.

• Place used syringes or needles in a puncture-proof container, along with other sharp or breakable items.

• Wear latex surgical gloves and a gown of low-permeability fabric with a closed front and cuffed long sleeves when mixing chemotherapeutic drugs. Change gloves every 30 minutes when working steadily with chemotherapeutic drugs. If you spill a drug solution, or puncture or tear a glove, remove your gloves immediately. Wash your hands before donning new gloves and any time you remove your gloves.

• If some of the drug comes in contact with your skin, wash the involved area thoroughly with soap (not a germicidal agent) and water. If eye contact occurs, flood the eye with water or an isotonic eyewash for at least 5 minutes while holding the eyelid open. Obtain a medical evaluation as soon as possible after accidental exposure.

• If a major spill occurs, use a chemotherapeutic spill kit to clean the area.

• Discard disposable gowns and gloves in an appropriately marked, waterproof receptacle whenever they become contaminated or whenever you leave the work area.

• Don't place any food or drinks in the same refrigerator as chemotherapeutic drugs.

• Become familiar with drug excretion patterns, and take appropriate precautions when handling a chemotherapy patient's body fluids. (See *Administration and excretion routes of alkylating agents,* page 122.)

• Provide male patients with a urinal with a tight-fitting lid. Wear disposable latex surgical gloves when handling body fluids. Before flushing the toilet, place a waterproof pad over the toilet bowl to avoid splashing. Wear gloves and a gown when handling linens soiled with body fluids. Place soiled linens in isolation linen bags designated for separate laundering.

• When caring for a patient in his home, empty waste products into the toilet close to the water to minimize splashing. Close the lid and flush two or three times. Place soiled linens in a washable pillowcase; then launder them twice, separately from other household linens. Wear gloves when handling contaminated linens, bedclothes, or other materials.

• Women who are pregnant, trying to conceive, or breast-feeding should exercise caution when handling chemotherapeutic drugs.

• Document each incident of exposure according to the policies at your health care facility.

Patient teaching

When teaching your patient about handling chemotherapeutic drugs, discuss appropriate safety measures. If the patient will be receiving chemotherapy at home, you'll need to teach him how to dispose of contaminated equipment. Tell the patient and his family to wear gloves whenever handling chemotherapy equipment or contaminated linens or bedclothes. Instruct them to place soiled linens in a separate washable pillowcase and to launder the pillowcase twice, with the soiled linens inside, separate from other household linens.

All materials used for the treatment should be placed in a leakproof container and taken to a designated disposal area. The patient or his family should make arrangements with either a hospital or a private company for pickup and proper disposal of contaminated waste.

Administering chemotherapeutic drugs

Some aspects of giving chemotherapeutic drugs are the same as for any other drug. For example, you'll still take care to check the doctor's order, prepare the proper dose, use aseptic technique, administer the drug properly, and know about the drug's potential adverse effects.

However, the administration of chemotherapeutic drugs requires additional skills. For example, some drugs require specialized equipment or must be given through an unusual route. Others become unstable after awhile, and still others must be protected from light. Finally, the drug dosage must be exact to avoid possibly fatal complications. For these reasons, only specially trained nurses and doctors should give chemotherapeutic drugs.

You may use a number of routes to administer chemotherapeutic drugs. Although the I.V.

Administration and excretion routes of alkylating agents

DRUG	ADMINISTRATION ROUTES	HOW DRUG IS EXCRETED
alfa-interferons	I.M., S.C.	Excretion through urine, amount unknown
asparaginase	I.V., I.M.	Excretion route and amount unknown
bleomycin	I.V., I.M., S.C.	50% of drug excreted in urine in 24 hours, mainly as metabolites
carboplatin	I.V.	71% of drug excreted in urine in 24 hours
cisplatin	I.V.	23% of drug excreted in urine in 24 hours; 27% to 45% in 5 days
dacarbazine	I.V.	30% to 46% of drug excreted in urine, half as metabolites
dactinomycin	I.V.	30% of drug excreted in urine and feces in 7 days
daunorubicin	I.V.	23% of drug excreted in urine and bile in 5 days; 40% in 7 days
doxorubicin	I.V.	4% to 5% of drug excreted unchanged in urine in 5 days; 40% to 50% excreted in bile or feces in 7 days
etoposide	I.V.	40% to 60% of drug excreted in urine in 72 hours; 2% to 16% excreted in feces in 72 hours
fluorouracil	I.V.	15% of drug excreted unchanged in urine in 6 hours; up to 80% excreted through lungs as carbon dioxide in 24 hours
hydroxyurea	P.O.	Excreted in urine and through lungs, 50% unchanged and 50% as urea and carbon dioxide
methotrexate	P.O., I.V., I.M., intrathecal	80% to 90% of drug excreted unchanged in urine in 24 hours
mitomycin	I.V.	10% to 30% of drug excreted in urine
mitoxantrone	I.V.	25% of drug excreted in bile in 5 days; 6% to 11% excreted in urine in 5 days
plicamycin	I.V.	40% of drug excreted in urine in 15 hours
procarbazine	P.O.	Excreted in urine, with less than 5% unchanged and 70% as metabolites within 24 hours
teniposide	I.V.	40% of drug excreted in urine in 72 hours, primarily as metabolites
vinblastine	I.V.	30% of drug excreted in urine within 72 hours; 20% excreted in feces within 72 hours
vincristine	I.V.	50% of drug excreted unchanged in urine and feces
vindesine	I.V.	Unknown amount excreted in feces

route is used most commonly, these drugs may also be given orally, through a central venous catheter, through an Ommaya reservoir into the spinal canal, or through a device implanted in a vein. They may also be administered into an artery, the peritoneal cavity, or the pleural space.

The administration route depends on the drug's pharmacodynamics and the tumor's characteristics. For example, if a malignant tumor has remained confined to one area, the drug may be administered through a localized, or regional, method. Regional administration allows you to deliver a high drug dose directly to the tumor. This is particularly advantageous because many solid tumors don't respond to drug levels that are safe for systemic administration.

You may administer chemotherapy to a patient whose cancer is believed to have been eradicated through surgery or radiation therapy. This treatment, called *adjuvant chemotherapy,* helps to ensure that no undetectable metastasis exists. A patient may also receive chemotherapy before surgery or radiation therapy. This is called *neoadjuvant chemotherapy,* or *induction* or *synchronous chemotherapy.* Induction chemotherapy helps improve survival rates by shrinking a tumor before surgical excision or radiation therapy.

In general, higher doses of chemotherapeutic drugs prove more effective than lower doses. Unfortunately, though, these drugs' adverse effects often limit the dosage. One exception to this rule is methotrexate. This drug is particularly effective against rapidly growing tumors, but it's also toxic to normal tissues that are growing and dividing rapidly. However, doctors have discovered that they can give a large dose of methotrexate to destroy cancer cells and then, before the drug has had a chance to permanently damage vital organs, give a dose of folinic acid antidote called leucovorin rescue factor. This antidote stops the effects of methotrexate, thus preserving normal tissue. (See *Leucovorin rescue.*)

Equipment

To give a chemotherapeutic drug, make sure you have the prescribed drug, the patient's medication record and chart, aluminum foil or a brown paper bag (if the drug is photosensitive), 0.9% sodium chloride solution, syringes and needles, an infusion pump or controller, gloves, and impervious containers labeled "Caution: Biohazard."

Insertion of the access device

Chemotherapy may be administered subcutaneously, intramuscularly, intravenously (using peripheral or central veins), intra-arterially, or into a body cavity. Each route, and the insertion of the necessary access device, is discussed thoroughly elsewhere in this book.

Leucovorin rescue

Methotrexate interferes with cell division in the *S* phase of the cell cycle by inhibiting dihydrofolate reductase, an enzyme involved in deoxyribonucleic acid (DNA) synthesis. (See *How chemotherapeutic drugs disrupt the cell cycle,* page 113.) High-dose methotrexate is most effective against cells that have a high metabolic rate, such as leukemia cells. Used alone, high-dose methotrexate eventually will affect normal cells as well, producing toxicity.

To protect normal cells, methotrexate commonly is prescribed with leucovorin (folinic acid). Leucovorin rescues cells by bypassing the S phase. For the drug to work efficiently, leucovorin must be administered exactly as prescribed—the proper doses must be given at the proper times, with no skipped doses. When given correctly, leucovorin rescues cells before they begin active growth and division.

Because leucovorin can't prevent methotrexate toxicity completely, you should closely monitor any patient on high-dose methotrexate therapy for bone marrow suppression, stomatitis, pulmonary complications, and renal damage (from drug precipitates in tubules). You should also maintain the patient's urine alkalinity to avoid drug precipitates in renal tubules and monitor his urine output closely.

Directions for administration

Before giving a chemotherapeutic drug, you'll assess the patient's physical condition and go over his medical history. Make sure you understand what needs to be given and by what route, and provide the necessary teaching and support to the patient and his family. You'll determine the best site to administer the drug and, finally, after giving the drug, you'll clean up carefully.

Getting ready

When you evaluate your patient's condition, pay particular attention to the results of recent laboratory studies, specifically his complete blood count, blood urea nitrogen level, platelet count, urine creatinine level, and liver function studies.

Review the patient's medical history for past chemotherapy, noting the severity of any adverse effects. Check his drug history for any medications that might interact with the chemotherapy. As a rule, you shouldn't mix chemotherapeutic drugs with any other medications. If you have any questions or concerns about administering the chemotherapeutic drug, talk with the patient's doctor before you give it.

Next, double-check the chart for the complete chemotherapy protocol order, including the patient's name; the drug's name and dosage; and the route, rate, and frequency of administration. See if the drug's dosage depends on certain laboratory values. Be aware that some health care facilities require two nurses to read the dosage order and to check the drug and the amount being administered.

Also check to see if the doctor has ordered an antiemetic, fluids, a diuretic, or electrolyte supplements to be given before, during, or after chemotherapy administration. Finally, talk with the patient and his family to evaluate their understanding of chemotherapy, and make sure that either the patient or a responsible family member has signed the consent form.

Next, don gloves. Keep them on through all stages of handling the drug, including preparation, priming the I.V. tubing, and administration.

Before giving the drug, you'll need to perform a new venipuncture proximal to the old site. Avoid giving chemotherapeutic drugs through an existing I.V. line. To identify an administration site, examine the patient's veins, beginning with his hand and proceeding to his forearm. When selecting a site, consider drug compatibilities, the frequency of administration, and the vesicant potential of the drug. For example, if the doctor has ordered the intermittent administration of a vesicant drug, you can give it by either instilling the drug into the side port of an infusing I.V. line or by direct I.V. push. If, however, the vesicant drug is to be infused continuously, you should administer it only through a central venous line or a vascular access device. On the other hand, nonvesicant agents (including irritants) may be given by direct I.V. push, through the side port of an infusing I.V. line, or as a continuous infusion.

Check the policy at your health care facility before administering a vesicant. Because vein integrity decreases with time, some facilities require that vesicants be administered *before* other drugs. Conversely, because vesicants increase vein fragility, other facilities require that vesicants be given *after* other drugs. (See *Classifying chemotherapeutic agents*.)

Implementing delivery

Once an appropriate line is in place, infuse 10 to 20 ml of 0.9% sodium chloride solution to test vein patency. Never test vein patency with a chemotherapeutic drug. Next, administer the drug as appropriate: nonvesicants by I.V. push or admixed in a bag of I.V. fluid; vesicants by I.V. push through a piggyback set connected to a rapidly infusing I.V. line.

During I.V. administration, closely monitor the patient for signs of hypersensitivity reaction or extravasation. Check for an adequate blood return after 5 ml of drug has infused, or according to guidelines. After infusion of the medication, infuse 20 ml of 0.9% sodium chloride solution. Do this between administrations of different chemotherapeutic drugs and before discontinuing the I.V. line.

Dispose of used needles and syringes carefully. To prevent aerosol dispersion of chemotherapeutic drugs, don't clip needles. Place them intact in an impervious container for incineration. Dispose of I.V. bags, bottles, gloves, and tubing in a properly labeled and covered trash container.

Wash your hands thoroughly with soap and warm water after giving any chemotherapeutic drug, even though you've worn gloves.

Complications

A common adverse effect of chemotherapy is nausea and vomiting, ranging from mild to debilitating. Nausea and vomiting may result from one of three causes. The first cause, which tends to trigger a milder form of nausea, is gastric irritation resulting from oral drug administration. A more severe form of nausea and vomiting may result if the chemotherapeutic drugs irritate the central nervous system.

Nausea and vomiting may also result from psychogenic causes originating in the cerebral cortex. Known as anticipatory emesis, this reaction can completely disable the patient. A patient who remembers the unpleasantness of previous chemotherapy may feel nauseated or even vomit when simply thinking about future treatments. Sights, sounds, and smells associated with treatment may even induce vomiting.

A major development in helping patients control nausea and vomiting is the drug ondansetron, or Zofran. This serotonin antagonist controls the emetic response without the extreme drowsiness and extrapyramidal adverse effects commonly associated with antiemetic medications. It's especially effective in reducing the nausea and vomiting induced by cisplatin. Other antiemetic medications that may be prescribed include metoclopramide, lorazepam, dexamethasone, prochlorperazine, diphenhydramine, droperidol, and dronabinol.

A second major complication is bone marrow suppression, leading to neutropenia and thrombocytopenia. An important method of treatment that reduces this risk is the use of colony-stimulating factors. Normally, T-lymphocytes, monocytes, endothelial cells, and fibroblasts produce colony-stimulating factors.

Other adverse effects of chemotherapy include intestinal irritation, stomatitis, pulmonary fibrosis, cardiotoxicity, nephrotoxicity, neurotoxicity, hearing loss, anemia, alopecia, urticaria, radiation recall (if drugs are given with or soon after radiation therapy), anorexia, esophagitis, diarrhea, and constipation. I.V. administration may also lead to extravasation, causing inflammation, ulceration, and necrosis, and loss of vein patency (leading to fibrosis). (See *Preventing and treating adverse reactions,* pages 126 and 127.)

Nursing considerations
• Observe the I.V. site frequently for signs of extravasation or allergic reaction (swelling, redness, urticaria). If you suspect extravasation, stop the infusion immediately. Leave the needle in place and notify the doctor. A conservative method for treating extravasation involves aspirating any residual drug from the tubing

Classifying chemotherapeutic agents

To administer a chemotherapeutic agent safely, you need to know whether it's a vesicant (capable of producing blisters), an irritant (capable of producing undue sensitivity), or a nonvesicant drug.

Vesicant agents	Irritant agents	Nonvesicant agents
• dacarbazine	• carmustine	• asparaginase
• dactinomycin	• etoposide	• bleomycin
• daunorubicin	• streptozocin	• carboplatin
• doxorubicin		• cisplatin
• mitomycin		• cyclophosphamide
• mitoxantrone		• cytarabine
• nitrogen mustards		• floxuridine
• plicamycin		• fluorouracil
• vinblastine		• ifosfamide
• vincristine		
• vindesine		

and needle, instilling an I.V. antidote, and then removing the needle. Afterward, you may apply heat or cold to the site and elevate the affected limb.
• During infusion, some drugs need protection from direct sunlight to avoid possible drug breakdown. If this is the case, cover the vial with a brown paper bag or aluminum foil.
• When giving vesicants, avoid sites where damage to underlying tendons or nerves may occur (veins in the antecubital fossa, near the wrist, or in the dorsal surface of the hand).
• If you're unable to remain with the patient during the entire infusion, use an infusion pump or controller to ensure delivery of the drug within the prescribed time and rate.
• Observe the patient at regular intervals and after treatment for adverse reactions.
• Monitor the patient's vital signs throughout infusion to assess any changes during chemotherapy administration.
• Maintain a list of the types and amounts of drugs the patient has received. This is especially important for drugs that have a cumulative effect and that can be toxic to certain organs, such as the heart, kidneys, or lungs.
• Record the location and description of the I.V. site before treatment or the presence of blood

Preventing and treating adverse reactions

Different chemotherapeutic drugs commonly cause similar adverse reactions. This chart will help you prevent or treat common adverse effects, including bone marrow suppression, anemia, and alopecia.

ADVERSE REACTIONS	PREVENTION AND TREATMENT
Bone marrow suppression The most common, and potentially the most serious, adverse reaction to chemotherapeutic drugs.	• Watch for the blood count nadir—when the patient has the greatest risk of leukopenia, thrombocytopenia, and anemia. • Plan a patient-teaching program that covers bone marrow suppression, including information about blood counts, potential sites of infection, and personal hygiene.
Leukopenia Places the patient at increased risk for infection, especially if the granulocyte count drops below 1,000/mm³.	• Provide information about good hygiene, and assess the patient frequently for signs and symptoms of infection. • Teach the patient to recognize and report the signs and symptoms of infection: fever, cough, sore throat, or a burning sensation on urination. • Teach the patient how to take his own temperature. • Caution the patient to avoid crowds and people with colds or the flu during the blood count nadir. • Remember that the inflammatory response may be decreased, and the complications of leukopenia more difficult to detect, if the patient is receiving a corticosteroid.
Thrombocytopenia May accompany leukopenia. When the platelet count drops below 50,000/mm³, the patient risks excessive bleeding. When it drops below 20,000/mm³, the patient has a severe risk of excessive bleeding and may require a platelet transfusion.	• Assess the patient for bleeding gums, increased bruising or petechiae, hypermenorrhea, tarry stools, hematuria, and coffee-ground vomitus. • Advise the patient to avoid cuts and bruises and to use a soft toothbrush and an electric razor. • Tell the patient to report sudden headaches, which could indicate potentially fatal intracranial bleeding. • Instruct the patient to use a stool softener, as prescribed, to prevent colonic irritation and bleeding. • Instruct the patient to avoid using a rectal thermometer or receiving I.M. injections, to prevent bleeding.

return during bolus administration. Also record the drugs and dosages administered; sequence of drug administration; needle type and size used; amount and type of flushing solution; and the site's condition after treatment. Document any adverse reactions, the patient's tolerance of the treatment, and the topics discussed with the patient and his family.

Patient teaching

First evaluate the patient's and family's desire for information and their level of understanding. Take the time to find out what they already know about chemotherapeutic drugs, and try to clear up any misconceptions they might have about the patient's disease or treatments. Then teach them specifically about the chemotherapeutic drug prescribed, the treatment protocol, and the schedule of administration. If the patient is experiencing pain, let him know that his pain can be treated and that he doesn't have to endure pain.

Your teaching should include a discussion of the potential adverse effects of chemotherapy.

ADVERSE REACTIONS	PREVENTION AND TREATMENT
Anemia Develops slowly over several courses of treatment.	• Assess the patient for dizziness, fatigue, pallor, and shortness of breath after minimal exertion. • Monitor the patient's hematocrit, hemoglobin level, and red blood cell counts. Remember that a patient dehydrated from nausea, vomiting, or anorexia may exhibit a false-normal hematocrit reading. • Be prepared to administer a blood transfusion to a symptomatic patient. • Instruct the patient to rest more frequently and to increase his dietary intake of iron-rich foods. Advise him to take a multivitamin with iron, as prescribed.
Nausea and vomiting May result from gastric mucosal irritation, chemical irritation of the central nervous system, or psychogenic factors.	• Control the chemical irritation by administering combinations of antiemetics, as prescribed. • Monitor the patient for signs and symptoms of aspiration because most antiemetics cause sedation. • Encourage the patient to express feelings of anxiety. • Encourage the patient to listen to music or engage in relaxation exercises, meditation, or hypnosis to promote feelings of control and well-being. • Adjust the drug administration time to meet the patient's needs. Some patients prefer treatments in the evening when they find sedation comfortable. Patients who are employed may prefer to receive their treatments on their days off.
Stomatitis Although this may occur on any mucous membrane, the most common site is the oral mucosa. Stomatitis, which is temporary, can range from mild and barely noticeable to severe and debilitating.	• Initiate preventive mouth care before chemotherapy to provide comfort and decrease the severity of stomatitis. • Provide therapeutic mouth care, including topical antibiotics, if prescribed.
Alopecia Patient may view alopecia as the most distressing adverse reaction.	• Prepare the patient for alopecia. Inform him that hair loss usually occurs gradually and reverses after treatment ends. • Inform the patient that alopecia may be partial or complete and that it affects both men and women. • Inform the patient that alopecia may affect the scalp, eyebrows, eyelashes, and body hair.

Patients and their families need to know which signs and symptoms warrant an immediate call to the doctor and which are considered normal. Reassure the patient that the adverse effects of treatment can be treated as well and that they won't last forever.

Teach the patient how to ward off certain adverse effects through such measures as good mouth care. Also, prepare the patient for alopecia. Inform him that hair loss is usually gradual and reversible. Instruct the patient and family about the use of wigs and scarves. If you can, provide the patient with the name of a store that specializes in these products.

If the patient is taking a narcotic, instruct him in the use of laxatives or stool softeners, as ordered, to relieve constipation. If the patient has leukopenia, emphasize the need to avoid crowds or people who have colds.

Throughout your teaching, maintain a supportive and nonjudgmental attitude. Encourage the patient and his family to express their fears and to ask questions. If appropriate, refer them to outside resources, such as support groups.

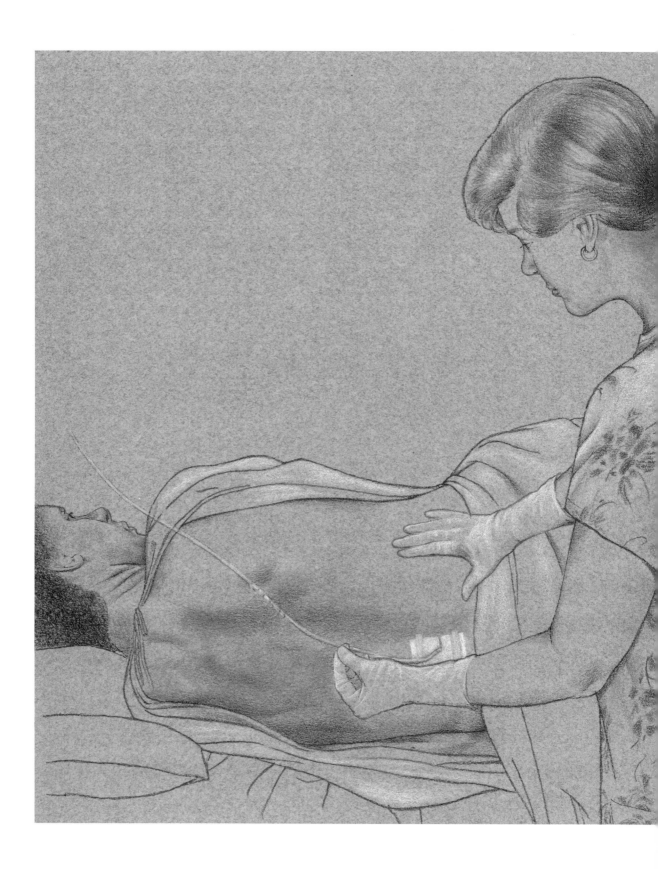

CHAPTER

Delivering drugs to the central nervous system

If your patient is in severe pain and doesn't get adequate relief from I.M. injections or oral medications, the doctor may order drugs to be injected or infused into the central nervous system (CNS). CNS injections give greater analgesia without causing the adverse systemic effects of large doses of opioids or multiple, painful injections. This route is commonly used to administer opioids, local anesthetics, and antineoplastic and anti-inflammatory drugs.

This chapter will help you master the specialized skills that you need to deliver drugs to the CNS. You'll start by reviewing the anatomy of this system and discussing how various drugs work within it. Then you'll learn about the most common administration techniques and nursing care before, during, and after treatment. With this knowledge, you'll be able to give quality nursing care and help relieve your patient's pain.

CNS anatomy

To better understand the principles underlying CNS administration, you'll need to review CNS anatomy. (See *CNS drug administration sites.*) The spinal cord and brain are protected by three layers of tissue collectively called the meninges. The dura mater—the thick, outer layer—lies closest to the skull. It creates two potential spaces: the epidural and the subdural, which may fill during an illness or injury, such as arterial bleeding. The ligamentum flavum encloses the epidural space posteriorly and contains fatty tissue, blood vessels, and extensions of nerves.

The middle layer of the meninges, known as the arachnoid, is a thin membrane containing a spidery vascular system. The subarachnoid space, or the space under the arachnoid, contains cerebrospinal fluid (CSF), which bathes and protects the spinal cord.

The innermost layer, the pia mater, is a thin membrane that adheres to the brain's surface.

Pharmacologic principles

You'll need to become familiar with the indications and dosage, pharmacokinetics, and other characteristics of the most commonly prescribed drugs.

Common drugs
Local anesthetics, opioids, corticosteroids, and antineoplastics are among the drugs commonly injected or infused into the CNS. Because preservatives in drugs can cause scarring, inflammation, and nerve-root destruction, hospitals use only preservative-free drugs. (See *Reviewing common CNS drugs,* pages 132 to 135.)

Anesthetics
Local anesthetics are given epidurally, intrathecally, or peripherally (directly into a nerve) to treat acute and chronic pain. They block the pain impulse by interfering with sodium conduction at the nerve site so that the action potential doesn't occur. They also block pain impulses before they reach the dorsal horn of the spinal cord. Low doses block sensory input; higher doses add a motor block. Local anesthetics may be given as a single injection or continuous infusion. The dosage reflects the desired effect (sensory or motor block) and the patient's weight, age, and overall condition. Drug selection depends on the desired duration of the block.

Opioids
Administered epidurally or intrathecally, opioids treat cancer pain, acute pain and, rarely, nonmalignant chronic pain. Epidural opioids diffuse slowly into the intrathecal space and then into the opioid receptors in the dorsal horn of the spinal cord.

Pain impulses arrive at the spinal column via the sensory root of a spinal nerve, which ends in the dorsal horn. When substance P, a neurotransmitter, exists in the dorsal horn, impulses move across and up the ascending fibers of the spinal cord to the brain, which interprets the impulses as painful. Morphine and other opioids block the discharge of substance P and the transmission of pain impulses to the brain.

Corticosteroids
These drugs reduce inflammation in irritated or compressed nerves. They're also given prophylactically for malignant CNS tumors and to treat irritation caused by such tumors. Corticosteroids may be administered epidurally, intrathecally, or peripherally.

Antineoplastics
Antineoplastic drugs can be injected intrathecally, allowing them to be placed directly on or close to a tumor site. Intrathecal injection also bypasses the blood-brain barrier. If given systemically, these drugs wouldn't cross this barrier in concentrations high enough to be effective. Once the drug is in the CSF, it's absorbed much more slowly than if given by other routes. These drugs are used prophylactically in disorders such as leukemia, where the chance of CNS involvement is high, and in the treatment of malignant CNS tumors.

(Text continues on page 134.)

CNS drug administration sites

Central nervous system (CNS) drugs are usually administered to relieve pain. Unlike drugs administered *peripherally,* which block the transmission of pain at its origin, CNS drugs are injected or infused directly into or around the central nervous system, which gives greater analgesia without causing the adverse effects of large systemic doses of opioids or multiple, painful injections.

This illustration shows the various sites at which CNS drugs can be injected, and how they block the pain impulse from traveling to the thalamus, the brain's pain center.

Drugs injected *epidurally* block the pain impulse at the nerve root as it enters the dura mater.

Drugs injected *intrathecally* go directly into the spinal canal and the cerebrospinal fluid. These drugs may act locally, blocking the pain impulse at the spinal cord, or they may migrate to the brain, modifying the response to pain.

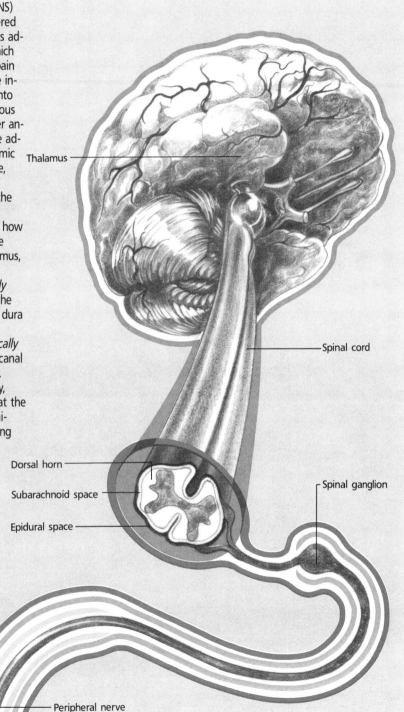

Thalamus

Spinal cord

Dorsal horn

Subarachnoid space

Epidural space

Spinal ganglion

Peripheral nerve

Reviewing common CNS drugs

DRUG	INDICATIONS AND DOSAGE	MECHANISM OF ACTION
Local anesthetics		
bupivacaine hydrochloride 0.25%, 0.5%, 0.75% (Marcaine, Sensorcaine); also available with epinephrine (Adrenaline) 1:200,000	Regional anesthesia. *Epidural:* If using 0.25% solution, dose is 25 to 50 mg. If using 0.5% solution, dose is 50 to 100 mg. *Intrathecal:* If using 0.75% solution, dose is 6 to 12 mg. *Peripheral nerve block:* If using 0.25% solution, dose is 12.5 mg. If using 0.5% solution, dose is 25 mg.	Local amide-type anesthetic; blocks depolarization by interfering with sodium-potassium exchange across nerve cell membrane, preventing generation and conduction of nerve impulses
chloroprocaine hydrochloride 1%, 2%; preservative-free 2%, 3% (Nesacaine, Nesacaine-CE)	Regional anesthesia. *Infiltration and peripheral nerve block:* If using 1% solution (60 to 80 ml), dose is 600 to 800 mg. If using 2% solution (2 to 40 ml), dose is 40 to 800 mg. Maximum adult dosage is 11 mg/kg/day or 14 mg/kg/day when used with epinephrine. *Caudal or epidural:* For 2% or 3% solution (15 to 25 ml), dose is 300 to 750 mg. May repeat with smaller doses every 40 to 50 minutes. Dose and intervals may be increased with epinephrine to a maximum adult dosage of 800 mg/day or 1 g/day.	Local ester-type anesthetic; blocks depolarization by interfering with sodium-potassium exchange across nerve cell membrane, preventing generation and conduction of nerve impulses
lidocaine hydrochloride 1%, 1.5%, 2%, 4%, 10%, 20% (Ardecaine, Xylocaine); also available with dextrose and epinephrine added	Regional anesthesia. *Infiltration and peripheral nerve block:* Use a 0.5% to 1% solution for percutaneous infiltration, or a 0.5% solution for I.V. regional (Bier) block. Use a 1% to 1.5% solution for peripheral nerve block. Most dental blocks use a 2% solution. The maximum single adult dose is 5 to 6 mg/kg. *Caudal:* For 1% solution (20 to 30 ml), dose is 200 to 300 mg. *Epidural:* If using 1.5% solution (15 to 20 ml), dose is 225 to 300 mg. If using 2% solution (10 to 15 ml), dose is 200 to 300 mg. *Spinal:* If using 5% with dextrose 7.5% in water (1.5 to 2 ml), dose is 75 to 100 mg. Dose and intervals increase with addition of epinephrine.	Local amide-type anesthetic; blocks depolarization by interfering with sodium-potassium exchange across nerve cell membrane, preventing generation and conduction of nerve impulses
Opioids		
fentanyl citrate (Sublimaze)	Moderate to severe pain. *Epidural:* 20 to 150 mcg/hour.	Binds with opioid receptors at many CNS sites (brain, brain stem, spinal cord), altering perception of pain and emotional response to it through an unknown mechanism
hydromorphone hydrochloride 1 mg/ml, 2 mg/ml, 3 mg/ml, 4 mg/ml, 10 mg/ml (Dilaudid, Dilaudid HP)	Moderate to severe pain. *Epidural:* 0.15 to 0.3 mg/hour. *Intrathecal:* 0.01 to 0.03 mg/hour. Titrate to effect if necessary.	Binds with opioid receptors at many CNS sites (brain, brain stem, spinal cord), altering perception of pain and emotional response to it through an unknown mechanism
meperidine hydrochloride 10 mg/ml, 25 mg/ml, 50 mg/ml, 75 mg/ml, 100 mg/ml (Demerol)	Moderate to severe pain. *Epidural:* 5 to 20 mg/hour. *Intrathecal:* 5 to 30 mg/hour.	Binds with opioid receptors at many CNS sites (brain, brain stem, spinal cord), altering perception of pain and emotional response to it through an unknown mechanism

NURSING CONSIDERATIONS

• A test dose verifies needle or catheter placement. Initially, 2 to 3 ml is given to check for intrathecal injection, which can cause extensive motor paralysis of the legs and sensory deficit. If no symptoms occur, a second, larger test dose of 5 ml is given 5 minutes later to check for intravascular injection, which can cause tinnitus, lip numbness, metallic taste, dysphoria, lethargy, and hypotension.
• Keep resuscitation equipment and drugs available.
• Use solutions containing epinephrine cautiously in patients with cardiovascular disorders and in body areas with limited blood supply (ears, nose, fingers, toes).
• Onset is 4 to 17 minutes; duration, 3 to 6 hours.

• Test dose checks for intrathecal or I.V. placement. Wait 5 minutes after test dose before proceeding.
• Keep resuscitation drugs and equipment available.
• Use solutions with epinephrine cautiously in patients with cardiovascular disorders.
• Onset is 3 to 6 minutes; duration, 30 to 60 minutes.

• Contraindicated in patients with inflammation or infection in puncture region, septicemia, severe hypertension, spinal deformities, and certain neurologic disorders.
• Use cautiously in elderly or debilitated patients.
• Keep patient off food for at least 6 hours before administering local anesthetics.
• Test dose of drug verifies placement of needle or catheter.
• Use epinephrine cautiously in patients with cardiovascular disorders.

• Keep resuscitation equipment and drugs available.
• After drug administration, monitor patient carefully for hypotension, seizures, loss of consciousness, myocardial depression, arrhythmias, respiratory arrest, and anaphylaxis. Monitor fetal heart tones of patient in labor.
• To treat overdose, check airway and administer oxygen, vasopressors, and I.V. fluids. Give anticonvulsants for seizures.
• Monitor blood pressure, electrocardiogram rhythm, oxygen saturation, and pulse rate.

• Monitor patient's circulatory and respiratory status. Immediately report a respiratory rate below 12 breaths/minute.
• Keep naloxone available.

• High doses can produce muscle rigidity. This effect can be treated with neuromuscular blocking agents.
• Monitor bladder function in postoperative patients.
• Onset is 5 minutes; duration, 4 to 6 hours.

• Monitor circulatory and respiratory status and bowel function.
• Keep naloxone available.
• Warn patient to avoid activities that require alertness.

• When hydromorphone is given postoperatively, encourage patient to turn, cough, and breathe deeply to avoid atelectasis.
• May worsen or mask gallbladder pain.
• Onset is 15 minutes; duration, 6 to 17 hours.

• Monitor patient's circulatory and respiratory status.
• Not recommended for treatment of chronic pain because meperidine and normeperidine accumulate and cause seizures.

• Keep naloxone available.
• Monitor bowel function. Give stool softener if necessary.
• Onset is 5 minutes; duration, 6 to 17 hours.

(continued)

Reviewing common CNS drugs (continued)

DRUG	INDICATIONS AND DOSAGE	MECHANISM OF ACTION
Opioids (continued)		
morphine sulfate (Astramorph, Duramorph [preservative-free solutions])	Moderate to severe pain. *Epidural:* 0.2 to 1.5 mg/hour. *Intrathecal:* 0.1 to 0.5 mg/hour. Dosages must be titrated to effect for cancer pain.	Binds with opioid receptors at many CNS sites (brain, brain stem, and spinal cord), altering perception of pain and emotional response to it through an unknown mechanism
Corticosteroids		
betamethasone (Betnelan, Celestone)	Sciatica and abdominal pain secondary to pancreatitis or pancreatic cancer. *Epidural and intrathecal:* 6 to 12 mg.	Decreases inflammation, mainly by stabilizing leukocyte lysosomal membranes
methylprednisolone (Depo-Medrol, Medrol)	Severe inflammation or immunosuppression. Deposit where slow-release characteristics are desired. *Epidural:* 40 to 120 mg.	Decreases inflammation, mainly by stabilizing leukocyte lysosomal membranes
Antifungal agent		
amphotericin B (Fungizone)	Systemic fungal infections and meningitis. *Intrathecal or intraventricular:* 25 mcg/0.1 ml. Initial dose shouldn't exceed 100 mcg.	Probably acts by binding to sterols in fungal cell membrane, altering cell permeability and allowing leakage of intracellular components
Antineoplastics		
cytarabine (ara-C) (Cytosar-U)	Meningeal leukemias and neoplasms. *Intrathecal:* 10 to 30 mg/m² every 4 days.	Inhibits DNA synthesis
methotrexate	Meningeal leukemias. *Intrathecal:* 10 to 15 mg/m² every 2 to 5 days until cerebrospinal fluid is normal.	Prevents reduction of folic acid to tetrahydrofolate by binding to dihydrofolate reductase

Other drugs

Some of the drugs described above may be given together to control pain. For example, a patient with intractable cancer pain may require both an opioid and a local anesthetic for adequate relief. A bulging or herniated disk that causes nerve irritation and back pain may be treated with a local anesthetic (to provide immediate relief) and a corticosteroid (to decrease nerve irritation).

Moreover, some drugs may be combined with epinephrine (Adrenaline), alkylating agents, and dextran (Macrodex). For example, epinephrine is often used with a local anesthetic to lengthen the duration of a nerve block. A vasoconstrictor, epinephrine prevents

Nursing considerations

• Monitor blood pressure, respirations, and level of sedation. • Keep naloxone available. • Initiate a continuous infusion by adding the number of mg used in 24 hours and dividing by 24. This number equals the hourly rate.	• Monitor bowel function, and give a stool softener if necessary. • When morphine is used postoperatively, encourage the patient to turn, cough, breathe deeply, and use the incentive spirometer to avoid atelectasis. • Onset for epidural injection is 30 minutes; duration, 6 to 24 hours. Onset for intrathecal injection is 15 minutes; duration, 8 to 24 hours.
• Don't use for long-term treatment. • Preparation should be compatible for intraspinal injection.	
• Don't use for long-term treatment. • Preparation should be compatible for intraspinal injection.	
• Use cautiously in patients with impaired renal function. • Monitor vital signs, and watch for fever and hypotension, which may appear 1 to 2 hours after infusion. • Monitor intake and output closely.	• Monitor complete blood count (CBC), blood urea nitrogen levels, and serum creatinine levels at least weekly. Test liver and renal function weekly. Also monitor potassium levels closely and make dosage adjustments as necessary.
• Reduced dosages may be needed in patients with leukopenia, thrombocytopenia, or renal or hepatic disease, and after chemotherapy or radiation therapy. • Watch for signs of infection and bleeding. Monitor CBC. • Monitor intake and output, and encourage adequate fluid intake.	• Assess patients receiving high doses for signs of neurotoxicity. • Modified dosages may be needed in patients with impaired hepatic or renal function, bone marrow suppression, aplasia, leukopenia, thrombocytopenia, or anemia. • Monitor laboratory values closely.
• Leucovorin calcium (Wellcovorin) rescue is necessary with high-dose protocols. This rescue is effective against systemic toxicity but doesn't interfere with tumor cells' absorption of methotrexate.	• Watch for bleeding (especially GI) and infection. • Take patient's temperature daily, and watch for cough, dyspnea, and cyanosis.

another drug from being absorbed and metabolized as quickly by the blood vessels. It also prolongs the local action and decreases the systemic effects of anesthetics. Studies are also being conducted on the use of epidural clonidine (Catapres) and its ability to reduce the narcotic dose needed. Intrathecal baclofen (Lioresal) is being tested on patients with muscle spasticity.

Epidural administration

A relatively new route, epidural administration has been proven effective. Drugs are injected or infused into the epidural space, from which they diffuse slowly through the dura mater into the intrathecal space, which contains CSF. The CSF carries the drug directly into the

Epidural catheter placement

This cross-sectional view shows the internal structures of the central nervous system (CNS), while the inset shows a catheter inserted into the epidural space. This catheter may exit directly over the spine or it can be tunneled subcutaneously to an exit site on the patient's side or abdomen, as shown.

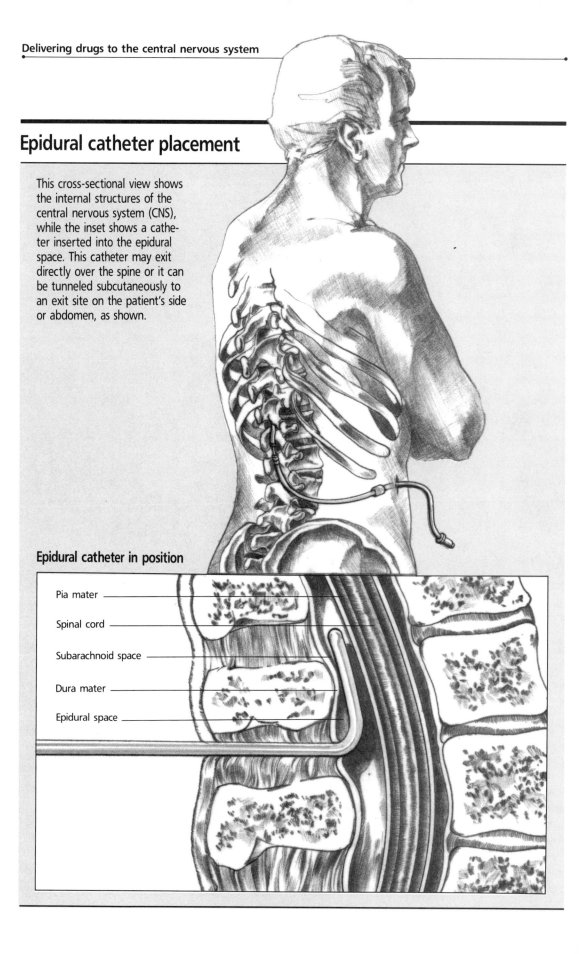

Epidural catheter in position

Pia mater

Spinal cord

Subarachnoid space

Dura mater

Epidural space

Comparing analgesic doses by route

This chart shows the usual drug doses given to achieve effective pain relief by the I.V., oral, epidural, and intrathecal routes.

DRUG	I.V. DOSE	ORAL DOSE	EPIDURAL DOSE	INTRATHECAL DOSE
morphine	10 mg	10 to 60 mg (immediate release) 30 to 60 mg (sustained release)	2 to 3 mg	0.2 mg
methadone (Dolophine, Methadose)	10 mg	15 mg	5 mg	Not usually given by this route
meperidine (Demerol)	75 to 100 mg	200 mg	15 to 20 mg	10 mg
hydromorphone (Dilaudid, Dilaudid HP)	1.5 to 2.5 mg	3 to 5 mg	0.75 mg	0.4 to 0.5 mg
fentanyl (Sublimaze)	70 to 100 mcg	Not given by this route	70 to 100 mcg	50 to 70 mcg
codeine	60 to 90 mg	180 mg	Not given by this route	Not given by this route

spinal cord, bypassing the blood-brain barrier. In some patients, the drug is injected directly into the intrathecal space.

Indications and contraindications

Drugs are given epidurally to treat moderate-to-severe acute and chronic pain from surgery, labor, cancer, reflex sympathetic dystrophy, degenerative joint disease, and spinal trauma. A single injection of a corticosteroid may be given to relieve nerve inflammation or reduce the pain of a bulging disk; a series of injections is commonly given for such conditions as low back pain or acute herpes zoster.

Contraindications for an epidural infusion or injection include systemic or insertion site infection, certain neurologic conditions, anticoagulant therapy, spinal arthritis or deformity, hypotension, marked hypertension, allergy to the prescribed drug, and chemotherapy that might interfere with the blood platelet count.

Advantages and disadvantages

The epidural route provides excellent analgesia with a relatively small dosage, so patients are more alert and have fewer adverse reactions with long-term use. (For example, 2 to 3 mg of morphine sulfate [Duramorph] given epidurally has the same effect as 10 mg given I.V.) Postoperative patients become ambulatory sooner; therefore, they have fewer pulmonary complications and shorter hospitalizations. Because a higher concentration of drug can be deposited closer to its intended site of action, pain relief occurs more quickly. (See *Comparing analgesic doses by route.*)

A continuous epidural infusion minimizes adverse cerebral and systemic effects and eliminates the risks of multiple I.M. injections. It also eliminates the peaks and valleys that occur with oral and intermittent I.M. regimens. Plus, this type of infusion can be used for days or weeks—for example, in a postoperative patient who needs 3 or 4 days of pain relief, or in a patient with chronic pain who must feel well enough to undergo intensive physical therapy.

Disadvantages of the epidural route include the risk of infection; respiratory depression; urine retention; pruritus; nausea and vomiting (from opioids); the risk of hypotension (from anesthetics); and, possibly, an allergic reaction to the drug.

Equipment

Use an I.V. pump for continuous epidural infusions. Avoid gravity-dependent devices because resistance of the epidural catheter prevents effective drug delivery. You'll also need an epidural filter (if one's not already on the catheter), nonsterile gloves, and alcohol sponges. The drug should be in a bag of I.V. 0.9% sodium chloride solution that's clearly labeled EPIDURAL USE ONLY. Use nitroglycerin tubing to connect the epidural catheter to the I.V. bag. To prevent accidental injections of other drugs into the epidural infusion line, use this type of tubing or a similar tubing with no side ports.

Although the setup described above is usually the least expensive and easiest to use, it may not be the safest. Open-faced, the pump can easily be manipulated by anyone, including the patient. The pump also has no bolus or patient-controlled analgesia (PCA) mode. In addition, the drug isn't secured in a locked chamber, so it might be removed accidentally. The best pump keeps the drug secured and the program locked in, allowing the patient to give either incremental or bolus doses as needed, such as the Pharmacia CADD-PCA.

Insertion

Depending on the patient's needs, drugs can be administered through an epidural needle, a temporary catheter, or a permanent catheter. (See *Epidural catheter placement,* page 136.)

Epidural needle or temporary catheter

Before the anesthesiologist arrives, place an epidural tray at the patient's bedside. The tray should contain a special epidural needle (a Tuohy or similar needle); a glass syringe; an epidural filter; 0.9% sodium chloride solution (preservative-free); a sterile drape; an epidural catheter; and sponges saturated with an antiseptic solution, such as povidone-iodine or chlorhexidine.

Have the patient sit on the edge of the bed with his chin pressed into his chest. This position flexes the neck vertebrae and opens the spaces between them so the needle can pass easily. If the patient can't sit, help him into a lateral decubitus position or fetal position (his chin tilted to his chest and knees drawn up toward his chest). Then expose his back.

Using sterile technique, the anesthesiologist prepares the insertion site and then inserts the epidural needle into the patient's lower back at an interspace between the 10th thoracic and 4th lumbar (T10 and L4) vertebrae, depending on the region to be anesthetized. He may insert the needle at the cervical level for arm pain. Once the needle enters the epidural space, it meets very little resistance, so injecting the 0.9% sodium chloride solution is easy. The catheter should thread easily into the epidural space.

To verify placement, the anesthesiologist injects a small test dose of 2 to 3 ml of 2% lidocaine (Xylocaine). If no loss of sensation occurs after 3 to 5 minutes, the ordered drug is administered. If loss of sensation does occur, the catheter is in the intrathecal space, not the epidural space, and the drug dose must be adjusted. (One-tenth of the epidural dose can achieve the same effect intrathecally.)

Catheter placement can also be verified by injecting dye into the catheter under fluoroscopy (epidurogram). This verifies that the catheter is in the epidural space, not in the intrathecal space or in a vein. If it's in a vein, the catheter must be removed and reinserted.

If the patient requires only one injection, the drug is given through the needle; then the needle is removed. If a continuous infusion is needed, a catheter is threaded through the needle 1¼" to 2" (3 to 5 cm) into the epidural space. Then the needle is removed and the catheter is left in place. The catheter is secured with Steri-Strips, and a transparent semipermeable dressing is applied to further secure it and to allow visualization of the site.

Permanent catheter

If the patient needs an epidural infusion for longer than 5 days, the anesthesiologist will insert a permanent catheter. Usually, he'll insert a temporary catheter first to determine the analgesia's effectiveness. Permanent placement is usually performed in the operating room under strict aseptic technique. The patient is positioned the same way as for insertion of a temporary catheter. Then the site is prepared and the patient is draped in standard surgical fashion. The anesthesiologist locates the epidural space with a large-bore epidural needle. He threads an epidural Silastic catheter through the needle into the epidural space and tunnels the catheter underneath the skin to the anterior portion of the costochondral cartilage. If an external catheter is used, it exits through the skin near the anterior axillary line.

If the patient is terminally ill and has intractable pain, the doctor may insert a permanent catheter with an implanted port. He makes a subcutaneous pocket over the ribs, places the port in it, and then connects the catheter to it.

Drug administration

A drug may be injected or continuously infused into an epidural catheter or continuously infused into an epidural implanted port. After catheter placement has been confirmed and the first dose has been given, you may give subsequent doses as ordered or initiate an infusion.

Injection into a catheter

To inject a drug through the temporary catheter, first fill the syringe with the ordered narcotic plus 1 cc of air. Disinfect the catheter hub and injection cap. Aspirate the catheter with an empty 3-ml syringe. Check for the return of clear fluid or blood. If you see blood, the catheter may be in the epidural blood vessels. If you see clear fluid, it's probably CSF because the catheter is in the subarachnoid space. In either case, don't inject the drug. Inform the doctor. If nothing is aspirated, remove the empty syringe, attach the drug-filled syringe, and infuse the drug.

Infusion through a catheter

To give a continuous infusion through a temporary epidural catheter using a bedside pump, first verify that the drug in the bag is for epidural use, is preservative-free, and is the correct drug and strength. Be sure that the catheter, medication bag, and pump are labeled EPIDURAL USE ONLY. Next, insert the nitroglycerin tubing in the medication bag and prime the tubing. Set the pump rate and ask another nurse to verify it with the order.

Use an alcohol sponge to clean the site where the cap connects to the epidural catheter. Let the site dry completely. Then remove the catheter cap and connect the nitroglycerin tubing to the catheter. Secure this connection with a piece of tape to prevent the catheter from separating and becoming contaminated. Tape all tubing connections. Make sure that the tubing is positioned correctly inside the pump and the rate is set correctly.

Follow the manufacturer's directions for setting up the infusion pump. Then open the clamp and start the infusion.

Infusion through a port

After washing your hands, gather a portable PCA infusion pump; extension tubing; a medication cassette; a 22G Huber needle; a transparent semipermeable dressing; a dressing kit with sterile gloves, sterile 2" × 2" gauze pads, three alcohol sponges, three povidone-iodine sponges, povidone-iodine ointment, and tape; and an extra pair of sterile gloves.

Next, prepare the pump, following the manufacturer's instructions. Open the packages for the Huber needle and transparent semipermeable dressing, and place the items on a sterile field. Put a sterile glove on your dominant hand. Hold the needle in your gloved hand, and remove the cap with your ungloved hand. Return the needle to the sterile field. Then pick up the wrapped extension tubing with your gloved hand, and remove the cap with your ungloved hand.

Connect the needle to the extension tubing, using your ungloved hand to hold the tubing and your gloved hand to pick up the needle. Then remove air from the tubing and needle. Return the needle to the sterile field

ADVANCED EQUIPMENT

Epidural port

If a patient is terminally ill and in intractable pain, the doctor may implant an epidural port. This device consists of a port with a self-sealing septum attached to a silicone catheter that terminates in the epidural space.

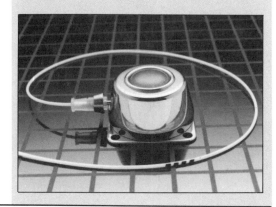

and place a clean glove on your other hand.

Clean the skin over the implanted port with an alcohol sponge, wiping in circles from the center outward. Do this three times, using a clean sponge each time. When the area is completely dry, repeat the process with the three povidone-iodine sponges. Again, let the area dry.

Remove the protective covering from the needle, and palpate the implanted port through the patient's skin. Stabilize the port with your thumb and index finger; then insert the needle into the center of the septum.

Apply povidone-iodine ointment to the needle insertion site. Place a sterile 2″ × 2″ gauze pad under the needle's butterfly wings, and cover it with the transparent semipermeable dressing. Secure all junctures with tape. Then set the pump on the appropriate lock code or level and start it. (See *Epidural port.*)

Complications

Infection is the most serious complication for the patient with a temporary or permanent catheter. So look for redness, tenderness, or drainage at the port site, catheter access site, or insertion site for the epidural needle on the patient's back. Also monitor him for fever and an increased white blood cell (WBC) count. Localized cellulitis can also appear at the exit site of a temporary catheter or at the needle exit site of the port, causing redness, tenderness, and a low-grade fever.

To help prevent infection, change the dressings using sterile technique. Securely tape all connections, and discard premixed epidural solutions after 48 hours. If cellulitis occurs, the catheter should be removed immediately and oral or, sometimes, I.V. antibiotics should be administered. If the patient has a permanent catheter, an effort may be made to salvage the port or catheter by removing the needle and giving I.V. antibiotics. Occasionally, epidural antibiotics are infused to try to maintain the epidural access.

If the patient develops meningitis, the catheter must be removed and I.V. antibiotics given immediately. Signs and symptoms of meningitis include fever, nuchal rigidity, malaise, and an elevated WBC count.

A post–spinal-puncture headache is another possible complication. (See *Treating a spinal headache.*)

Catheter occlusion can occur if the catheter develops a kink or becomes compressed between vertebrae. The catheter can also migrate into the tissue of the patient's back. Fortunately, this problem doesn't occur often and can be checked by infusing a contrast medium into the catheter under fluoroscopy.

An expanding hematoma in the epidural space can cause back pain or leg weakness. Report these symptoms to the doctor immediately so that he can intervene to prevent permanent nerve damage.

Catheter migration into the subarachnoid space can occur if the tip of the catheter punctures the dura mater and becomes lodged in the intrathecal sac. Because a smaller drug dose is needed intrathecally, the patient will have signs and symptoms of an overdose, including unilateral analgesic effect, changes in respiration, hypotension, weakness in the extremities, and nausea. If any of these occur, the doctor will probably discontinue the drug;

if respirations decrease, he'll ask you to administer oxygen and I.V. fluids. To prevent catheter migration, securely tape the catheter at its exit site, and keep checking the hash marks that indicate how far it's inserted.

Catheter erosion through the skin may result when skin over the implanted port is fragile. This rare complication usually occurs in patients who have lost weight after port insertion and in cancer patients or others with poor nutritional status.

Respiratory depression may result from administering opioids through an epidural catheter. Watch closely for signs and symptoms, which can appear up to 24 hours after opioid administration. This rare complication is dose-related, occurring most often with drugs that are less lipid-soluble, and is treated with 0.2 to 0.4 mg I.V. of naloxone.

Some patients with epidural catheters develop urine retention, although the cause is unknown. Treatment consists of naloxone or bethanechol (Duvoid), which can cause spontaneous voiding. Urinary catheterization may also be required.

Also, some patients develop pruritus. This was once thought to result from preservatives in the solution, but itching still occurs with preservative-free solutions. Unfortunately, this problem doesn't respond well to treatment with naloxone or antihistamines.

Nausea and vomiting can occur from increased blood levels of the opioid or from an interruption of CSF flow. Some patients get relief from antiemetics, but these can cause drowsiness. Small doses of naloxone I.V. also reduce nausea.

Hypotension may occur when a patient who's been bedridden with chronic pain becomes pain-free and tries to walk. Blood and fluid shifts occur when he sits upright after being in bed for a long time.

Nursing considerations
• Before an epidural access device is inserted, a consent form must be signed.
• Have the following items on hand for emergency use during insertion: 0.4 mg I.V. of naloxone (Narcan), 50 mg I.V. of ephedrine sulfate (Ephed II), oxygen, an intubation set, and a hand-held resuscitation bag.

COMPLICATIONS

Treating a spinal headache

A spinal headache occurs when the dura mater is torn and cerebrospinal fluid leaks out of the intrathecal space. The tear may be caused by the needle during epidural catheter insertion, or by the catheter migrating from the epidural space through the dura mater into the intrathecal space. The patient will complain of an intense headache that increases when he sits up or tries to walk. He may also experience nausea and vomiting, muscle aches, vision changes (difficulty focusing, spots, or blurred or double vision), and hearing problems (buzzing, roaring, or popping).

Using a blood patch
Treatment usually consists of an epidural blood patch. About 15 to 20 ml of the patient's own blood is drawn from a peripheral vein and then injected into the epidural space. When the epidural needle is withdrawn, the patient is instructed to sit up. Because the blood clots and seals off the leaking area, the headache should subside immediately. The patient can resume his regular activity after this procedure.

Monitoring the patient
Nursing interventions include increasing fluid intake, decreasing caffeine and sugar intake, and providing a quiet, dimly lit environment. Maintaining adequate fluid intake and lying flat for 8 hours after catheter insertion can help prevent a spinal headache.

• During catheter insertion and while the patient is in the recovery room, monitor and record his blood pressure, pulse, arterial oxygen saturation, and respirations every 15 minutes.
• Document the drug, route, and rate used when the catheter was inserted. Note that aseptic technique was used. If the pump has a special lock to prevent unauthorized manipulation, record the lock code or level and whether a key was used. Document the exit site for the epidural port or catheter. If anything was done to the site — for example, if it was reinforced or the needle was changed — document this too.

Caring for an epidural catheter site

Using aseptic technique, change the dressing over the catheter exit site every 24 to 48 hours, or as needed. Follow these steps.
• Wash your hands, and gather the following equipment: sterile gloves, three alcohol sponges, three povidone-iodine sponges, povidone-iodine ointment, a transparent semipermeable dressing, compound benzoin tincture, Steri-Strips, and tape.
• Put on sterile gloves, and remove the old dressing carefully.
• Clean the exit site three times with the alcohol sponges, wiping in concentric circles, moving outward from the site about 2″ to 3″ (5 to 8 cm). Use a clean sponge each time. Let the site dry for about 2 minutes.
• Clean the site three times with the povidone-iodine sponges, using the same technique. Again, let

the site dry completely. Because alcohol, povidone-iodine, and hydrogen peroxide (used by some hospitals) are potentially neurotoxic, make sure the exit site is thoroughly dry before accessing the port or covering the site.
• Apply a small amount of povidone-iodine ointment to the area. Cover it with a transparent semipermeable dressing to allow inspection of drainage. (The dressing will normally look moist or slightly blood-tinged.)
• To prevent a temporary catheter from dislodging, use one of these methods: Spray the skin with compound benzoin tincture to make it tacky; secure the catheter with Steri-Strips; or loop part of the catheter under the dressing or under some tape.

Record the name and dose of the drug, the time, and the patient's response every time you give a drug.
• After starting a continuous infusion, monitor the patient's blood pressure and respirations every hour for the next 8 hours, then every 4 hours for the next 16 hours.
• Make sure that the patient has I.V. access either through a continuous infusion or a heparin lock to allow for immediate administration of emergency drugs, if necessary.
• If the patient has lung cancer or other respiratory problems, or is already receiving oxygen therapy, the doctor may order bedside pulse oximetry for the first 24 hours. Call the doctor if you notice a respiratory rate of less than 8 breaths/minute, a systolic blood pressure of less than 90 mm Hg, or a diastolic blood pressure of less than 60 mm Hg. If the patient's baseline vital signs change more than 30%, notify the doctor.
• Assess the patient's level of sedation, mental status, and level of pain relief every hour initially, then every 2 to 4 hours until adequate pain control is achieved. Many hospitals use the Visual Analog Scale, which measures pain severity on a scale of 1 to 10. Even if the pa-

tient can't assign a number to his pain, he can usually assess relief in terms of a percentage. For example, he may say "The pain is 50% better now."
• Assess the patient's extremities for weakness every 2 to 4 hours for the first 24 hours. If the catheter is in the cervical or upper thoracic area, his arms may be weak; if it's in the lumbar area, his legs may be weak. Epidural opioids don't cause motor weakness, but local anesthetics can, so patients need help walking. Dosage adjustment can decrease weakness or numbness.
• Notify the doctor if the patient feels pain or if he has any of these common narcotic adverse reactions: anuria, nausea and vomiting, drowsiness, or itching. The doctor may increase or decrease the dosage, prescribe another drug, or take other measures to alleviate the signs and symptoms. Remember that epidural drugs diffuse slowly and that adverse reactions may occur up to 12 hours after an infusion is discontinued.
• If your patient is receiving epidural opioids, question any order for a narcotic by a different route. An opioid given systemically along with an epidural opioid can potentiate the effect of

the epidural opioid, making assessment difficult and increasing the chance of adverse reactions. If the patient has a PCA pump, advise him to push the incremental dose button to control breakthrough pain.
• Change dressings only every 7 days as long as the transparent semipermeable dressing is dry and intact. Change the tubing on a closed system every 7 days at the same time you change the dressing; also change the medication cassette and filter at this time. (See *Caring for an epidural catheter site.*)

Patient teaching
Teach the patient and family about the epidural route of drug administration, its possible complications and expected outcome, and how it will affect their life-style. Explain the procedure thoroughly, using an illustrated information booklet from the equipment company. Tell the patient that he'll feel some pain when the catheter's inserted. Then demonstrate the pump that he'll be using. Allow plenty of time for questions.

Home care
Home use of epidural analgesia is possible only if the patient and family are willing and able to provide the care needed. Warn the patient to abstain from alcohol and illicit drugs because these substances potentiate opioid action. He should also check with the doctor before taking any over-the-counter drugs.
If the patient is to be discharged with an epidural catheter or port, help the family arrange for home care. Be sure that the visiting nurses are qualified to care for the port and that they reinforce your patient teaching. The home health care agency should have skilled nurses and pharmacists on call 24 hours a day to handle unexpected occurrences.

Intrathecal administration

In intrathecal drug administration, drugs are injected or infused via one of two access routes:

directly into the subarachnoid space or into the ventricle of the brain.
The first access route is made by inserting the catheter into the space between L3 and L4. The equipment is the same as for an epidural infusion. The insertion technique is also the same, except that the catheter tip is placed in the intrathecal sac. The catheter can be tunneled to an exterior exit site and capped for intermittent injections or connected to a pump for continuous infusion. Also, a port can be used for intermittent injections or continuous infusions.
The second access route is through an Ommaya reservoir, which allows delivery of long-term drug therapy to the CSF via the brain's ventricles. (See *Ommaya reservoir,* page 144.)
Because the first access route is similar to that used for an epidural infusion, the following discussion will focus only on the Ommaya reservoir.

Indications and contraindications
The intrathecal route is an effective way to administer opioids and other analgesics, antineoplastic agents for CNS tumors, and antibiotics and antifungal agents. Local anesthetics like lidocaine can also be given intrathecally to achieve regional anesthesia as in spinal anesthesia or epidural block.
The intrathecal route is used to administer water-soluble drugs, which can't cross the blood-brain barrier if given I.V.
Patients who shouldn't receive intrathecal injections include those with inflammation or infection at the puncture site, septicemia, and spinal deformities.

Advantages and disadvantages
The intrathecal route has the same advantages and disadvantages as the epidural route, but drugs given by this route have longer half-lives. They're injected directly into the CSF, so lower doses are required, causing fewer systemic adverse effects because of less diffusion into fewer capillaries. This route also provides access to CSF for sampling and, if a catheter is inserted, spares the patient repeated lumbar punctures. It permits consistent and predictable drug distribution and monitoring of drug

Ommaya reservoir

The Ommaya reservoir (also called the Rickham reservoir and the subcutaneous cerebrospinal fluid reservoir) is a mushroom-shaped device with an attached catheter. It's implanted in the lateral ventricle of the patient's brain through a burr hole drilled in the nondominant frontal lobe. The reservoir has a silicone injection dome that rests over the burr hole under a scalp flap, causing a small bulge. Drugs can be injected into the dome with a syringe.

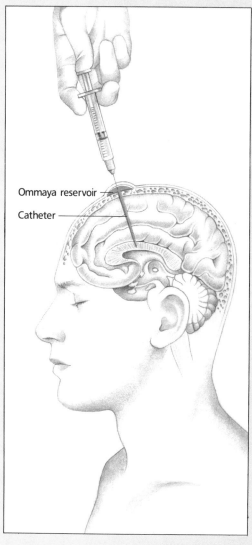

Ommaya reservoir

Catheter

levels throughout the intrathecal space and CNS. The Ommaya reservoir has the added advantage of allowing measurement of intracranial pressure (ICP) and tumor or cyst drainage. And, in patients with acute lymphoblastic leukemia, the reservoir prevents the disease from spreading to the brain.

Equipment

Much of the equipment needed is the same as for an epidural injection: an epidural tray that includes a Tuohy needle (special needle), a glass syringe, sterile drapes, sterile gloves, a 0.22-micron filter, a catheter (either a small-bore plastic catheter included on the tray for a temporary placement or a Silastic catheter for permanent placement). Depending on the access route, an Ommaya reservoir may also be necessary. As indicated, intrathecal injections also may require the following supplies: preservative-free drug for injection; sterile gloves; three alcohol sponges; three povidone-iodine sponges; a sterile towel; two 3-ml syringes; a 25G needle or 22G Huber needle; a sterile gauze pad; collection tubes for CSF samples, if ordered; and a vial of bacteriostatic 0.9% sodium chloride solution.

Insertion

The Ommaya reservoir is usually inserted in the operating room. After the doctor evaluates ventricular size using a computed tomography (CT) scan, he makes an incision in the right frontal region. He tunnels a subgaleal pocket and places the reservoir in it. Next, he makes a burr hole just anterior to the coronal suture. He cauterizes the dura mater and opens it to allow catheter insertion. Then, he cauterizes the pia mater, opens the cortex, and introduces the catheter with its stylet into the nondominant frontal horn. He positions the catheter at the foramen of Monro and confirms its position by X-ray. Finally, he connects the catheter to the reservoir, sutures the system to the edge of the burr hole, and closes the wound.

A pressure dressing remains in place for 24 hours, then a gauze dressing for 1 or 2 days. The reservoir is usually ready for use by the 3rd postoperative day.

Drug administration

A doctor usually injects drugs into an Ommaya reservoir with a nurse's assistance. However, some specially skilled nurses may perform this procedure.

If you're assisting, shampoo the patient's hair with chlorhexidine, as ordered. Then shave the area over the port. After obtaining baseline vital signs, position the patient so he's either sitting or reclining. Establish a sterile field near the patient. Prepare a syringe with the drug to be instilled and place the syringe, the CSF collection tubes, and the vial of sodium chloride solution within reach of the sterile field.

Next, wash your hands, put on the gloves, and prepare the patient's scalp with the alcohol sponges, wiping with each sponge in a circular motion from the center outward. Let the area dry for 1 or 2 minutes. Repeat the process with the three povidone-iodine sponges and, again, let the area dry completely.

If the doctor is injecting the drug, assist him. If you're injecting it, place the 25G needle at a 45-degree angle, insert it into the reservoir, and gently aspirate 3 ml of CSF into the syringe. If the aspirate isn't clear, consult the doctor before continuing.

Some health care facilities advise using CSF instead of a preservative-free diluent to deliver the drug. If your facility does this, continue to aspirate as many milliliters of CSF as you will instill of the drug. Then detach the syringe from the needle hub, attach the drug syringe, and slowly inject the drug, monitoring the patient for headache, nausea, and dizziness.

Cover the site with the sterile gauze pad, and apply gentle pressure for a minute or two until superficial bleeding stops.

Complications

One serious complication, infection at the reservoir site, can usually be treated successfully by injecting antibiotics directly into the reservoir. However, chronic infection may require removal of the system.

Catheter migration or blockage can cause symptoms of increased ICP, such as headache and nausea. To confirm this problem, the doctor gently pumps (pushes and releases) the reservoir several times. Then he places his finger on the patient's scalp to feel the reservoir refill. Slow filling suggests migration or blockage, which can be confirmed by a CT scan, and requires surgical correction.

Another potential complication is an inadvertent injection of local anesthetic into the CSF, which can cause spinal block.

Nursing considerations

• Before the reservoir is inserted, make sure that the consent form has been properly signed. Also check the patient's chart to make sure that laboratory work is complete. Prerequisites for the procedure include a normal complete blood count; a WBC count greater than 2,500/mm^3; a stable platelet count, preferably greater than 100,000/mm^3; and the absence of sepsis.
• If the doctor orders an antiemetic, administer it 30 minutes before reservoir insertion to control nausea and vomiting.
• After insertion, instruct the patient to lie still for 15 to 30 minutes. This helps prevent meningeal irritation leading to nausea and vomiting.
• Before administering any drug into the reservoir, ask the patient how his health has been since his last visit, taking special note of colds, fevers, headaches, nausea or vomiting, or other signs of infection.
• Record the appearance of the reservoir insertion site before and after access, the amount of CSF withdrawn and its appearance, and the name and dose of the drug instilled.
• Monitor the patient for adverse drug reactions and signs of increased ICP, such as nausea, vomiting, pain, and dizziness. Assess him for adverse reactions every 15 to 30 minutes for 2 hours and then every 4 hours.

Patient teaching

Before the procedure, carefully explain how the reservoir is inserted and used. Make sure that the patient and his family understand the potential complications, and answer any questions they have. Reassure the patient that hair shaved for the implant will grow back and that only a coin-sized patch must remain shaved for injections.

Nerve block for chronic pain

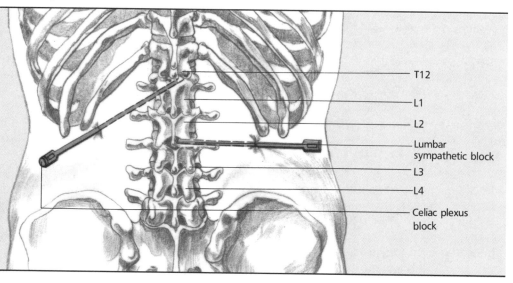

This illustration shows the needle positions for the celiac plexus block and the lumbar sympathetic block. Although the exact needle-entry sites may vary, the target areas are the anterolateral aspects of the 12th thoracic-1st lumbar (T12-L1) junction for the celiac plexus block, and the anterolateral aspect of the L2, L3, or L4 vertebra for the lumbar sympathetic block.

T12
L1
L2
Lumbar sympathetic block
L3
L4
Celiac plexus block

Teach the patient and his family the signs and symptoms of local infection (swelling, redness, tenderness, and drainage at the site) and of systemic infection (fever, headache, and neck stiffness). Tell them to notify the doctor if these problems develop.

Tell the patient that he can resume normal activities within a few days after the reservoir is implanted. But warn him to avoid bumping the infusion site until the incision heals. Explain that if no complications develop, the reservoir may function for years.

Nerve blocks

A doctor may decide to perform a nerve block using a less common access route. For example, he may do a celiac plexus block to treat pancreatic cancer or a lumbar sympathetic block for persistent leg pain that has a sympathetic component. In patients with extreme pain, he may perform a neurolytic block, which permanently destroys pain pathways.

A nerve block may be performed by an anesthesiologist or a neurosurgeon. Depending on the pain site, he injects a local anesthetic into the spine (as in epidural or intrathecal blocks), into a peripheral nerve (as in a celiac plexus block), or into a major nerve plexus (as in a lumbar sympathetic block). (See *Nerve block for chronic pain*.)

Nerve blocks are being used more frequently and, like other pain-control methods, require a nurse's participation. Although nerve blocks are performed by the doctor, you'll need to assist him and monitor the patient during and after the procedure. You may also be required to give sedatives and subsequent doses of anesthetics.

Indications and contraindications
Nerve blocks can provide short-term pain relief for patients with pancreatitis, costochondritis, renal colic, and other conditions that respond poorly to narcotic and other analgesics. Although single-treatment relief rarely lasts more than 8 hours, repeated nerve blocks can produce progressively longer relief periods for some patients, such as those with musculoskeletal pain. In some patients, pain relief lasts for months or even years.

Nerve blocks can also be used diagnostically and prognostically. Diagnostic nerve blocks help to identify pain pathways and involved structures and to separate the physical and emotional components of pain. Prognostic blocks help a doctor determine the probable effect of a neurolytic block by temporarily producing the same effects as that procedure. This allows the patient and doctor to weigh the advantages and disadvantages before deciding on an irreversible procedure.

Because administration of nerve blocks requires verbal feedback from patients, nerve blocks are contraindicated for patients who aren't fully alert, such as heavily medicated patients.

Advantages and disadvantages
Advantages of nerve blocks include dense analgesia and selective blockade of a specific nerve. Nerve blocks can also help diagnose the affected nerve in a painful condition.

Disadvantages include infection and the risk of temporary loss of function in nearby structures, such as the lungs and vascular structures. In a neurolytic block, the patient permanently loses sensation or function in the tissues and organs served by the blocked nerve.

Equipment
The equipment you'll need depends on the type of block but, generally, you'll need a specialized tray for the particular block; two 25G needles and two 3-ml syringes for injecting the drug locally; sterile gloves; povidone-iodine or a similar antiseptic solution; the preservative-free drug to be injected; a sedative, if ordered; and any other specialized equipment necessary for the procedure (for example, a nerve stimulator).

Drug administration
Start an I.V. line for all invasive nerve blocks except local field blocks. A heparin lock is acceptable if no I.V. sedation is ordered. Then help the patient into the appropriate position for the particular block.

To perform a nerve block, the doctor injects a local anesthetic into the spine, into or around a peripheral nerve, or into a major nerve plexus. To induce a neurolytic block, he first verifies needle placement under fluoros-

copy, then injects a caustic substance, such as alcohol or phenol, into the affected nerve. Unlike a therapeutic block, this procedure permanently destroys nerve tissue.

Complications
An I.V. injection of a local anesthetic can cause adverse effects including a metallic taste, tinnitus, slurred speech, decreased sensorium, seizures, and cardiac arrest. Numbness or a painful inflammatory response may also occur and may be more unpleasant than the patient's original complaint.

Nursing considerations
• Before the nerve block, make sure the consent form has been properly signed.
• During the procedure, monitor the patient's vital signs and check his position. Monitor his electrocardiogram and pulse oximetry measurements (especially if he's sedated). Administer more sedation, if ordered. Typical sedatives are 1 to 3 mg I.V. of midazolam (Versed) and 500 to 1,000 mg I.V. of alfentanil (Alfenta). Sedatives calm the patient and decrease apprehension.
• Afterward, record the outcome of the block, and document the names and routes of all drugs administered. A flow sheet specifically designed for block procedures is helpful.
• Be aware of the policy of your health care facility before administering sedatives or subsequent doses of local anesthetics. State guidelines also vary, so make sure that your state's nurse practice act permits you to give these injections.

Patient teaching
Instruct the patient not to eat or drink for 6 hours before the procedure. Warn the outpatient in advance that he'll need someone to drive him home. Explain to him and his family how the block is performed and which adverse reactions are possible.

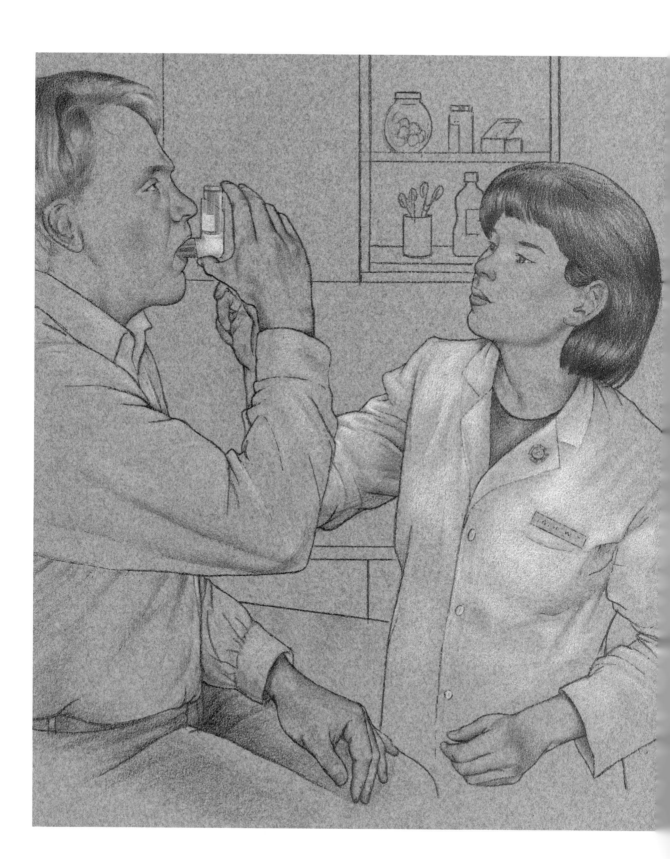

CHAPTER

7

Giving drugs through the respiratory system

Any patient, regardless of his diagnosis, may develop respiratory complications and need drug therapy. This therapy may be delivered nasally through inhalers and nebulizers or orally through nebulizers, metered-dose inhalers, and turbo-inhalers. An alternative method, using an endotracheal tube, allows emergency drug administration when an I.V. line isn't readily available.

Giving respiratory drugs isn't complicated, once you learn how to use the equipment. But because many patients who receive these drugs in an acute care setting continue to need them after they're discharged, thorough patient teaching plays a vital role in promoting compliance.

This chapter will help you gain skill and confidence in giving respiratory drugs and in teaching patients about their use. First, the chapter reviews respiratory anatomy and physiology, pharmacologic principles, and commonly ordered respiratory drugs. Next, it discusses advanced drug administration routes, covering the equipment used, the administration procedure, the potential complications, and the nursing considerations for each route. You'll also find what you need to teach your patient before discharge to ensure that he continues to receive proper treatment at home.

Anatomy and physiology

The respiratory organs permit the exchange of gases between the air and the blood, thereby serving as the body's lifeline. If any disorder seriously impairs this exchange, death may follow quickly.

The respiratory system consists of two distinct parts: the upper tract, including the nose, sinuses, mouth, larynx, and pharynx; and the lower tract, including the trachea and lungs (bronchi, bronchioles, and alveoli). The upper respiratory tract filters, humidifies, and warms inspired air. The lower respiratory tract is the prime area for drug absorption because of the lungs' vast alveolocapillary bed. (See *Intrapulmonary circulation.*)

Respiration has three phases. First, gases are exchanged between the air and the blood. Next, gases are transported between the lungs and the body tissues. Finally, gases are exchanged between the blood and body tissues. The first and second phases are vital only because they make the third phase possible.

Pharmacologic principles

Drugs may be administered into the respiratory tract by inhalation, instillation, or injection. Absorption into the alveoli occurs rapidly because only a thin, permeable membrane separates the air and the drug in each alveoli from the capillary blood flow. Absorption is also facilitated because the lungs provide a large surface area for absorption to take place.

Once drugs reach the surface of the lower respiratory tract, they produce a pharmacologic effect on special target cells. In asthma, for example, the smooth muscle cells will relax in the lower airways, and the cell activity that pro-

duces allergic reactions and inflammation will decrease.

Particle size must be considered when choosing a drug to be administered into the respiratory tract. It determines how the drug travels through the respiratory tract and where it falls within the tract. Drug particles must be between 0.5 and 10 micrometers for the drug to be delivered and deposited adequately in the lower respiratory tract. Larger particles usually collect in the upper tract only, and smaller particles are exhaled.

Several classes of drugs are given through the respiratory system. These include sympathomimetics, methylxanthines, corticosteroids, respiratory stimulants, anticholinergics, antibiotics, mast-cell stabilizers, and oxygen. (See *Giving common respiratory drugs,* pages 152 to 155.)

Sympathomimetics
Also called adrenergics, sympathomimetics stimulate the sympathetic nervous system to produce bronchodilatory effects. Bronchodilator therapy either stimulates the production of adenosine 3',5'-cyclic monophosphate (cyclic AMP) or decreases its breakdown. These drugs also help improve mucociliary clearance. They're used alone or in conjunction with methylxanthines.

Sympathomimetics may be given orally, parenterally, or by inhalation. However, inhalation is preferred because it produces a greater bronchodilation with fewer cardiac effects (such as beta$_1$ stimulation) and fewer systemic effects (such as nausea or tremor). Although many sympathomimetics are available, the longer-acting agents with beta$_2$ selectivity are the most effective. The most commonly used sympathomimetics include isoetharine (Bronkosol), metaproterenol (Alupent), albuterol (Ventolin), and terbutaline (Bricanyl).

Glucocorticoids
The main effect of glucocorticoids is to reduce airway inflammation. These drugs are given along with bronchodilators, and although they're beneficial and effective, their adverse effects are significant. They're usually given

(Text continues on page 154.)

Intrapulmonary circulation

In the illustration at right, you'll see the major respiratory structures. Inhaled air is filtered, humidified, and heated in the upper respiratory tract. Gas exchange takes place in the lower respiratory tract, as does drug absorption. This absorption occurs rapidly through the alveoli, where only a thin membrane separates gas and drug from the capillary blood flow. The inset shows alveolar circulation.

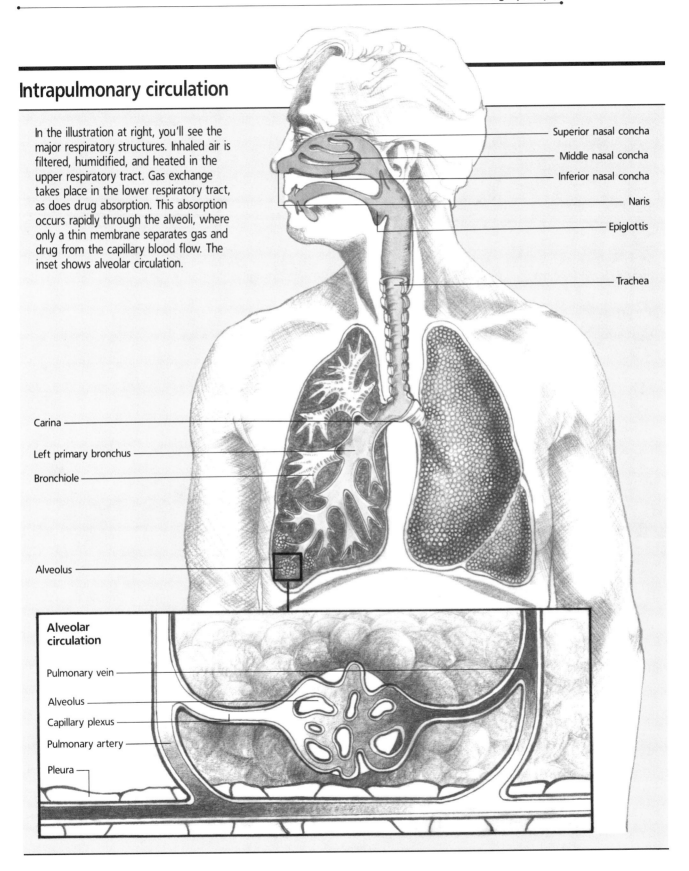

Superior nasal concha

Middle nasal concha

Inferior nasal concha

Naris

Epiglottis

Trachea

Carina

Left primary bronchus

Bronchiole

Alveolus

Alveolar circulation

Pulmonary vein

Alveolus

Capillary plexus

Pulmonary artery

Pleura

Giving common respiratory drugs

DRUG	INDICATIONS AND DOSAGE	MECHANISM OF ACTION
Anticholinergics		
atropine sulfate	Short-term treatment and prevention of bronchial spasm associated with brochial asthma, bronchitis, and chronic obstructive pulmonary disease (COPD). *Usual adult dosage:* 0.025 mg/kg diluted with 3 to 5 ml of 0.9% sodium chloride solution; administer by nebulizer three or four times daily.	Inhibits acetylcholine at the parasympathetic neuroeffector junction
ipratropium bromide (Atrovent)	Maintenance treatment of bronchospasm associated with COPD. *Usual adult dosage:* 2 inhalations (36 mcg) 3 or 4 times daily to a maximum dosage of no more than 12 inhalations every 24 hours	Inhibits vagally mediated reflexes by antagonizing acetylcholine
Antiprotozoal		
pentamidine isethionate (Pentam 300)	Prevention of *Pneumocystis carinii* pneumonia in high-risk patients. *Usual adult dosage:* 300 mg by nebulizer every 4 weeks	Interferes with biosynthesis of deoxyribonucleic acid, ribonucleic acid, phospholipids, and proteins in susceptible organisms
Glucocorticoids		
beclomethasone dipropionate (Beclovent, Vanceril)	Treatment of corticosteroid-responsive asthma. *Usual adult dosage:* 2 to 4 inhalations at 1-minute intervals 3 or 4 times daily, to a maximum dosage of 20 inhalations daily	Decreases inflammation by stabilizing leukocyte lysosomal membranes; may also directly act as a bronchodilator; may enhance bronchodilating action of beta-adrenergic agonists
dexamethasone sodium phosphate (Decadron Turbinaire, Respihaler)	Treatment of corticosteroid-responsive asthma. *Usual adult dosage:* 2 to 4 inhalations at 1-minute intervals 3 to 4 times daily, to a maximum dosage of 20 inhalations daily; 3 inhalations 3 or 4 times daily to a maximum dosage of 12 inhalations daily	Reduces inflammation, mainly by stabilizing leukocyte lysosomal membranes; may also directly act as a bronchodilator; may enhance bronchodilating action of beta-adrenergic agonists
Expectorant and antitussive		
acetylcysteine (Mucomyst)	Adjunctive treatment of pneumonia, bronchitis, tuberculosis, cystic fibrosis, emphysema, and atelectasis. *Usual adult dosage:* 6 to 10 ml of 10% solution by inhalation three or four times daily	Diminishes the viscosity of respiratory secretions
Nasal drugs		
beclomethasone dipropionate (Beconase Nasal Inhaler, Vancenase Nasal Inhaler)	Relief of seasonal or perennial rhinitis symptoms; prevention of recurrence of nasal polyps after surgical removal. *Usual adult dosage:* one spray (42 mcg) in each nostril two to four times daily to a maximum dosage of 168 to 336 mcg/day.	Reduces inflammation by stabilizing leukocyte lysosomal membranes; may also directly act as a bronchodilator; may enhance bronchodilating action of beta-adrenergic agonists
flunisolide (Nasalide)	Relief of seasonal or perennial rhinitis. *Usual adult dosage:* two sprays (50 mcg) in each nostril twice daily to a maximum dosage of four sprays in each nostril (200 mcg)	Decreases inflammation by stabilizing leukocyte lysosomal membranes; may also directly act as a bronchodilator; may enhance bronchodilating action of beta-adrenergic agonists

Nursing considerations

• Monitor the patient for tachycardia. • Keep in mind that other anticholinergic drugs may increase vagal blockage. • Do not exceed a total daily dosage of 2.5 mg.	• Because the drug causes urine retention and urinary hesitancy, monitor intake and output closely.
• Not effective in acute episodes of bronchospasm where rapid response is required. • Be sure that the patient uses the inhaler correctly. • Drug is largely free of systemic adverse effects.	• If accidentally sprayed into eyes, temporary blurring of vision may occur. • Safe and effective for patients with heart disease. • Enhances effects of sympathomimetics.
• May cause fatigue, dizziness, or anxiety. If these symptoms occur, stop treatment and allow patient to rest a few minutes; then resume therapy.	• May cause throat irritation or burning. If so, stop treatment and have the patient drink water; then resume therapy. • May cause bronchospasm or excessive coughing. Most patients use a bronchodilator before treatment to minimize bronchospasm.
• When changing from oral therapy to inhaled therapy, taper oral drug slowly to prevent acute adrenal insufficiency. • Tell the patient to inhale a bronchodilator several minutes before taking beclomethasone. • Have patient rinse his mouth with water after inhalations to prevent oral infections. Check his mouth regularly for signs of fungal infection.	• Keep inhaler clean and unobstructed. • Contraindicated in status asthmaticus. • Allow 1 minute to elapse before administering subsequent puffs of drug. Tell patient to hold his breath for a few seconds to enhance drug action.
• When changing from oral therapy to inhaled therapy, taper oral drug slowly to prevent acute adrenal insufficiency. • Use inhaled bronchodilators several minutes before taking dexamethasone. • Have patient rinse his mouth with water after inhalations to prevent oral infections. Check his mouth regularly for signs of fungal infection.	• Keep inhaler clean and unobstructed. • Contraindicated in status asthmaticus. • Allow 1 minute to elapse before administering subsequent puffs of drug. Tell patient to hold his breath for a few seconds to enhance drug action.
• Administer with nonreactive metal, glass, or plastic nebulizer. Don't use bulb nebulizers because particle size is too large and output too small. • Have the patient cough to clear airway before administration.	• Warn the patient that the drug smells like sulphur and may cause nausea or vomiting. • It is irritating to bronchial smooth muscle, so always give after a bronchodilator such as a beta-adrenergic agonist.
• Drug effects may take 2 to 3 weeks. • Effective only if used exactly as prescribed.	• Observe the patient for signs of fungal infection, which occurs rarely. • Be sure the patient uses the inhaler correctly.
• Use when conventional treatment, such as antihistamines or decongestants, fails. • For maximum effectiveness, use exactly as prescribed.	• Maximum effects may not occur for 2 to 3 weeks. • Be sure the patient uses the inhaler correctly and rinses it after each use.

(continued)

Giving common respiratory drugs *(continued)*

DRUG	INDICATIONS AND DOSAGE	MECHANISM OF ACTION
Sympathomimetics		
albuterol (Proventil, Ventolin)	Prevention and treatment of bronchospasm in patients with reversible obstructive airway disease. *Usual adult dosage:* (inhaler) one to two inhalations at 2-minute intervals every 4 to 6 hours; (nebulizer) 0.25 to 0.5 ml in 3 ml of 0.9% sodium chloride solution; prevention of exercise-induced asthma: two inhalations 15 minutes before exercise	Acts on beta$_2$-adrenergic receptors to relax bronchial smooth muscles
epinephrine (Bronkaid Mist, Medihaler-Epi, Primatene Mist)	Treatment of bronchospasm. *Usual adult dosage:* one to two inhalations every 1 to 5 minutes until relief occurs	Stimulates alpha- and beta-adrenergic receptors within the sympathetic nervous system; when inhaled, it acts primarily on beta receptors and the respiratory tract
metaproterenol sulfate (Alupent, Metaprel)	Treatment of acute episodes of bronchial asthma and reversible bronchospasm. *Usual adult dosage:* (inhaler) 2 to 3 inhalations every 3 to 4 hours, to a maximum of 12 inhalations daily; (nebulizer) 0.2 to 0.3 ml in 3 ml of 0.9% sodium chloride solution.	Relaxes bronchial smooth muscle by acting on beta$_2$ adrenergic receptors
Uncategorized drug		
cromolyn sodium (Intal, Nasalcrom)	Adjunct treatment for severe perennial bronchial asthma. *Usual adult dosage:* two metered sprays four times daily. Also available as an aqueous solution to be administered through a nebulizer. Prevention and treatment of allergic rhinitis. *Usual adult dosage:* one spray in each nostril three to four times daily, to a maximum of six times daily. Prevention of exercise-induced bronchospasm. *Usual adult dosage:* two metered sprays inhaled 1 hour before exercise.	Inhibits degranulation of sensitized mast cells that occurs after exposure to specific antigens; also inhibits release of histamine and slow-reacting substance of anaphylaxis

orally, but several inhalable steroids are also available. When inhaled, the drugs have a high topical potency and ease withdrawal from oral drugs—without causing the adverse effects of hyperadrenocorticism and adrenal suppression. Inhaled drugs also reduce airway reactivity. Two widely used inhaled steroids are triamcinolone acetonide (Kenalog) and beclomethasone dipropionate (Vanceril).

Respiratory stimulants

The usefulness of these stimulants has been under investigation for several years. Formerly, ethamivan (Emivan) and nikethamide (Coramine) were given because they stimulate the central nervous system to initiate respiration. Unfortunately, they also cause muscle twitching, sneezing, facial irritation, and anxiety. Carbonic anhydrase inhibitors may be beneficial,

especially in patients who are alkalotic from diuretic therapy. However, the carbonic anhydrase inhibitor acetazolamide (Diamox) proves ineffective for the patient whose blood pH is below 7.35.

Anticholinergics

Use of anticholinergics increased during the 1980s. Currently available anticholinergics include atropine sulfate and ipratropium bromide (Atrovent). When inhaled, these drugs inhibit cholinergics in the bronchial smooth muscle, producing bronchodilation. Then acetylcholine is blocked, reducing cyclic guanosine monophosphate (GMP), which normally acts as a bronchoconstricting agent.

Studies show that inhaled anticholinergics cause greater improvements in pulmonary function tests than sympathomimetics; how-

• Produces less cardiac stimulation than other sympathomimetics.
• Elderly patients may require a lower dosage.
• Be sure the patient uses the inhaler correctly.
• Allow 2 minutes between inhalations.
• Use cautiously in patients with hypertension, coronary artery disease (CAD), hyperthyroidism, and diabetes.
• Watch for paradoxical bronchospasm, and caution patient about this adverse effect.

• If patient is using a corticosteroid inhaler, tell him to use the bronchodilator first, then to wait 5 minutes before using the corticosteroid. This allows the bronchodilator to open air passages for maximum penetration of corticosteroid.

• Use with extreme caution in patients with heart disease resulting from chronic obstructive pulmonary disease.

• Don't mix with alkaline solutions.
• Use cautiously in patients with hypertension, CAD, hyperthyroidism, and diabetes.

• Use cautiously in patients with hypertension, CAD, hyperthyroidism, and diabetes.
• Allow 2 minutes between inhalations.
• Warn the patient that the drug can cause paradoxical bronchospasm.

• If patient is using a corticosteroid inhaler, tell him to use the bronchodilator first, then to wait 5 minutes before using the corticosteroid. This allows the bronchodilator to open air passages for maximum penetration of corticosteroid.

• Contraindicated in acute asthma attacks.
• Remind the patient that the drug is most effective with continued use. It may not exhibit maximum effectiveness for 6 to 8 weeks of daily therapy.

• Be sure the patient uses the inhaler correctly.

ever, using these two types of drugs together increases bronchodilation. (Sympathomimetics have a more rapid onset and are given first.) Anticholinergics are administered with a hand-held nebulizer (atropine) or a metered-dose inhaler (ipratropium bromide).

Antibiotics
Acquired immunodeficiency syndrome (AIDS) has prompted an increased use of inhaled antibiotics. Pentamidine isethionate (Pentam 300), an antiprotozoal drug, is commonly used with tobramycin (Tobrex) for the prophylaxis and treatment of *Pneumocystis carinii* pneumonia.

Mast-cell stabilizers
These drugs appear to prevent mediator release from mast cells of histamine and slow-

reacting substance of anaphylaxis. Most mast-cell stabilizers are used to manage asthma. They have no bronchodilator, antihistamine, or anti-inflammatory activity. Several weeks of therapy are usually required before the severity of asthma symptoms decreases noticeably. The most common adverse effects of these drugs include throat irritation, cough, wheezing, and nausea.

Oxygen
Oxygen therapy has been used for many years to treat advanced chronic obstructive pulmonary disease (COPD) and other disorders. In COPD, low-flow oxygen (1 to 2 liters/minute) for at least 15 hours a day decreases the number of hospitalizations and improves the patient's quality of life.

Oxygen delivery is categorized two ways.

Low-flow oxygen meets the patient's inspiratory demand via nasal cannula or oxygen mask. High-flow oxygen meets or exceeds the patient's inspiratory demand and supplies an exact percentage of oxygen via a Venturi mask or high concentration of oxygen via partial rebreather or nonrebreather mask.

Nasal inhalation

Drugs may be inhaled through the nose into the respiratory system via a device that delivers a spray (nasal inhaler) or an aerosol (nasal nebulizer). These delivery methods diffuse drugs throughout the nasal passages, with most drugs producing local rather than systemic effects. Only small doses are needed for maximum benefit.

Most nasal drugs, such as phenylephrine (Neo-Synephrine), are vasoconstrictors that relieve nasal congestion by coating and shrinking swollen mucous membranes. Because vasoconstriction occurs rapidly, few systemic adverse effects occur.

Other types of nasal drugs include antiseptics, anesthetics, and corticosteroids. Local anesthetics may be administered to decrease discomfort during nose and throat examinations, laryngoscopy, bronchoscopy, and endotracheal intubation. Corticosteroids reduce inflammation in allergic or inflammatory conditions and in nasal polyps. Adrenergic agonists and epinephrine are used to relieve swelling of the larynx and subglottic area.

Equipment
You'll use a hand-held inhaler to administer a nasal spray, and a hand-held nebulizer to administer a nasal aerosol. Both devices deliver a metered dose of the drug.

Before administering a nasal spray or aerosol, gather the following equipment: the prescribed drug, a nasal inhaler (if giving a spray) or a nasal nebulizer (if giving an aerosol), facial tissues, 0.9% sodium chloride solution, and an emesis basin.

Drug administration
You'll administer a nasal spray or an aerosol at the patient's bedside. (If his condition permits, he can be taught to give himself the drug.) You'll use different techniques to administer each type of drug.

Nasal spray
To administer a nasal spray, first have the patient gently blow his nose to clear his nostrils of mucus. Wash your hands. Then shake the medication cartridge and insert it into the adapter. (When inserting a refill cartridge, first remove the protective cap from the stem.) Remove the protective cap from the adapter tip.

Hold the inhaler with your index finger on top of the cartridge and your thumb under the nasal adapter. The adapter tip should be pointing toward the patient.

Have the patient tilt his head back. Place the adapter tip into one nostril, pointing away from the septum, while occluding the other nostril with your finger.

Instruct the patient to inhale gently while you press the adapter and the cartridge together firmly to release a measured dose of the drug. Be sure to follow the manufacturer's instructions. With some drugs, such as dexamethasone sodium phosphate (Decadron Turbinaire), inhaling during administration isn't desirable. Tell the patient to exhale through his mouth.

If ordered, spray the nostril again. Then shake the inhaler, and repeat the procedure in the other nostril.

Instruct the patient to keep his head tilted back for several minutes and to breathe slowly through his nose so the drug has time to work. Tell him not to blow his nose for several minutes.

Have the patient gargle with 0.9% sodium chloride solution to remove medication from the mouth and throat and expectorate the solution into the emesis basin. Use a facial tissue to wipe any excess medication from his nostrils and face.

Remove the medication cartridge from the nasal inhaler, and wash the nasal adapter in lukewarm water.

Nasal aerosol

To administer a nasal aerosol, first instruct the patient to blow his nose gently to clear his nostrils of mucus.

Insert the medication cartridge according to the manufacturer's directions. With some models, you'll fit the cartridge over a small hole in the adapter. When inserting a refill cartridge, first remove the protective cap from the stem.

Shake the aerosol well immediately before each use, and remove the protective cap from the adapter tip. Hold the aerosol between your thumb and index finger with your index finger positioned on top of the medication cartridge.

Tilt the patient's head back, and carefully insert the adapter tip in one nostril while sealing the other nostril with your finger. Press the adapter and cartridge together firmly to release one measured dose of the drug. Shake the aerosol and repeat the procedure to instill the drug into the other nostril.

Have the patient gargle with 0.9% sodium chloride solution to remove medication from the mouth and throat and expectorate the solution into the emesis basin. Use a facial tissue to wipe any excess medication from his nostrils and face.

Remove the medication cartridge and wash the nasal adapter in lukewarm water daily. Allow the adapter to dry thoroughly before reinserting the cartridge.

Complications

Potential complications result from the particular drug being given, not from the route of administration. Some nasal drugs may cause restlessness, palpitations, nervousness, and other systemic effects. For example, excessive use of corticosteroid aerosols may cause hyperadrenocorticism and adrenal suppression.

Nursing considerations

• To prevent the spread of infection, label the medication bottle so it will be used only for that patient.
• Record the medication instilled, its concentration, the number of instillations, and whether it was given in one or both nostrils. Also note the time, date, and any adverse effects.

• Never puncture or incinerate a pressurized aerosol cartridge. Store the medication cartridge at temperatures below 120° F (48.9° C).

Patient teaching

Teach the patient how to instill nasal drugs correctly so he can continue treatment after discharge, if necessary.

Caution the patient against using these drugs longer than prescribed because they may cause his condition to worsen. Explain that this rebound effect occurs when the drug loses its effectiveness and relaxes the vessels in the nasal turbinates, producing stuffiness that can be relieved only by discontinuing the drug.

Inform the patient of possible adverse reactions. If he's taking aerosol corticosteroids, explain that therapeutic effects may not appear for up to 2 weeks.

Instruct the patient to store the inhaler or nebulizer in a plastic bag to keep it clean. Tell him to remove the medication cartridge once a day and rinse the plastic adapter thoroughly with warm water.

Oral inhalation

Some respiratory drugs may be inhaled through the mouth into the respiratory system. The most common oral inhalation devices include metered-dose inhalers, compressed air or oxygen nebulizers, and turbo-inhalers. These hand-held devices deliver topical drugs to the respiratory tract, producing local and systemic effects. They use air under pressure to create a mist containing tiny droplets of the drug. The droplets travel deep into the lungs and are absorbed by the mucosal lining almost immediately. As with the nasal route, small doses of orally inhaled drugs can provide maximum benefit with few adverse effects.

Oral inhalers may be contraindicated in patients who can't form an airtight seal around the device, and in those who lack the coordination and clear vision necessary to assemble a turbo-inhaler. Contraindications may also exist for specific inhalant drugs.

Equipment

Each oral inhalation device uses different equipment. A metered-dose inhaler contains a disposable, pressurized canister of the drug with a Freon propellant. The canister holds drugs in liquid or powder form, and these drugs are propelled from the canister and inhaled into the bronchioles. An attachment called an extender (or spacer) may be used with children or patients who have coordination problems and cannot inhale efficiently.

An oral nebulizer is powered by an air compressor or attached by a connecting tube to an oxygen outlet. It delivers a measured aerosolized spray of the drug.

Instead of a drug canister, a turbo-inhaler holds capsules that, when punctured, release the drug into the respiratory system.

Metered-dose inhaler

Before drug administration, gather the following equipment: a metered-dose inhaler (consisting of a mouthpiece and cap), the prescribed drug (contained in a disposable medication canister with an adapter), an extender (if indicated), 0.9% sodium chloride solution, facial tissues, and an emesis basin.

Oral nebulizer

To use this device, you'll need the following equipment: an oral nebulizer (consisting of a mouthpiece, T-adapter, corrugated tubing reservoir, nebulizer cup, and connecting tube); an air compressor; the prescribed drug; 0.9% sodium chloride solution; facial tissues; and an emesis basin.

Turbo-inhaler

Before administering the drug, gather this equipment: a turbo-inhaler (consisting of a mouthpiece, a sleeve, and a can); prescribed drug capsules; 0.9% sodium chloride solution; facial tissues; and an emesis basin.

Drug administration

You'll administer drugs at the patient's bedside. Each oral inhalation device requires a different administration technique.

Metered-dose inhaler

To use a metered-dose inhaler, first remove the cap from the mouthpiece and from the extender attachment, if you're using one. Insert the metal stem on the canister into the small hole on the flattened portion of the mouthpiece. If you're using an extender, insert the canister into the end of the attachment opposite the mouthpiece. Then turn the canister upside down. Shake the inhaler to mix the drug and aerosol propellant.

Tell the patient to exhale normally and hold his breath. Then place the mouthpiece well into his mouth and have him close his lips around it. Tell him not to block the opening of the inhaler with his tongue or teeth.

Instruct the patient to begin a slow, deep inhalation through his mouth. At the same time, depress the metal canister once. Inhaling slowly and deeply draws the drug into the lungs and ensures maximum drug delivery. Check to see if mist or vapor is escaping from the patient's mouth; if so, repeat the procedure.

Remove the mouthpiece from the patient's mouth and tell him to hold his breath for 5 to 10 seconds to allow the drug to reach the alveoli. Then tell him to exhale slowly through his nose or pursed lips.

If you're using an extender, have the patient inhale once or twice to ensure that all the drug is used. (See *Using an extender attachment.*)

If another puff is ordered, wait 1 to 3 minutes (2 to 3 minutes if an extender is used). Then repeat the procedure.

Have the patient gargle with 0.9% sodium chloride solution to remove medication from the mouth and throat and expectorate the solution into the emesis basin. Use a facial tissue to wipe any excess medication from his nostrils and face.

Oral nebulizer

To administer drugs with an oral nebulizer, first wash your hands thoroughly. Then twist off the nebulizer cup from the nebulizer, T-adapter, and mouthpiece. Place the ordered amount of the drug in the nebulizer cup. (See *Giving drugs with an oral nebulizer,* page 160.)

ADVANCED EQUIPMENT

Using an extender attachment

Children or older patients with coordination problems often have trouble using metered-dose inhalers. They may inhale drug particles inefficiently, or larger particles may be deposited in the mouth or throat instead of in the respiratory tract. For such patients, the addition of an extender, or spacer, attachment may make the inhaler easier to use.

Newer models, such as the Inspir-Ease extender shown at right, provide more dead-air space for mixing medication and have a reservoir bag that keeps the aerosolized drug suspended in the air for several seconds after activation of the inhaler. This provides more effective inhalation and ensures that the larger particles are deposited in the respiratory tract, not in the mouth or throat.

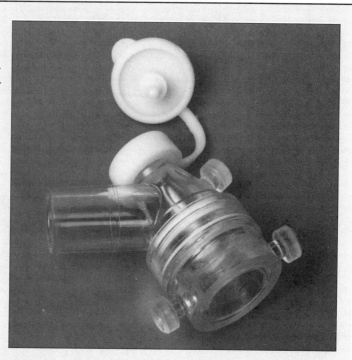

Next, reconnect the nebulizer and the nebulizer cup. Attach one end of the connecting tube to the nebulizer cup and the other end to the air compressor outlet or oxygen outlet.

Turn the power switch for the air compressor or oxygen to "on." You should see a fine mist of the drug escaping through the mouthpiece.

Place the mouthpiece between the patient's teeth and instruct him to close his lips tightly around it to form a seal. Tell him to inhale slowly through the mouthpiece and hold his breath for 2 to 3 seconds before exhaling. If the patient is dyspneic, instruct him to take a deep breath and hold it for 5 to 10 seconds every four to five breaths. The inspiratory hold allows for greater aerosol deposition in the lower respiratory tract and prevents hyperventilation, tingling in the fingers, and light-headedness.

Continue this procedure until all the drug is inhaled. Periodically tap the side of the nebulizer cup during the treatment to release particles clinging to the side.

Have the patient gargle with 0.9% sodium chloride solution and expectorate the solution into an emesis basin. Use facial tissues to remove excess drug from his mouth and face.

After completing the treatment, rinse the used equipment in warm water and allow it to air dry on a clean towel.

Turbo-inhaler

Hold the mouthpiece in one hand, and with the other hand, slide the sleeve away from the mouthpiece as far as possible. Unscrew the tip of the mouthpiece by turning it counterclockwise.

Firmly press the colored portion of the drug capsule into the propeller stem of the

Giving drugs with an oral nebulizer

An oral nebulizer delivers small, measured doses of medication through the mouth and into the respiratory tract. It can either be powered by an air compressor or plugged into an oxygen outlet in the patient's room. As shown in the illustration at right, the patient places her lips firmly around the mouthpiece. She inhales slowly through the mouthpiece and holds her breath for 2 to 3 seconds before exhaling.

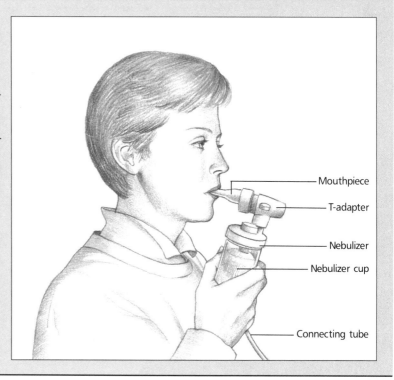

Mouthpiece

T-adapter

Nebulizer

Nebulizer cup

Connecting tube

mouthpiece. Screw the inhaler together again securely.

Holding the inhaler with the mouthpiece at the bottom, slide the sleeve all the way down and then up again to puncture the capsule and release the drug. Do this only once.

Have the patient exhale completely and tilt his head back. Then place the mouthpiece in his mouth, and tell him to close his lips around it and inhale once — quickly and deeply. Instruct the patient to hold his breath for 5 to 10 seconds to allow the drug to reach the alveoli. Tell him not to exhale through the mouthpiece. Remove the inhaler from the patient's mouth, and tell him to exhale as much air as possible.

Repeat the procedure until all the drug in the device is inhaled. Then, have the patient gargle with 0.9% sodium chloride solution and expectorate the solution into an emesis basin. Use facial tissues to remove any excess drug from his mouth and face.

Discard the empty drug capsule, put the inhaler in its can, and secure the lid. Rinse the inhaler with warm water at least once a week.

Complications

Potential complications result from the particular drug being given, not from the route of administration. Some oral respiratory drugs may cause restlessness, palpitations, nervousness, and other systemic effects. They can also cause hypersensitivity reactions such as rash, urticaria, or bronchospasm.

Administer oral respiratory drugs cautiously to patients with heart disease because these drugs may potentiate coronary insufficiency, cardiac arrhythmias, or hypertension. If paradoxical bronchospasm occurs, discontinue the drug and call the doctor. He'll prescribe another drug.

Nursing considerations

• To prevent the spread of infection, label the drug bottle so it will be used only for that patient.
• If the patient hears a whistling sound through his extender, he's inhaling too quickly.
• Record the drug instilled, its concentration, the number of instillations and, with metered-dose inhalers, whether oxygen or compressed air was used. Also note the time, date, and any adverse effects.
• When using an aerosol, be careful not to puncture or incinerate the pressurized cartridge. Store it at temperatures below 120° F (48.9° C).

Patient teaching

Teach the patient to administer drugs himself so he'll stay symptom-free after discharge. Instruct him to take the drug only as ordered. Taking more than the prescribed amount can lead to a tolerance of the drug so it no longer provides adequate symptom relief. If appropriate, also teach him to determine how much drug is left in a used drug canister. (See *How full is the canister?*)

Teach the patient how to care for his drug administration equipment. If the patient is too tired or dyspneic to clean his equipment every day, advise him to clean it only once a week. A once-a-week cleaning doesn't increase the infection rate. However, the patient who's pressed to clean too often may neglect to clean at all, increasing his chance of infection.

If the patient is using an oral nebulizer, instruct him to soak the nebulizer parts weekly in a vinegar and water solution for 10 to 20 minutes; then rinse with clean water and allow to air dry. Equipment should be replaced monthly or more often, depending on how frequently it's used.

If the patient is using a turbo-inhaler, show him how to take it apart and rinse it thoroughly with warm water. It should be completely dry before reassembling. Tell him to prevent capsules from deteriorating by leaving them wrapped until needed. Instruct him to put the entire inhaler in a plastic bag to keep it clean. He should also remove the drug car-

How full is the canister?

If your patient doesn't know how to estimate the amount of medication left in a canister, he'll end up with a collection of partially used canisters. Here's an easy method to teach him how to avoid this problem at home.

Remove the inhaler canister from the plastic sleeve and place it in a large container or sink filled with water. If the canister is full, it will sink to the bottom of the container. If the canister is three-quarters full, it will float upside down near the bottom. If it floats upside down and extends one-quarter of the way out of the water, it's one-half full. If it leans toward the surface of the water, it's one-quarter full. If it floats almost horizontally, the canister is empty.

Tell the patient to refill his prescription or to contact the doctor for a renewal when the canister is one-quarter full.

tridge once a day and thoroughly rinse the plastic adapter with warm water.

Endotracheal administration

When an I.V. line isn't readily available, drugs can be administered into the respiratory system through an endotracheal tube. This route allows uninterrupted resuscitation efforts and avoids such complications as coronary artery laceration, cardiac tamponade, or pneumothorax, which can occur when emergency drugs are given intracardially.

When giving drugs by this route, remember that the duration of action is usually longer than if the drug were given I.V. This is due to sustained absorption in the alveoli. So you'll need to adjust repeat doses and continuous infusions to prevent adverse effects. Drugs commonly given by this route include naloxone

Administering endotracheal drugs

In an emergency, some drugs may be given through an endotracheal tube if I.V. access isn't available. They may be given using the syringe method or the adapter method. Before injecting any drug, however, check for proper placement of the endotracheal tube.

Checking tube placement
With your stethoscope, check placement of the endotracheal tube, as shown below. Make sure the patient is supine and the head is level with or slightly higher than the trunk.

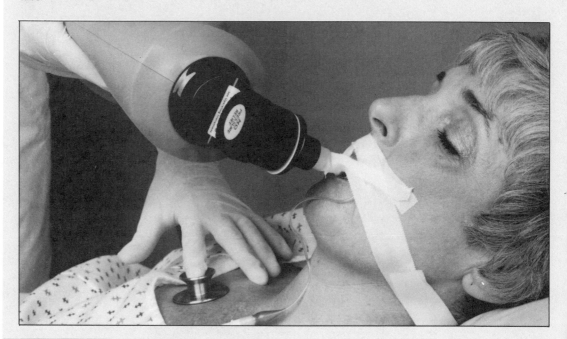

(Narcan), atropine, diazepam (Valium), epinephrine (Adrenalin), and lidocaine (Xylocaine solution 4%).

Equipment
Before drug administration, collect the following equipment: an endotracheal tube, gloves, stethoscope, hand-held resuscitation bag, ordered drug, syringe, and sterile water or 0.9% sodium chloride solution.

Drug administration
Endotracheal drugs are usually given in emergency situations by a doctor, emergency medi-

cal technician, or critical care nurse. Although guidelines may vary depending on state, county, or city regulations, the basic administration method is the same. (See *Administering endotracheal drugs.*)

To give drugs through an endotracheal tube, first put on gloves. Check tube placement by using a hand-held resuscitation bag and stethoscope. Now, move the patient into the supine position with his head level with or slightly higher than his trunk.

Calculate the drug dose. Adult Advanced Cardiac Life Support guidelines recommend that drugs be administered at 2 to 2½ times the recommended I.V. dose.

Using the syringe method
Remove the needle before injecting medication into the endotracheal tube. Insert the tip of the syringe into the endotracheal tube, and inject the drug deep into the tube, as shown at right.

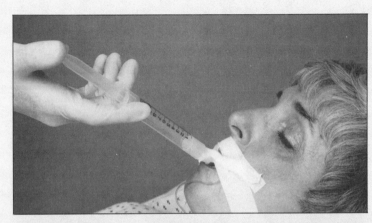

Adapter method
A recently developed device for endotracheal drug administration, shown at right, provides a more closed system of drug delivery than the syringe method. A special adapter placed on the end of the endotracheal tube allows needle insertion and drug delivery through the closed stopcock.

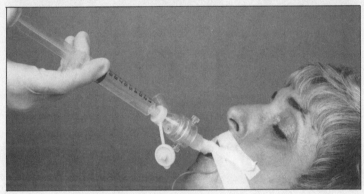

Ventilate the patient three to five times with the resuscitation bag. Remove the bag.

Remove the needle from the syringe. Insert the tip of the syringe into the endotracheal tube. Inject the drug deep into the tube.

After injecting the drug, reattach the resuscitation bag and ventilate the patient briskly, five or six times. This propels the drug into the lungs, oxygenates the patient, and clears the tube. Prevent drug reflux by briefly placing your thumb over the tube opening.

An endotracheal drug device offers an alternative to a syringe for delivering endotracheal drugs. Usually used for bronchoscopy suctioning, this swivel adapter can be placed on the end of the tube, and while ventilation continues through a bag-valve device, the drug can be delivered with a needle through the closed stopcock.

Complications
Potential complications would result from the prescribed drug, not the administration route.

Nursing considerations
• Document the drug administration procedure and monitor the patient's response.
• Be prepared: The drug's onset of action may be quicker than it would be by I.V. administration. If the patient doesn't respond quickly, the doctor may order a repeat dose.

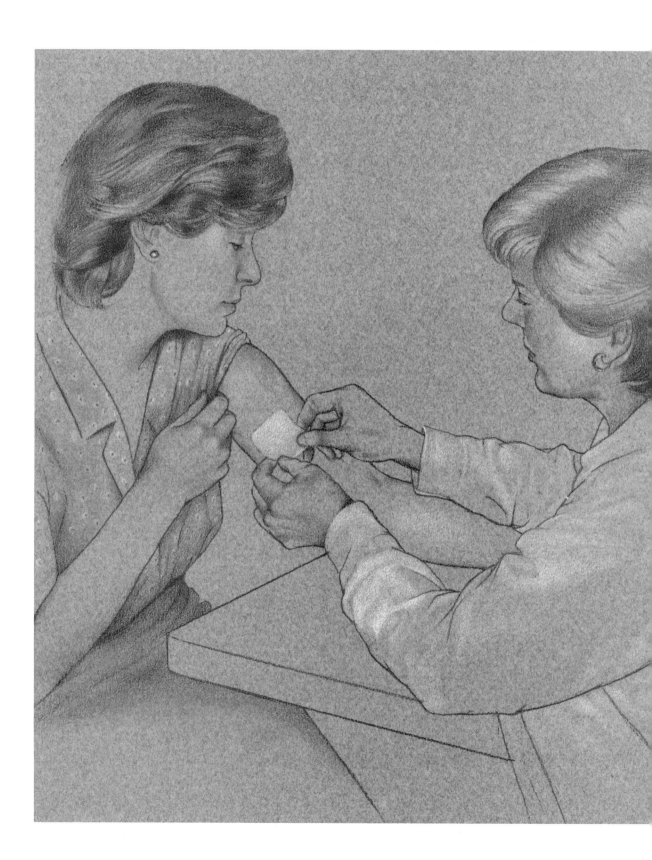

CHAPTER 8

Giving drugs through the skin

Technological advances have greatly expanded the possibilities for giving drugs through the skin. In the past, dermal drug delivery was limited to creams and ointments. But new methods have been developed for administering drugs across the skin layers, both subdermally and subcutaneously.

As you use these drug delivery methods, you'll find they provide accurate doses to better meet your patient's needs. And these methods are fairly simple to use—once you know how. Frequently, the patient or caregiver himself can use the delivery method or monitor the dose.

This chapter covers the newest and most advanced forms of drug delivery: the transdermal patch or disk; subdermal, radiation, and subcutaneous implants; and subcutaneous infusion. For each delivery method, you'll find an overview of essential information. Next comes a discussion of the equipment you'll need, followed by an explanation of drug administration. Then you'll find complications, nursing considerations, and patient-teaching information.

Before covering the drug delivery methods, however, the chapter reviews the skin's anatomy and physiology and explains how drugs are absorbed from the skin layers.

Anatomy and physiology

The body's largest organ, the skin consists of two layers: the outer layer of stratified squamous epithelium, called the epidermis, and the inner layer, or dermis. The epidermis serves as a protective barrier against mechanical injury and foreign material and prevents loss of tissue fluid. The dermis harbors the superficial blood vessels, cutaneous nerves, sweat glands, sebaceous glands, and hair follicles—all held together by connective tissue. Regulation of body temperature (thermoregulation) and participation in the inflammatory process are two key functions of the superficial vascular network.

During resting conditions, the skin receives about 8% of the cardiac output through a highly resistant vascular bed. With hypotension or blood loss, blood flow to the skin diminishes and the skin becomes cold and clammy. When body temperature rises, the blood vessels in the hands, feet, and face dilate. The resulting fall in total peripheral resistance causes a rise in cardiac output. The resulting increase in skin blood flow enhances heat exchange between the blood and external environment.

Pharmacologic principles

With the newer delivery methods, drugs can be delivered at a controlled rate over a specific duration. The absorption rate depends on the method and on the skin area used. The skin's structure makes it an ideal distribution site for many drugs.

Drug delivery
With the transdermal method, the drug contained in an adhesive patch or disk penetrates the stratum corneum, or outer layers of the epidermis, by passive diffusion. After penetrating the dermis, the drug is absorbed into the systemic circulation during a plateau phase of sustained release from the adhesive patch or disk. Drugs that are available in transdermal patches and disks include clonidine, estradiol, nitroglycerin, scopolamine, fentanyl, and nicotine. (See *Understanding transdermal drug delivery*.)

In subdermal drug delivery, the drug is enclosed in a flexible capsule that is inserted below the dermis in an area having an extensive superficial network of arterioles, capillaries, and venules. A continuous low dose of the drug gradually diffuses through the capsule wall.

Radiation implant therapy, or brachytherapy, destroys malignant cells or curtails their growth. Encapsulated in small pellets, needles, or sutures, implants of radioactive isotopes deliver ionizing radiation within a body cavity or interstitially near or within tumor tissue. Radiation implants deliver a continuous radiation dose over several hours or days, minimizing exposure to adjacent tissues.

In subcutaneous implant therapy, a drug pellet is placed in the subcutaneous tissue. Subcutaneous infusion, another form of therapy, delivers a continuous dose of a drug such as heparin, insulin, or an opioid. Here, the skin is pierced with a needle that's fixed in the subcutaneous tissue. The drug is then delivered continuously and directly into connective tissue or fat, away from bone and major blood vessels. A subcutaneous infusion allows slower, more sustained drug absorption than a subcutaneous implant, and it causes minimal tissue trauma. It also carries minimal risk of trauma to large blood vessels and nerves.

Transdermal drug delivery

This delivery method ensures a constant blood level of a drug. Thus, unlike the oral and parenteral routes, the transdermal route reduces the risk of adverse effects caused by a high blood level of a drug, such as aminophylline,

Understanding transdermal drug delivery

This illustration shows how medication from a transdermal skin patch diffuses passively through the outer layers of the epidermis and penetrates the dermis. Note the route that medication takes from the skin surface to the bloodstream.

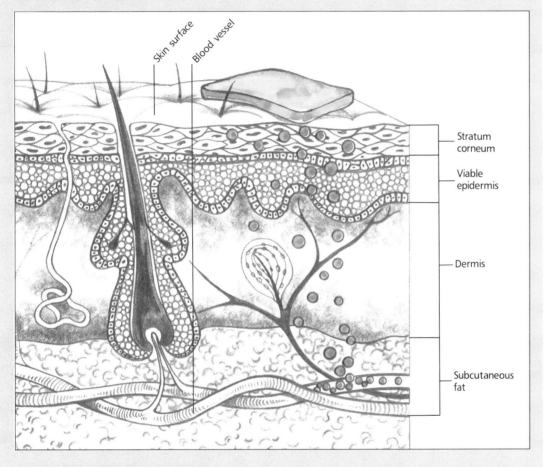

Skin surface

Blood vessel

Stratum corneum

Viable epidermis

Dermis

Subcutaneous fat

which can cause palpitations, sinus tachycardia, dizziness, and seizures.

Transdermal drug delivery has some disadvantages, however. Often, the onset of action is slow. Several hours may elapse between the time you apply the patch or disk and the time a steady blood level is achieved. What's more, a patch or disk may be easily bumped and dislodged. And, finally, reversing the toxic effects of transdermal drugs may be difficult. (See *Reviewing transdermal drugs,* pages 168 and 169.)

Equipment

Before applying a disk or patch, make sure you have the patient's medication record and chart. Besides the prescribed disk or patch, you'll also need to gather adhesive tape, a transparent semipermeable dressing, and disposable gloves.

Reviewing transdermal drugs

DRUG	INDICATIONS AND DOSAGE	MECHANISM OF ACTION
clonidine (Catapres)	Treatment of moderate hypertension. *Usual adult dosage:* 0.1-, 0.2-, or 0.3-mg patch once every 7 days.	Central-acting sympathetic nervous system inhibitor reduces sympathetic activity and thus decreases arteriolar constriction. Absorbed well from the skin, distributed widely, metabolized in the liver, and excreted primarily in the liver.
estradiol (Estrace)	Estrogen replacement therapy. *Usual adult dosage:* 0.05 to 0.1 mg/day.	Estrogens are absorbed well and distributed throughout the body. Metabolism occurs in the liver, and the metabolites are excreted primarily by the kidneys. Drug increases the synthesis of deoxyribonucleic acid, ribonucleic acid, and protein in responsive tissues. It also reduces release of follicle-stimulating and luteinizing hormones from the pituitary gland.
nitroglycerin (Nitrodisc, Nitro-dur, Transderm Nitro)	Angina prophylaxis. *Usual adult dosage:* once daily.	Nitrates diminish preload and myocardial oxygen demand by dilating veins. They decrease afterload and may increase myocardial oxygen supply by dilating arteries. In coronary circulation, nitrates redistribute the circulating blood flow, thereby improving myocardial perfusion.
scopolamine (Transderm-Scōp)	Prevention of nausea and vomiting related to motion. *Usual adult dosage:* one patch for 3 days.	Cholinergic blocking agent that blocks action of acetylcholine at muscarinic receptors in the parasympathetic nervous system. Absorbed more readily and distributed more widely in the body than other anticholinergics. Scopolamine crosses the blood-brain barrier and strongly affects the eye and its secretory glands. Drug binds with serum proteins, is metabolized in the liver by hydrolysis, and is excreted by the kidneys as unchanged drug and metabolites.
fentanyl (Duragesic)	Management of chronic pain. *Usual adult dosage:* one patch every 3 days.	Distributed widely throughout the body. Drug has a relatively low plasma protein-binding capacity. Metabolized extensively in the liver; metabolites excreted by the kidneys. Small amount excreted in the feces via the biliary tract. Drug binds with opiate receptors at many sites in the CNS—brain, brain stem, and spinal cord—altering both perception of and emotional response to pain through an unknown mechanism.
nicotine (Nicoderm, ProStep, Habitrol, Nicotrol)	Smoking cessation. *Usual adult dosage:* one patch daily; start with 21 mg/day and taper to 7 mg/day.	Absorbed well and distributed widely. Metabolized in the liver and excreted in the urine. Drug stimulates receptors in the CNS and causes the release of catecholamines from the adrenal medulla.

Drug administration

Open the package and remove the patch or disk. Without touching the adhesive surface, remove the clear plastic backing. Then apply the patch or disk to a dry, clean, hairless area. Depending on patch size, select an appropriate site, such as the upper arm, chest, back, or the area behind the ear.

Complications

Skin irritation, such as pruritus or a rash, is perhaps the most common complication of transdermal delivery. The patient may also suffer other adverse reactions from the drug. For instance, transdermal nitroglycerin may cause headaches and, in the elderly patient, postural hypotension. Scopolamine produces various un-

NURSING CONSIDERATIONS

• An erythematous, pruritic rash develops beneath the patch in 12% to 50% of patients. Use aerosolized beclomethasone as preventive treatment for rash.
• Monitor patient's blood pressure. Dermatitis may impair absorption and lead to rebound hypertension.

• Observe for rare adverse reactions, such as nausea, fatigue, headache, nervousness, and orthostatic symptoms.
• Apply to a hairless area of intact skin on the upper arm or torso.

• Use estrogen cautiously in smokers and women with an increased metabolic rate because they metabolize estrogen more rapidly than normal.
• Drug poses risks of endometrial cancer, gallbladder disease, thromboembolic disease, hepatic adenoma, and hypertension.

• Check for redness and irritation at the site, genitourinary changes, headache, and dizziness.
• Teach diabetic patients to report elevated blood glucose levels so that antidiabetic dosage can be adjusted.
• Teach women to perform regular breast self-examinations.

• Patient will develop tolerance to the drug.
• Erythema may develop under the patch because the drug is a vasodilator. Rotate application sites.

• Observe patient for headaches and hypotension.
• Remove the patch before defibrillation.

• Advise patient to apply the patch 12 hours before experiencing motion.
• Teach him to apply the patch to postauricular area to enhance absorption.
• Caution patient to wash hands after applying the patch. Otherwise, he may touch his eye, causing pupil dilation.

• Warn patient against driving until central nervous system (CNS) effects are known. These may include hallucinations, agitation, drowsiness, confusion, dry mouth, and visual disturbances.

• Use only in patients who can tolerate opioids. Drug is contraindicated in patients who've received monoamine oxidase inhibitors within 14 days and those who have myasthenia gravis.
• When converting from I.V., I.M., or oral morphine, calculate dose based on equianalgesic conversion table.
• Instruct patients not to shave skin before patch application because the absorption ratio can be altered.
• Observe patient for lethargy, decreased level of consciousness, decreased respiratory rate, hyperventilation,

hypotension, urinary retention, nausea, vomiting, constipation, confusion, and somnolence.
• Dispose of patch according to hospital guidelines.
• Monitor patient for 12 to 17 hours after discontinuing the patch because the drug's blood levels decline gradually. Some patients may experience pain after 48 hours and will need a new patch.
• Make sure oral and injectable opioids are available for breakthrough pain.

• This drug delays healing in patients with peptic ulcer disease.
• Teach patient to rotate skin sites.

• Advise patient to keep used and unused patches out of the reach of children. Tell patient to handle the patch carefully to avoid unnecessary contact with drug.

---

toward effects, including dry mouth and drowsiness. Transdermal estradiol raises the risk of endometrial cancer, thromboembolic disease, and birth defects. Clonidine may cause severe rebound hypertension, especially if withdrawn suddenly.

Nursing considerations
• Apply the patch or disk at the same time each day to ensure consistent therapeutic effects. Apply a new patch about 30 minutes before removing an old one.
• Apply the patch or disk to unbroken, hairless skin. Clip hair at the application site. (Shaving alters the skin's integrity and allows the drug

Avoiding problems with transdermal delivery

With some precautions, a patient may avoid problems with his transdermal patch or disk. Advise him not to touch the gel because medication may rub off onto his fingers. Remind him to wash his hands after application to remove medication that may have rubbed off inadvertently. To avoid skin irritation, remind him to use a different site for each application. To avoid uneven absorption, he shouldn't place the patch or disk on a skin fold, scar, callus, or any irritated or damaged skin area.

to penetrate too fast.)
• Document the time of administration, the drug, the dose, and the initial application site. Also document any adverse reactions, such as postural hypotension or a headache.

Patient teaching
Talk with your patient before you apply the first patch or disk and make sure he understands the benefits and risks. The patient or his caregiver may be in charge of applying the new patches or disks and removing the old ones after discharge. So make sure the appropriate person knows how to apply the patch or disk. Also make sure he knows the appropriate skin areas to use. Remind him to wash his hands after application to remove any medication that may have rubbed off. (See *Avoiding problems with transdermal delivery*.)

Warn your patient not to allow the patch or disk to get wet. If it leaks or falls off, he should discard it, clean the site, and apply a new patch or disk at a new site.

Instruct the patient or caregiver to apply the patch or disk at the same time of day and at the prescribed interval. Bedtime application is ideal because of diminished body movement during the night.

If your patient will be wearing a scopolamine patch or disk, instruct him not to drive or operate machinery until his response to the

drug has been evaluated. Warn a patient wearing a clonidine patch or disk to check with his doctor before using any over-the-counter cough or cold preparations because they may counteract clonidine's effects.

Subdermal implants

When placed under the skin, these flexible capsules can't break or migrate in the body. Explain to the patient that bumping the area or putting pressure on it won't harm the capsules. Once the drug implants lose their effectiveness, they should be removed.

Levonorgestrel (Norplant System), a synthetic hormone used as a long-term contraceptive, is the drug most commonly administered by this method. Small silastic capsules filled with the hormone are inserted just under the skin of the patient's upper arm in a fanlike pattern. The drug then diffuses through the capsule walls continuously, with an average daily dose of 30 mcg. The blood level maintained with levonorgestrel capsules suppresses ovulation in most women and makes the cervical mucus thick and viscous, preventing sperm penetration into the cervical canal.

The procedure for inserting a subdermal implant can be performed by a doctor with a nurse assisting him, or by a specially trained nurse.

Equipment
Before the doctor begins the insertion procedure, you should gather the equipment he'll need. Make sure you have sterile surgical drapes, sterile gloves, antiseptic solution, and a local anesthetic. The doctor will also need a set of implants, needles, syringe, scalpel (#11), trocar (#10), forceps, sutures, sterile gauze, and tape.

Drug administration
Before the procedure, tell the patient what will happen and let her see a set of implants. Also explain to her the benefits and risks of the procedure. Then assist her into a supine position on the examination table. Stay with her

during the procedure and provide support as necessary.

After anesthetizing the upper portion of the nondominant arm, the doctor will use a trocar to insert each capsule through a 2-mm incision. After positioning the capsules correctly, he'll remove the trocar and palpate the area. He'll then close the incision and cover it with a dry compress and sterile gauze. (See *Inserting subdermal implants,* pages 172 and 173.)

Complications
Possible complications of levonorgestrel include hyperpigmentation at the insertion site, menstrual irregularities, headache, nervousness, nausea, dizziness, adnexal enlargement, dermatitis, acne, appetite changes, weight changes, mastalgia, hirsutism, and alopecia. Some women suffer more serious reactions, including breast abnormalities and mammographic changes; diabetes; elevated cholesterol or triglyceride levels; hypertension; seizures; depression; or gallbladder, heart, or kidney disease.

Nursing considerations
Document the name of the drug, the insertion site, the date and time of insertion, and the patient's response to the procedure. Also note the date the implants should be removed and a new set inserted.

Patient teaching
Explain the procedure to the patient and tell her how long it will take. Explain that the procedure is painless except for the injection of the local anesthetic. Make sure she understands that the incision leaves a small scar.

Tell the patient that after the implantation she can resume her normal activities, although she should use extra caution during the first few days. Advise her not to bump the insertion site and to keep the area dry and covered with a gauze bandage for 3 days. Also tell her not to smoke after the implants are in place. Smoking increases the risk of serious cardiovascular adverse effects from implanted as well as oral contraceptives.

Tell the patient to report severe lower abdominal pain, heavy vaginal bleeding, arm pain, or signs of bleeding or infection at the insertion site. She should also call the doctor or nurse if a capsule is expelled or if episodes of migraine, severe headache, or delayed menstrual period occur.

Explain that periodically she must have the old implants removed and new ones inserted. Tell her to call the doctor or nurse for a referral if she'll be moving to another area.

Radiation implants

These implants may be temporary or permanent. Common sites for radiation implants include the brain, mouth, neck, breasts, lungs, cervix, endometrium, vagina, and prostate gland. Implants with a short half-life may be placed inside a body cavity, into a tumor, on the surface of a tumor, or in the area from which a tumor has been removed.

Permanent implants include iodine 125 for lung and prostate tumors and gold 198 for oral and ocular tumors. Sealed temporary implants, which have a longer half-life, are inserted into body tissue for a specified amount of time. They include radium 226 and cesium 137 for tongue, lip, and skin therapy as well as iridium 192.

During treatment, the patient is usually placed in a private room (with its own bathroom) as far away from high-traffic areas as possible. If monitoring indicates an increased radiation hazard, adjacent rooms and hallways may also need to be restricted.

Because sealed permanent implants decay rapidly, patients can be discharged within a few days of implantation. Before discharge, dose levels must be less than 30 millicuries. After removal of a temporary implant, radiation precautions are no longer necessary.

Radiation implants are put in place by a doctor trained in radiation oncology, usually in an operating room or radiation oncology suite. The radiation source may be loaded at that time or when the patient is back in his room. Follow the policy of the health care facility for the nurse's role during insertion and in caring for a patient with a radiation implant. Also re-

Inserting subdermal implants

The illustrations below show how levonorgestrel subdermal contraceptive implants are inserted.

Have the patient lie supine on the examination table and flex the elbow of her nondominant arm so that her hand is opposite her head, as shown.

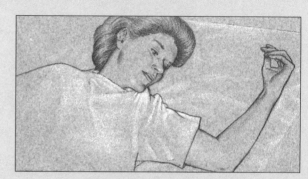

Swab the insertion site with antiseptic solution. (The ideal insertion site is inside the upper arm about 3" to 4" [8 to 10 cm] above the elbow.) Cover the arm above and below the insertion site with sterile cloths.

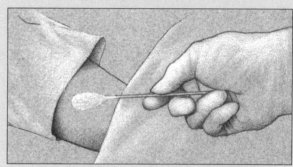

The doctor fills a 5-ml syringe with a local anesthetic, then inserts the needle under the skin and injects a small amount of anesthetic into several areas, each about 1½" to 2" (4 to 4.5 cm) long, in a fanlike pattern.

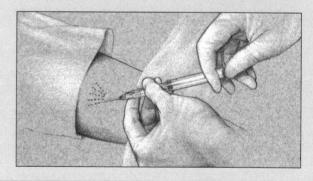

view your facility's radiation safety manual.

Brachytherapy is commonly combined with external radiation therapy (teletherapy). (See *Understanding radiation implants,* page 174.)

Equipment

Because excessive radiation can be harmful to the patient and to others nearby, make sure you have the necessary precaution signs and labels. You'll need a RADIATION PRECAUTION sign for the patient's door and warning labels for his wristband and personal belongings. You'll also need a film badge or pocket dosimeter, lead-lined container, long-handled forceps, masking tape, and a portable lead shield.

Place the lead-lined container and long-handled forceps in a corner of the patient's

The doctor uses the scalpel to make a small, shallow incision (about 2 mm) through the skin.

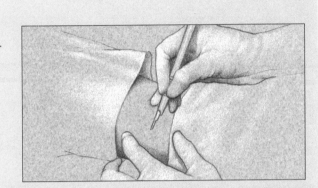

Next, he inserts the tip of the trocar through the incision at a shallow angle beneath the skin. He makes sure the trocar bevel is up so he can place the capsules in a superficial plane. To avoid placing the capsules too deep, he tents the skin with the trocar. He advances the trocar slowly to the first mark near the hub of the trocar. The tip of the trocar should now be about 1½" to 2" from the incision site. The doctor then removes the obturator and loads the first capsule into the trocar.

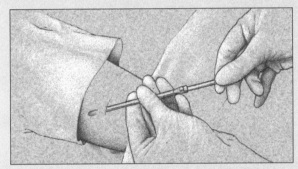

He gently advances the capsule with the obturator toward the tip of the trocar until he feels resistance. Next, he inserts each succeeding capsule beside the last one in a fanlike pattern. With the forefinger and middle finger of his free hand, he fixes the position of the previous capsule, advancing the trocar along the tips of his fingers. This ensures a suitable distance of about 15 degrees between capsules and keeps the trocar from puncturing any of the previously inserted capsules.

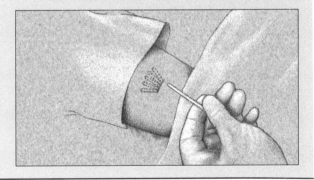

room. With masking tape, mark a safe line on the floor 6' (1.9 m) from the patient's bed to warn visitors of the danger of radiation exposure. Also place the lead shield in the back of the room to wear when providing care.

Place an emergency tracheotomy tray in the room if an implant will be inserted in the patient's mouth or neck.

Drug administration

To insert the implant, the doctor makes a small incision in the skin and creates a pocket in the tissue. He puts the implant in position and closes the incision. If the patient is being treated for tonsillar cancer, he'll undergo a bronchoscopy, during which radioactive pellets will be implanted in tonsillar tissue.

Your role in the implant procedure is to ex-

Understanding radiation implants

ISOTOPE AND INDICATIONS	DESCRIPTION	NURSING CONSIDERATIONS
cesium 137 • Gynecologic cancers	• 30-year half-life • Emits gamma rays • Encased in steel capsules that are placed temporarily in the patient in the operating room	• Elevate the head of the bed no more than 45 degrees. • Encourage fluids and implement a low-residue diet. • Encourage quiet activities; enforce strict bed rest as ordered.
gold 198 • Oral and ocular tumors and localized male genitourinary tumors	• 3-day half-life • Emits gamma rays • Permanently implanted as tiny seeds directly in the tumor or tumor bed	• If the seed is dislodged and found, call the radiation oncology department for disposal.
iodine 125 • Localized or unresectable tumors • Slow-growing tumors • Recurrent disease	• 60-day half-life • Emits gamma rays • Used in lung and prostate tumors • Permanently implanted as tiny seeds or sutures directly in the tumor or tumor bed	• Because seeds may become dislodged, no linens, body fluids, instruments, or utensils should leave the patient's room until they're monitored. • If the seed is dislodged and found, call the radiation oncology department; use long-handled forceps to put the implant into a lead-lined container in the room. • Monitor body fluids to detect displaced seeds. Give the patient a 24-hour urine container that can be closed.
iridium 192 • Localized or unresectable tumors	• 74-day half-life • Emits gamma rays • Temporarily implanted as seeds strung inside special catheters that are implanted around the tumor	• If a catheter is dislodged, call the radiation oncology department; use long-handled forceps to put the implant into a lead-lined container in the room.
palladium 103 • Superficial, localized, or unresectable intrathoracic or intra-abdominal tumors	• 17-day half-life • Emits gamma rays • Permanently implanted as seeds in the tumor or tumor bed	• Because seeds may become dislodged, no linens, body fluids, instruments, or utensils should leave the patient's room until they're monitored. • If the seed is dislodged and found, call the radiation oncology department; use long-handled forceps to put the implant into a lead-lined container in the room. • Monitor body fluids to detect displaced seeds. Give the patient a 24-hour urine container that can be closed.

plain the treatment and its goals to the patient. Review radiation safety procedures and visitation policies. Talk with the patient about long-term physical and emotional aspects of the therapy, and discuss home care.

Complications
Depending on the implant site and radiation dosage, complications may include dislodgment of the implant, tissue fibrosis, xerostomia, radia-tion pneumonitis, muscle atrophy, sterility, vaginal dryness or stenosis, fistulas, altered bowel habits, hypothyroidism, infection, airway obstruction, diarrhea, cystitis, myelosuppression, neurotoxicity, and secondary cancers.

If an implant becomes dislodged, notify the radiation oncology department staff and follow their instructions. Typically, the dislodged implant should be collected with long-handled forceps and placed in a lead-lined container.

(For more information on complications, see *Radiation implants: Code precautions,* page 176.)

Make sure your patient understands the potential long-term adverse reactions, such as tissue necrosis, skin hyperpigmentation, and impaired healing of the implanted area.

A patient who undergoes radiation implant therapy may feel isolated, contaminated, or unclean. Explore your patient's feelings about his therapy and discuss what he can do while the implant is in place. Because he can't socialize during this time, the patient needs to anticipate solitary activities, such as writing letters, reading, watching television, or drawing.

Nursing considerations

• Make sure informed consent has been obtained before the implantation.
• Before treatment, ensure that all laboratory tests have been performed. If laboratory work is required during treatment, a technician wearing a film badge will obtain the specimen, affix a RADIATION PRECAUTION label to the specimen container, and alert laboratory personnel. If urine tests are needed, ask the radiation oncology department or laboratory technician how to transport the specimens safely.
• Place a RADIATION PRECAUTION sign on the door of the patient's room. Affix a RADIATION PRECAUTION label to the patient's wristband and to any specimens. Also affix warning labels to the patient's chart and Kardex.
• Minimize your own exposure to radiation. Wear a personal, nontransferable film badge or dosimeter at waist level during your entire shift. Turn in the film badge regularly. Pocket dosimeters measure immediate exposures. In many health care facilities, these measurements aren't part of the permanent exposure record but are used to ensure that nurses receive the lowest possible exposure.

Use the three principles of time, distance, and shielding: *Time:* Plan to give care in the shortest time possible. Less time equals less exposure. *Distance:* Work as far away from the radiation source as possible. Give care from the side opposite the implant or from a position allowing the greatest working distance possible. Prepare the patient's meal trays outside his

room. The intensity of radiation exposure varies inversely with the square of the distance from the source. *Shielding:* Wear a portable shield, if necessary.

Give only essential nursing care; omit bed baths. If ordered, provide perineal care, making sure that wipes, sanitary pads, and similar items are disposed of correctly and monitored. (Refer to the policy of the health care facility.)
• Remember that dressing changes over an implanted area must be supervised by the radiation technician or a designated caregiver.
• Ensure that the patient's room is monitored daily by the radiation oncology department, and that disposable items are monitored and removed according to the facility's guidelines.
• Keep staff members and visitors who are pregnant or trying to conceive or father a child away from the patient. The gonads and a developing embryo or fetus are highly susceptible to the damaging effects of ionizing radiation.
• If you must take the patient out of his room, notify the appropriate department of the patient's status to allow time for the necessary preparations. When transporting the patient, make sure the route is clear of equipment and other people. If you must use an elevator, make sure it's been called and is ready to receive the patient. Transport the patient in a bed or wheelchair, accompanied by two caregivers, each wearing a film badge. If the patient is delayed along the way, stand as far away from the bed as possible until you can continue.
• If a patient with an implant dies on the unit, notify the radiation oncology staff so they can remove a temporary implant and store it properly. If an implant was permanent, they will determine which precautions to follow before postmortem care can be provided and before the body can be taken to the morgue.
• Before discharge, a patient's temporary implant must be removed and stored properly by the radiation oncology department. A patient with a permanent implant may not be released until his radioactivity level is less than 5 millirems/hour at a distance of about 3' (1 m).
• Upon discharge, instruct the patient and family members to call the radiation oncology doc-

Radiation implants: Code precautions

If a code is called on a patient with an implant, follow the code procedure of your health care facility as well as the steps listed here.
• Notify the code team of the patient's radioactive status to exclude any team member who's pregnant or trying to conceive or father a child.
• Notify the radiation oncology department.
• Cover the implant site with a strip of lead shielding, if possible.
• Don't allow anything to leave the patient's room until it's monitored for radiation.
• If you're the patient's primary care nurse, remain in the room as far away from the patient as possible. As the patient's resource person, you'll provide film badges or dosimeters to code-team members.

tor immediately if physical changes or other problems develop.
• Document radiation precautions taken during treatment, adverse reactions to therapy, instructions given to the patient and family and their responses, the patient's tolerance of isolation procedures and the family's compliance with procedures, and referrals to local cancer services.

Patient teaching

Tell a patient who has received a cervical implant to expect slight to moderate vaginal bleeding after discharge. The color of the bleeding may change from pink to brown to white. Instruct her to notify the doctor if bleeding increases, persists for more than 48 hours, or develops a foul odor. Tell the patient that she may resume most normal activities but should avoid sexual intercourse and the use of tampons until after her follow-up visit (about 6 weeks after she leaves the health care facility). Instruct her to take showers rather than baths for 2 weeks, to avoid douching unless permitted by the doctor, and to avoid activities that cause abdominal strain for

6 weeks. Refer the patient for sexual or psychological counseling, if necessary.

A patient who has had radioactive implants placed in the head or neck needs a special diet because the implants inhibit chewing. Advise him to eat only eggs; hot cereals, such as oatmeal; milk and cream; high-calorie liquid supplements; puddings; custards; jello; milk shakes; ice cream; yogurt; soufflés; soft cheeses, such as Brie; soup; mashed potatoes; gravies; honey; jam; and pureed fruits, vegetables, and meats.

When a patient is to receive a facial implant, tell him to anticipate temporary changes in his appearance. These changes include an enlarged tongue, which results from manipulation during implantation. Before the procedure, also tell the patient that he'll feel pain and that he'll receive parenteral or transdermal analgesia.

Subcutaneous implants

In subcutaneous implant therapy, drug pellets are injected into the skin's subcutaneous layer. The drug is then stored in one area of the body, which is called a *depot*.

A new treatment for prostate cancer calls for implants of goserelin acetate (Zoladex), a synthetic form of the luteinizing hormone. By inhibiting pituitary gland secretion, goserelin implants reduce serum testosterone to levels previously achieved only through castration. This reduction causes tumor regression and, in many patients, a suppression of symptoms.

A specially skilled nurse or doctor may inject the implant into the patient's upper abdominal wall. After injection, the implant begins releasing a 3.6-mg dose of the drug. The goserelin pellet degrades slowly over 28 days when a new implant can be injected.

Goserelin implants have advantages over other treatments for prostate cancer. A nonsurgical procedure, goserelin implant therapy is as effective as an orchiectomy and, to many patients, more acceptable. The implant seems to cause fewer of the complications produced by oral drug treatments, such as nausea and abdominal cramping. Also, patient compliance is better because treatment requires an injection once a month rather than every day.

The effectiveness of the goserelin implant is measured by the suppression level of the patient's serum testosterone and the speed with which the disease progresses.

Equipment

To insert a subcutaneous implant, you'll need an alcohol sponge and the drug implant in a preloaded syringe. A local anesthetic may be required for some patients.

Drug administration

Help the patient into the supine position and drape him so that his abdomen is accessible. Remove the syringe from the package and make sure you can see the drug in the chamber. Clean a small area on the patient's upper abdominal wall with the alcohol sponge.

As you stretch the skin at the injection site with one hand, grip the needle with the fingers of your other hand around the barrel of the syringe. Insert the needle into subcutaneous fat. Don't attempt to aspirate. If blood appears in the syringe, withdraw the needle and inject a new, preloaded syringe and needle at another site.

Next, change the direction of the needle so it's parallel to the abdominal wall. With the barrel hub touching the patient's skin, push the needle in. Then withdraw it about ½" (1 cm), creating a space in which to discharge the drug. Depress the plunger. Withdraw the needle and bandage the site.

Inspect the tip of the needle. If you can see the metal tip of the plunger, the drug has been discharged.

Complications

At the beginning of therapy, goserelin may cause symptoms of prostate cancer to worsen because the drug initially raises the serum testosterone level. But reports of exacerbation of the disease, resulting in spinal cord compression or ureteral obstruction, are rare.

Subcutaneous goserelin implants may produce anemia, lethargy, pain, dizziness, insomnia, anxiety, depression, headache, chills, fever, edema, congestive heart failure, arrhythmias, cerebrovascular accident, hypertension, peripheral vascular disease, nausea, vomiting, diarrhea, decreased number of erections, renal insufficiency, urinary obstruction, rash, sweating, hot flashes, gout, hyperglycemia, weight increase, and breast swelling and tenderness.

Nursing considerations

• If the package for the preloaded syringe is damaged or if you can't see the drug in the translucent chamber, don't use the syringe.
• If an implant must be removed, a doctor will order an X-ray to locate it.
• Document the name of the drug, the dose, the date, the site of administration, and the date of the next administration.

Patient teaching

Before your patient receives his first implant of goserelin, explain the implantation procedure to him and answer his questions. Make sure he understands the importance of keeping to a 28-day dosage schedule. (A few days delay between doses is acceptable, but he should try to adhere to the prescribed regimen.) Also teach him to check the administration site between injections for signs of infection or bleeding.

Subcutaneous infusion

Used for cancer patients, this technique provides a reliable method of delivering narcotic analgesics. Subcutaneous infusion is also used to administer insulin to diabetic patients.

To use this technique, a nurse or doctor inserts a needle into the subcutaneous tissue beneath the skin at a 35- to 45-degree angle. The needle is then attached to tubing and an infusion pump that delivers continuous medication. Appropriate injection sites include the supraclavicular area, abdomen, and thighs. Using these areas provides ample subcutaneous tissue, causes the patient minimal discomfort, and allows him to see the infusion site. The site can also be used to administer a loading dose and any subsequent doses.

With a continuous subcutaneous infusion, the patient can actively participate in his therapy. Plus, he feels less anxiety because regular injections aren't necessary. Patients also find this technique easier to learn than others, making the transition from health care facility to home easier for them and their families.

Subcutaneous infusions are recommended for cancer patients who can't receive drugs via the GI route because of GI obstruction, malabsorption syndrome, confusion, depression, dysphagia, or nausea. This technique is also suitable for diabetic patients whose blood glucose levels fluctuate despite optimal insulin and dietary regimens, those with irregular work schedules or irregular mealtimes, pregnant diabetic patients who benefit from more precise blood glucose level control, and children entering puberty whose blood glucose levels fluctuate.

Equipment

Make sure the infusion pump closely matches the patient's needs. The pump should deliver accurate doses and should be easy for the patient or caregiver to use. For safe, accurate delivery, the pump should have an alarm and a lock-out time if analgesics are to be delivered. The pump should also permit the administration of a loading dose, and it should have a sufficient reservoir capacity.

Analgesia pumps

To initiate a subcutaneous infusion of a narcotic, you'll need a 25G to 27G needle, a portable infusion pump filled with the prescribed amount of narcotic, alcohol sponges, waterproof tape to hold the needle in place, and an initial bolus of the drug. In some cases, you may use a three-way stopcock or T-connector to administer extra doses.

The most convenient pump for the patient is probably the Travenol infusor—a small, disposable plastic cylinder that may be clipped to the patient's clothes. This pump measures about 6" × 1" (16 × 3 cm) and weighs about 3 oz (90 gm) when full, making it a portable infusion device. The device delivers a total volume of 48 ml in 24 hours at a fixed rate of 2 ml/hour, with a reserve of 12 ml. A patient can inject extra medications, such as analgesics for breakthrough pain, without removing the infusor. (See *Giving a bolus dose with an infusor*.) Both morphine sulfate and hydromorphone (Dilaudid) remain stable for at least 1 week in the Travenol infusor. The pump's main drawback is that it can only be used for 24 hours.

The computerized, battery-operated Pharmacia 5200 pump was designed specifically for pain control in ambulatory patients. This device delivers a continuous infusion and allows the patient to administer extra injections at a preset interval and volume. The pump can be used with 50- or 100-ml cassettes. The drawbacks of the Pharmacia 5200 pump include its price and its weight and bulk. (The patient must carry this pump in a holster.) The device is also complicated and may be difficult for some patients or caregivers to use. A nurse specially skilled in its use should be available for troubleshooting.

The Cormed pump, another battery-operated narcotic infusion device, was originally developed to administer chemotherapy. Although the Cormed pump is simpler and less expensive than the Pharmacia 5200, a nurse or another health professional skilled in its use should be available.

Insulin pump

For a subcutaneous insulin infusion, you'll need an infusion set attached to an insulin pump. You'll also need a 25G to 27G subcutaneous needle, alcohol sponges, and waterproof tape. Sites for needle placement include the abdomen, upper hip, lower back, and thigh. By delivering basal insulin doses every few minutes and bolus doses at mealtimes, an insulin infusion pump helps a diabetic patient achieve better control over blood glucose levels and minimizes long-term complications. The pump holds a syringe filled with regular insulin. Insulin is infused in doses of 0.1 units or more continuously over a 24-hour period from a syringe pushed by a mechanical driver in the pump. The bolus mode of the pump is used to deliver a dose calculated to maintain normal glucose levels after meals and during illness. The battery-operated MiniMed insulin infu-

ADVANCED EQUIPMENT

Giving a bolus dose with an infusor

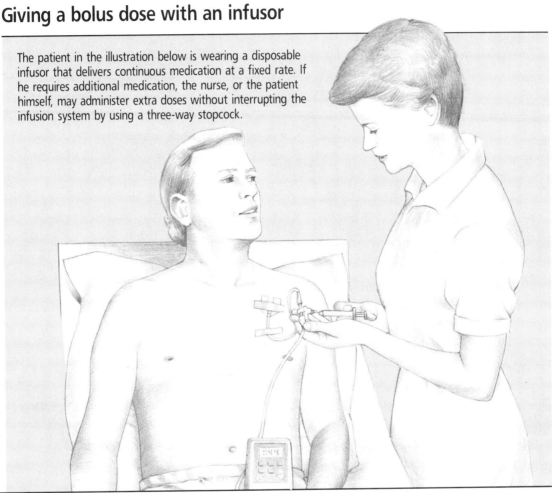

The patient in the illustration below is wearing a disposable infusor that delivers continuous medication at a fixed rate. If he requires additional medication, the nurse, or the patient himself, may administer extra doses without interrupting the infusion system by using a three-way stopcock.

sion pump, which is about the size of a beeper, delivers up to four different basal rates a day. (See *Using an insulin infusion pump,* page 180.)

Drug administration
Clean the insertion site by rubbing it with alcohol. Let it dry for at least 30 seconds. Then insert the needle at a 30- to 45-degree angle. Cover the area with a transparent semipermeable dressing.

Complications
Subcutaneous narcotic infusions can cause constipation, drowsiness, urinary retention, pruritus, plaque formation, and nausea. Irregular absorption may also occur, especially in a cachectic patient with little subcutaneous tissue. Other complications include redness or swelling at the infusion site and respiratory depression, particularly in patients with compromised renal function and metabolic disorders.

In insulin-dependent diabetic patients, hypoglycemia or hyperglycemia may result if the patient uses an insulin pump incorrectly. Ketoacidosis may result from a pump malfunction.

As with other subcutaneous infusions, infection or inflammation may occur at the infusion site, particularly if it's not rotated.

ADVANCED EQUIPMENT

Using an insulin infusion pump

There are several insulin infusion pumps on the market. The MiniMed pump is shown here. Roughly the size of a deck of cards, the MiniMed pump resembles a beeper. Three disposable batteries power the pump, and a syringe inside holds regular insulin. A tiny computer inside the pump controls the action of the syringe and precisely regulates how much insulin the pump delivers. The pump can deliver up to four different basal rates in a 24-hour period. These rates and their associated delivery times are called profiles. Insulin is delivered through an infusion set and exits through a needle inserted under the skin.

The MiniMed pump has four buttons and a display screen. These buttons are used to program the pump:
• M button. Meal bolus—used to set the amount of insulin given before a meal
• B button. Basal rate—used to set the amount of insulin delivered every hour during a 24-hour period.
• A button. Activates the pump to carry out the selected program.
• T button. Time of day—used to set the time of day the insulin is to be delivered.

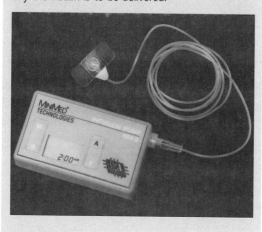

Routine maintenance is crucial to ensure that the pump functions properly. Each day, batteries must be changed or charged, and infusion syringes must be replaced and correctly primed to prevent air from getting into the system. Air in the system can lead to a reduction in the amount of insulin delivered. The infusion set should be changed every other day. Once the pump is running, it should be attached to the body using a belt loop or a pocket.

Nursing considerations
• Patients who won't benefit from a subcutaneous analgesic infusion include those with pain from nerve damage and those with incidental pain (no pain while resting and excruciating pain upon movement). Diabetic patients with severe complications—advanced renal disease, proliferative retinopathy, or severe autonomic neuropathy—may not benefit from a subcutaneous insulin infusion.
• Short-acting opioids, such as morphine and hydromophone, are the first choice for pain control via subcutaneous infusion. Although drugs with a longer half-life, such as methadone (Dolophine) and levorphanol (Levo-Dromoran), may also be prescribed, they don't control pain as well or as quickly.
• For a patient requiring analgesia via a subcutaneous infusion, determine the average daily dose he's currently receiving. Then use an equivalency table to convert the daily dose to the same dose in milligrams of parenteral morphine or hydromorphone. Assuming that the patient is receiving adequate pain control, divide the total daily dose by 24 hours and administer this amount per hour subcutaneously.
• Patients with portable pumps need a very slow infusion rate of a highly concentrated and stable solution such as hydromorphone.
• When giving an analgesic, assess the patient regularly for pain. Ask him to rate the severity of his pain on a scale of 0 to 10.
• Assess the infusion site for erythema, chemical irritation, and inflammation.
• Inspect the equipment regularly. Make sure the infusion rate is correct.
• Rotate the injection sites periodically (every 2 to 7 days). Patients with thrombocytopenia or neutropenia need more frequent changes.
• Document the drug used. Record the dosage given in the bolus dose as well as the dose delivered via the infusion. Record the date and time and injection site of the initial dose. At

each visit, record the date and time, injection site, and patient's reaction to the drug.

Patient teaching

Before a patient is discharged with an infusion pump, make sure that he and his caregiver thoroughly understand what subcutaneous infusion is and how the pump works. Demonstrate all techniques on a model, and have the patient or caregiver, or both, perform a return demonstration. If brochures or other printed materials describing the pump are available, give them to your patient.

One patient receiving a subcutaneous infusion may need more support than another. The amount of intervention necessary depends on the patient's alertness and independence, as well as on the complexity of the infusion pump he's using. Discuss with the patient and his caregiver the kind of support he'll need.

Advise the patient and his caregiver to inspect the infusion site every 4 to 6 hours and tell them how to recognize signs of infection. Also make sure the patient and his caregiver can change the infusion pump, tubing, or cassette. They should be familiar with the storage and, if necessary, disposal of pumps or cassettes.

Make sure the patient and his caregiver know who to call with questions or problems 24 hours a day.

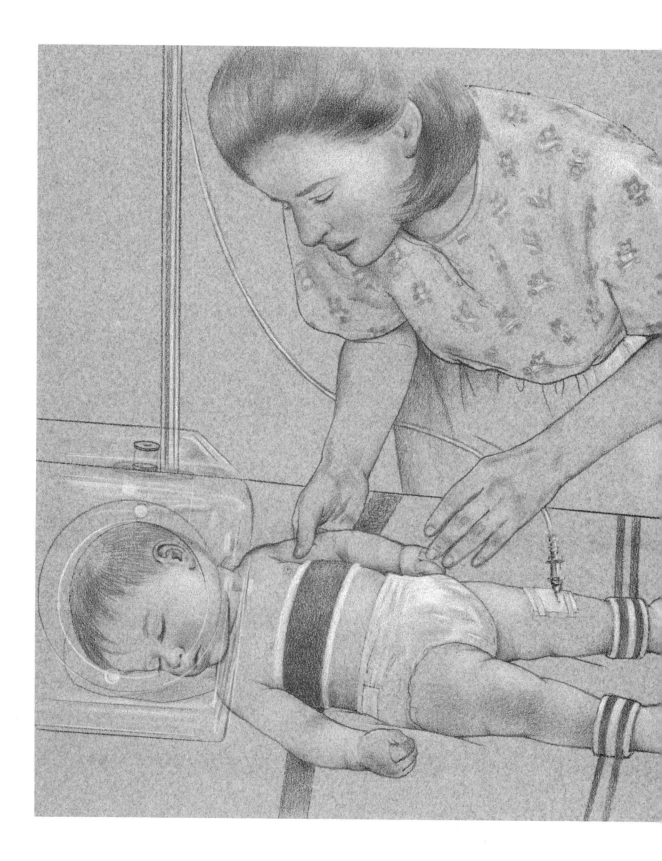

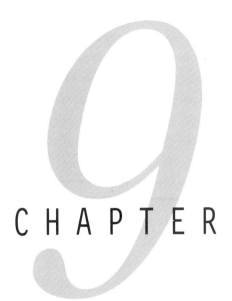

CHAPTER 9

Understanding other types of advanced drug delivery

As drug therapy has become more advanced, specialized techniques and devices have been developed to implement delivery. These include intra-articular, intraosseous, intraperitoneal, and intrapleural administration, the gastrostomy button, and the intraocular disk. With most of these techniques, the doctor injects or infuses the drug into a sterile access device.

With all six techniques, you're responsible for assembling the appropriate equipment, positioning the patient correctly, helping to insert the access device and maintain its patency, managing complications, and providing patient teaching. At times, you may also be responsible for giving the drug.

In this chapter, you'll find the information you need to meet these responsibilities. You'll learn about the pharmacologic principles underlying each administration method, as well as the advantages, disadvantages, and contrain-

Reviewing common intra-articular drugs

Drugs administered by intra-articular injection are typically corticosteroids. This chart presents important information about the four corticosteroids most commonly injected into the joint cavity.

DRUG	INDICATIONS AND DOSAGE	MECHANISM OF ACTION
dexamethasone sodium phosphate (Decadron Phosphate, Hexadrol Phosphate)	Inflammatory conditions requiring an immediate, short-term effect *Adult dosage:* 2 to 4 mg injected into large joints; 0.8 to 1 mg injected into small joints	A synthetic glucocorticoid, the drug decreases inflammation by stabilizing leukocyte lysosomal membranes. It also suppresses pituitary release of corticotropin, thereby halting adrenocortical secretion of corticosteroids and suppressing the immune response. Dexamethasone is absorbed rapidly and completely (because sodium phosphate is a freely soluble salt). It binds weakly to plasma proteins and is distributed by the bloodstream, metabolized in the liver, and excreted by the kidneys. Plasma level peaks in 1 hour.
hydrocortisone acetate (Hydrocortone Acetate)	Severe inflammation or lesion in a joint, ganglion, or bursa *Adult dosage:* 25 to 50 mg injected into large joints; 10 to 25 mg injected into small joints or ganglia	A naturally occurring corticosteroid, hydrocortisone affects virtually all body systems. Given systemically, it decreases inflammation by stabilizing leukocyte lysosomal membranes. It also suppresses pituitary release of corticotropin so that the adrenal cortex stops secreting corticosteroids. The drug is absorbed slowly but completely (because acetate is a poorly soluble ester). It binds extensively to plasma proteins and is distributed by the bloodstream, metabolized in the liver, and excreted by the kidneys. Plasma level peaks in 24 to 48 hours.
methylprednisolone acetate (Depo-Medrol, Medrol)	Inflammation and conditions requiring immunosuppression *Adult dosage:* 4 to 80 mg injected into a joint	A synthetic glucocorticoid, methylprednisolone suppresses pituitary release of corticotropin, preventing adrenocortical secretion of corticosteroids. As a result, the drug suppresses immune responses, stimulates bone marrow, and alters protein, fat, and carbohydrate metabolism. It also decreases inflammation by stabilizing leukocyte lysosomal membranes. The drug is absorbed slowly but completely (because acetate is a poorly soluble ester). It binds to plasma proteins and is distributed by the bloodstream, metabolized in the liver, and excreted by the kidneys. Plasma level peaks in 24 to 48 hours.
prednisolone sodium phosphate (Hydeltrasol)	Inflammation and conditions requiring immunosuppression *Adult dosage:* 2 to 30 mg injected into a joint; repeat dose every 3 days to 3 weeks	A synthetic glucocorticoid, prednisolone decreases or prevents inflammation by inhibiting phagocytosis, lysosomal enzyme release, and the synthesis and release of several chemical mediators of inflammation. The drug is thought to suppress the immune response by preventing or suppressing cell-mediated immune reactions (delayed hypersensitivity). Prednisolone also stimulates protein catabolism, increases glucose availability, enhances lipolysis and mobilization of fatty acids from adipose tissue, decreases bone formation and increases bone reabsorption, and suppresses pituitary release of corticotropin. The drug is absorbed rapidly and completely. It binds extensively to plasma proteins and is distributed by the bloodstream, metabolized in the liver, and excreted by the kidneys. Plasma level peaks in 1 hour.

dications for each one. You'll find out which equipment to gather and what procedure the doctor uses to insert the access device and administer the drug. You'll also learn about related complications, nursing considerations, patient teaching, and home care.

Intra-articular administration

An intra-articular injection delivers a drug directly into the synovial cavity of a joint to suppress inflammation, relieve pain, help preserve joint mobility, prevent contractures, and delay

NURSING CONSIDERATIONS

• Contraindicated in patients with systemic fungal infection or known hypersensitivity to any drug component. • Use cautiously in patients with GI ulcers, renal disease, hypertension, osteoporosis, varicella inoculata,	exanthema, diabetes mellitus, hypothyroidism, thromboembolic disorders, seizures, myasthenia gravis, congestive heart failure (CHF), tuberculosis, ocular herpes simplex, hypoalbuminemia, emotional instability, or psychosis.
• Contraindicated in patients with systemic fungal infection or known hypersensitivity to any drug component. • Use cautiously in patients with GI ulcers, renal disease, hypertension, osteoporosis, varicella inoculata, exan-	thema, diabetes mellitus, hypothyroidism, thromboembolic disorders, seizures, myasthenia gravis, CHF, tuberculosis, ocular herpes simplex, hypoalbuminemia, emotional instability, or psychosis.
• Contraindicated in patients with systemic fungal infection or known hypersensitivity to any drug component. • Use cautiously in patients with GI ulcers, renal disease, hypertension, osteoporosis, varicella inoculata, exan-	thema, diabetes mellitus, hypothyroidism, thromboembolic disorders, seizures, myasthenia gravis, CHF, tuberculosis, ocular herpes simplex, hypoalbuminemia, emotional instability, or psychosis.
• Contraindicated in patients with systemic fungal infection or known hypersensitivity to any drug component. • Use cautiously in patients with GI ulcers, renal disease, hypertension, osteoporosis, varicella inoculata, exan-	thema, diabetes mellitus, hypothyroidism, thromboembolic disorders, seizures, myasthenia gravis, CHF, tuberculosis, ocular herpes simplex, hypoalbuminemia, emotional instability, or psychosis.

muscle atrophy. Providing a local, short-term effect, this route is most commonly used to treat rheumatoid arthritis, gout, systemic lupus erythematosus, osteoarthritis, and other joint disorders.

Intra-articular injection sites include the shoulder, elbow, wrist, finger, knee, ankle, and toe. Most drugs administered intra-articularly are corticosteroids, anesthetics, and lubricants. (See *Reviewing common intra-articular drugs.*)

Intra-articular drugs must be absorbed into tissues or cells before they can exert an effect. Like other parenterally administered drugs, they have fewer barriers to overcome than oral drugs. However, doctors use the intra-articular route sparingly because of the greater risk of

Intra-articular injection sites

When injecting an intra-articular drug, the doctor may use one of the sites shown here. Note that the affected joint determines how you should position your patient and, in some cases, which needle gauge to use.

Knee
The patient lies supine with the knee fully extended or bent about 20 degrees over a rolled towel. If he can't extend his knee he can sit with his legs hanging over the edge of the examination table. The doctor uses an 18G to 20G 1½" needle.

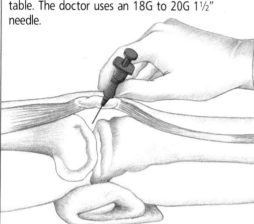

Shoulder
The patient sits with the affected arm at his side, his shoulder rotated externally. The doctor uses a 20G to 22G 1½" needle.

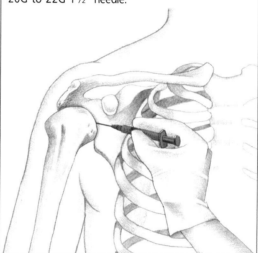

Wrist
The patient sits with his palm down and wrist flexed 20 to 30 degrees over a rolled towel. Have him turn his hand slightly toward the ulna. The doctor uses a 24G to 26G ⅝" needle.

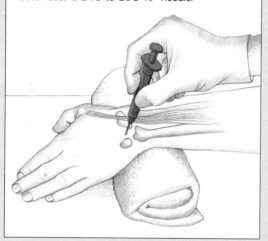

Finger
The patient sits with his palm flat on a table and his affected finger flexed slightly, or with his palm flat and traction applied to the affected finger. The doctor uses a 22G to 26G ⅝" to 1" needle.

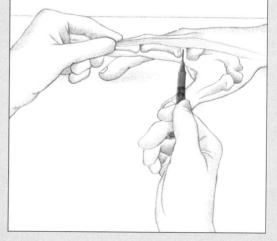

Elbow
The patient sits with his affected elbow flexed 90 degrees and his palm flat on a table. The doctor uses a 20G to 22G 1½″ needle.

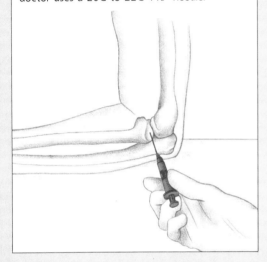

Ankle
The patient lies supine, with his sole flexed downward. The doctor uses a 20G to 22G 1½″ needle.

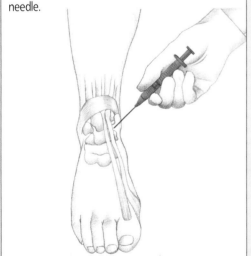

infection and potential problems accessing synovial joints. Intra-articular administration is contraindicated in patients with joint infection, instability, or fracture; systemic fungal infection; psoriasis around the injection site; bacteremia; bleeding disorders; and total arthroplasty.

Equipment
The doctor simply injects the drug into the synovial cavity using a standard needle and syringe. No access device is used.

For aspiration or injection, assemble the following sterile equipment: 18G 1½″ to 26G ⅝″ needle (depending on the affected joint); the prescribed medication; 3-ml and 5- or 10-ml syringes; sterile towels; pillows; 10- or 20-ml syringe; gauze pads; gloves; emesis basin; povidone-iodine or other antiseptic cleaning solution; drape; 1% lidocaine, ethyl chloride, or other local anesthetic; adhesive bandage; test tubes for synovial fluid, with appropriate additives and specimen labels; and glass slides and coverslips, if necessary.

Drug administration
The medication is injected at the patient's bedside, with the nurse assisting. Before the injection, the doctor may withdraw synovial fluid to relieve pain and inflammation and improve the patient's range of motion. By removing lysosomal enzymes and other causes of inflammation, fluid aspiration allows the injected drug to work more effectively. Aspirated fluid may also be cultured or examined under a microscope to help diagnose joint effusion, infection, or trauma.

Wash your hands. Then draw the prescribed amount of medication into the 5- or 10-ml syringe. Label the syringe with the name and amount of medication and take the medication container into the patient's room so the doctor can verify the syringe contents. Position the patient appropriately and stabilize the affected joint, supporting it with pillows, if necessary. Expose the joint completely. (See *Intra-articular injection sites*.)

Using aseptic technique, create a sterile field by opening a sterile towel. Place the appropriate-sized needles and syringes and the gauze pads onto it.

After putting on sterile gloves, the doctor picks up the gauze pads and holds them over the emesis basin. Pour the antiseptic cleaning solution over the gauze pads to saturate them.

The doctor cleans the injection site with the gauze pads, then drapes the site. He fills the 3-ml syringe with a local anesthetic while you hold the bottle upside down. Then he anesthetizes the skin and subcutaneous tissue at the injection site, using a needle.

If the doctor will aspirate synovial fluid, place the sterile test tubes and slides in the correct order. The doctor withdraws fluid with the appropriate needle and syringe, then sets the syringe aside until after the procedure. He leaves the needle in the joint for later medication injection.

If synovial fluid was aspirated, hand the doctor the filled medication syringe so he can attach it to the needle lodged in the joint. Otherwise, hand him the medication syringe with the appropriate needle attached. He then injects the medication into the synovial cavity.

Apply pressure to the injection site and, if necessary, massage the area gently for 1 to 2 minutes to promote drug absorption. Then apply an adhesive bandage.

Attach a needle to the specimen syringe and insert appropriate specimens into the test tubes, or make slides. Label the test tubes or slides appropriately and send them to the laboratory.

Complications
Local joint pain may increase for 24 to 48 hours after injection if the medication infiltrates and irritates surrounding tissue. Contamination may cause septic arthritis, a serious complication. Signs and symptoms of septic arthritis include fever, persistent and increased pain, redness, and swelling. Other potential complications are tendon rupture, tissue atrophy, steroid arthropathy, fat necrosis, calcification, and nerve damage.

Nursing considerations
Document the dosage, date, time, and site of the injection and the doctor's name. Record

the amount of synovial fluid aspirated (if any), laboratory studies requested, and the patient's tolerance of the procedure. Also document any patient teaching, such as instructions to rest the joint.

Patient teaching
Explain the aspiration or injection procedure to the patient and allow time for him to ask questions. Instruct him to rest the joint for 24 to 48 hours after the injection because medication may mask pain.

Teach the patient about the signs and symptoms of infection — fever and redness, swelling, and persistent pain at the injection site — and tell him to call the doctor if these occur.

Intraosseous administration

First used in the 1940s, intraosseous administration is making a comeback. Fast and temporary, it allows delivery of fluids, drugs, or whole blood into the bone marrow when I.V. access is difficult or impossible. Usually, the infusion site is the anteromedial surface of the proximal tibia. (See *Intraosseous infusion site*, page 190.)

With intraosseous administration, drugs enter the circulation within 3 minutes, providing rapid delivery if the patient is being resuscitated (when a cutdown or central line would take too much time). It's preferred over the endotracheal route, which is limited to administration of epinephrine, atropine, lidocaine, and naloxone and can't be used for blood or fluid infusion.

Most commonly used in infants and children under age 6, intraosseous administration avoids the problems that arise with traditional access routes in small children, who have extensive subcutaneous fat and small, empty, more collapsible veins. (In adults, intraosseous infusion through the femur has had limited success because adult bones lack the rich vascular network needed to carry drugs into the circulation.)

Intraosseous administration is especially valuable during an emergency, such as cardio-pulmonary arrest or circulatory collapse, hypo-kalemia from traumatic injury or dehydration, status epilepticus, status asthmaticus, burns, near drowning, and overwhelming sepsis. However, prolonged intraosseous therapy can cause serious complications, so expect the doc-tor to change to a more conventional drug de-livery route as soon as possible.

After intraosseous administration in chil-dren, a drug or solution moves through the rich vascular network of a long bone into the systemic circulation. Marrow within a bone's central cavity (medullary cavity) contains a dense network of sinusoids that drain into large venous channels. These channels, in turn, empty into veins that retrace the path of nu-trient arteries in marrow, then exit the bone and enter the systemic circulation.

Drugs and solutions instilled into the mar-row are absorbed as quickly as those adminis-tered I.V. But unlike peripheral veins, osseous vessels are protected by bony walls and won't collapse if the patient goes into shock. Thus, intraosseous infusion serves as a form of I.V. in-fusion through vessels within the marrow.

Contraindications to intraosseous adminis-tration include leg fracture or trauma (which can allow fluid or drugs to extravasate into the subcutaneous tissue), infected burns, cellulitis, and bone disorders, such as osteoporosis and osteogenesis imperfecta.

Equipment
Intraosseous infusion requires one of two types of disposable needles — a bone marrow biopsy needle or a special intraosseous infusion nee-dle. Bone marrow biopsy needles have a stylet to prevent them from becoming plugged with bone and a short shaft that bars accidental dislodgment. One brand also has a screw cap that prevents the stylet from retracting during insertion and an adjustable guard to add stabil-ity when the needle is lowered to the skin.

Intraosseous infusion needles have a can-nula and an obturator. One type has a screw handle that secures the stylet during insertion;

when the needle is removed, a lightweight cannula stays in place. To help you determine needle depth, the cannula is marked "1 cm" near the tip. It's available in 15G, 16G, or 18G and in 3- or 4-cm length. An optional silicone molnar disc stabilizes the needle at skin level. Use an 18G needle for infants up to 8 months old and a 15G to 16G needle for older infants and children.

Insertion of access device
The doctor inserts the access device under emergency conditions, with help from a nurse. If you're assisting with the insertion, gather the following sterile equipment: gloves, povi-done-iodine sponges, drape, 3- to 5-ml syringe, 1% lidocaine, appropriate-sized bone marrow biopsy needle or intraosseous infusion needle, bone marrow set with two 5-ml syringes, and heparinized saline flush solution.

If ordered, give the patient a sedative. Posi-tion him appropriately, depending on the se-lected puncture site. If an extremity will be used, secure it in a comfortable, stable, depen-dent position.

Wash your hands and put on gloves. Using sterile technique, clean the puncture site with a povidone-iodine sponge and let it dry. Cover the area with a sterile drape.

Hand the doctor the 3- to 5-ml syringe with 1% lidocaine so he can anesthetize the infusion site. The doctor inserts the cannula and obturator through the skin and into the bone at a 10- to 15-degree angle. Using a to-and-fro rotary motion, he advances it through the periosteum until the needle penetrates the marrow cavity. On entering the marrow, the needle will give suddenly, making a popping sound, and will stand erect when released.

The doctor removes the obturator from the needle and attaches a 5-ml syringe. He aspi-rates some bone marrow to confirm needle placement, then replaces this syringe with one containing 5-ml of heparinized saline flush so-lution. He flushes the cannula to confirm nee-dle placement and to clear the cannula of clots and bone particles.

Intraosseous infusion site

An intraosseous drug is usually infused at the anteromedial surface of the proximal tibia, about 1″ (2.5 cm) below the tibial tuberosity. (See the large illustration below.) Alternate infusion sites include the distal tibia, distal femur, iliac crest, and spinous process. The upper anterior portion of the sternum is rarely used because injection here can cause complete bone perforation.

Because the bone marrow acts as a noncollapsible vein, drugs infused into the marrow cavity enter the circulation rapidly via an extensive network of medullary sinusoids. (See the inset.)

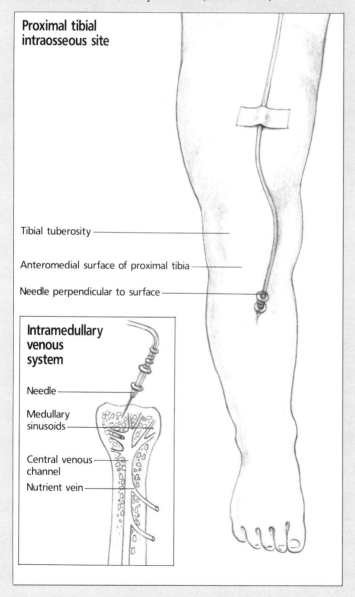

Proximal tibial intraosseous site

Tibial tuberosity

Anteromedial surface of proximal tibia

Needle perpendicular to surface

Intramedullary venous system

Needle

Medullary sinusoids

Central venous channel

Nutrient vein

Drug administration

If you're assisting the doctor with administration, gather the following sterile equipment: gloves, I.V. fluids and tubing, povidone-iodine sponges, gauze dressings, and tape. Once you're ready, the doctor removes the heparinized flush solution from the syringe and attaches I.V. tubing to the cannula. Then he infuses the medication and any fluids.

When the infusion ends, put on gloves and clean the infusion site with povidone-iodine sponges. Secure the site with tape and a sterile gauze dressing, then apply firm pressure to it for 5 minutes. Monitor the site for bleeding, extravasation, and signs of infection.

Complications

Common complications of intraosseous infusion include fluid extravasation into subcutaneous tissue (from incorrect needle placement); subperiosteal effusion (from failure of the fluid to enter the marrow space); and needle clotting (from delayed infusion or failure to flush the needle after placement). Other potential complications include subcutaneous abscess, osteomyelitis, and epiphyseal injury.

Nursing considerations

• Make sure the patient or a family member has signed the consent form.
• Document the date, time, and infusion site and the patient's tolerance for the procedure. Record the amount of fluid infused on the intake and output record.
• Be aware that intraosseous flow rates hinge on needle size and flow through the bone marrow. If needle placement is correct, fluid should flow freely. (A 0.9% sodium chloride solution has been administered through a 13G needle at a rate of 600 ml/hour by gravity and up to 2,500 ml/hour under 300 mm Hg of pressure.)
• To prevent infection from long-term intraosseous therapy, discontinue the infusion within 4 hours, or as soon as conventional vascular access is possible.

Patient teaching

Explain intraosseous infusion to the patient or family, discussing reasons for the procedure and the need to discontinue the infusion promptly. Describe signs and symptoms of infection at the access site (redness, swelling, exudate, and pain) and instruct them to report any of these problems to the doctor right away.

Intraperitoneal administration

An intraperitoneal catheter can deliver chemotherapeutic agents, antibiotics, and dialyzing solution to the peritoneal cavity. After administration, drugs are absorbed across the peritoneal membrane; dialyzing solution causes diffusion of fluid, electrolytes, and waste products. After a prescribed period, the drug or solution drains from the peritoneal cavity.

Intraperitoneal chemotherapy
Intraperitoneal chemotherapeutic agents can be delivered directly to a tumor in extremely high concentrations — up to 1,000 times the safe systemic dose. This technique inhibits cancer cell growth, kills tumor cells, and helps prevent tumor cell spread after resection of a primary tumor. (See *Reviewing common intraperitoneal drugs,* pages 192 and 193.)

The intraperitoneal route is especially useful in treating ovarian cancer because most ovarian tumors have metastasized to peritoneal surfaces by the time of diagnosis. It's also used to treat cancers of the colon, fallopian tubes, endometrium, gastric lining, bladder, and breast as well as cancers of unknown primary origin that have spread to the peritoneum.

Intraperitoneal chemotherapy has many benefits. It promotes drug penetration, enhances cytotoxic effects on cancer cells, and limits systemic toxicity (because the peritoneal cavity has a natural cellular barrier). It also maintains high drug levels in the portal vein, helping to prevent liver metastases. The liver absorbs most abdominal cavity fluid and detoxifies intraperitoneal drugs before releasing them into the bloodstream. This helps keep systemic drug concentrations low and reduces systemic adverse effects.

When given intraperitoneally, chemotherapeutic drugs are absorbed across the peritoneal membrane, either by passing through intracellular pores or by transcellular migration. A drug's molecular size affects its passage through pores, whereas its lipid solubility influences cellular transport. Large molecular size favors intraperitoneal retention, and high lipid solubility favors intraperitoneal escape. Thus, the ideal intraperitoneal drug has high systemic clearance but low peritoneal clearance — it has a hard time leaving the peritoneal cavity but is eliminated easily once it does.

Peritoneal dialysis
Using the peritoneal membrane as a semipermeable dialyzing membrane, peritoneal dialysis removes toxins from the blood of a patient with acute or chronic renal failure. A hypertonic dialyzing solution (dialysate) instilled through a peritoneal catheter draws excessive serum electrolytes and uremic toxins across the peritoneal membrane into the dialysate.

By the same route, excess water in the blood moves into the dialysate by osmosis. After an appropriate dwell time, the dialysate is drained, removing wastes, toxins, excess fluid, and electrolytes with it. This procedure is repeated, using new dialysate, until wastes are removed completely and fluid, electrolyte, and acid-base balance have been restored. (See *How peritoneal dialysis works,* page 194.)

Peritoneal dialysis may be performed in three ways: manually, with an automatic or a semiautomatic cycler machine, or as continuous ambulatory peritoneal dialysis (CAPD). In manual dialysis, the nurse, doctor, patient, or family member instills dialysate through a catheter into the peritoneal cavity, where it dwells for a specified time. A cycler machine accomplishes dialysis automatically but requires a sterile setup and connection technique.

The patient performs CAPD himself. Using aseptic technique, he instills dialysate from a special plastic bag through a catheter into the peritoneal cavity. While the solution dwells, he

(Text continues on page 194.)

Reviewing common intraperitoneal drugs

The intraperitoneal route is ideal for administering chemotherapy because it allows peak drug levels at the tumor site far beyond those your patient could tolerate systemically. The chart below presents the drugs most often administered intraperitoneally.

DRUG	INDICATIONS AND DOSAGE	MECHANISM OF ACTION
cisplatin (cis-platinum [Platinol])	Adjunctive therapy in metastatic ovarian tumors; treatment of metastatic testicular cancer and bladder, head, neck, and lung cancers (in combination with other chemotherapeutic agents) *Adult dosage:* 50 mg/m² every 3 to 4 weeks, as part of combination therapy; 100 mg/m² every 4 weeks, as a single agent. Alternatively, 30 to 120 mg/m² every 4 to 5 weeks	Precise mechanism of action is unknown, but the drug may cross-link strands of deoxyribonucleic acid (DNA) material, inhibiting DNA synthesis and leading to cell death. The drug distributes throughout body fluids and tissues, with the highest levels in the liver, kidneys, intestines, and prostate. Cerebrospinal fluid concentrations are low. It readily crosses the blood-brain barrier and apparently crosses the placenta. It binds extensively to plasma proteins. Metabolized rapidly, it's converted nonenzymatically to inactive metabolites. It's excreted by the kidneys, mainly by glomerular filtration, with 15% to 50% excreted within 48 hours. Extensive protein binding prolongs excretion; 27% to 45% remains in the body for 3 to 10 days. Whether the drug appears in breast milk is unknown. Initial half-life is roughly 75 hours. Plasma level peaks at the end of infusion. Duration of action is several days.
etoposide (VP-16 [VePesid])	Induces remission of refractory testicular cancer, small-cell lung cancer, and other malignant neoplasms *Adult dosage:* 300 to 800 mg/m²/day for 3 days (high-dose regimens)	Etoposide inhibits or alters DNA synthesis. It arrests the cell cycle at the G_2 phase, killing cells in that phase or in the late S phase. The drug is distributed minimally into pleural fluid, the liver, spleen, kidneys, and central nervous system and apparently crosses the placenta. It binds extensively (94%) to plasma proteins. Presumably metabolized in the liver, it's excreted mainly by the kidneys; 40% to 60% of a dose is excreted unchanged in 48 to 72 hours. A smaller portion (2% to 16%) is excreted in feces in 72 hours. Plasma level peaks at the end of infusion.
fluorouracil (5-FU [Adrucil])	Treatment of many solid tumors, including GI tract and breast tumors *Adult dosage:* initially, 12 mg/kg daily for 4 days; maximum daily dosage, 800 mg. If no toxicity occurs, 6 mg/kg is given on days 6, 8, 10, and 12. Maintenance dosage: initial dose repeated in 30 days, then 10 to 15 mg/kg weekly.	This antimetabolite interferes with DNA synthesis by inhibiting thymidylate synthetase. Drug also incorporates in ribonucleic acid (RNA), producing a fraudulent RNA. It inhibits utilization of preformed uracil in RNA synthesis by blocking uracil phosphatase. Drug distributes to all body areas containing water. In the liver, up to 80% of dose is detoxified rapidly by metabolic degradation to an active metabolite. About 60% to 80% is eliminated through the lungs as carbon dioxide. A small portion (roughly 15%) is eliminated unchanged in urine within 6 hours. The half-life is 10 to 20 minutes. Whether the drug appears in breast milk is unknown. Plasma level peaks immediately after injection.

NURSING CONSIDERATIONS

• Before the first infusion and each new course, measure the patient's serum magnesium, potassium, calcium, creatinine, and blood urea nitrogen (BUN) levels, and his creatinine clearance.
• Perform audiometric testing before each course to detect high-frequency hearing loss.
• Don't use aluminum needles for reconstituting or administering cisplatin because the drug will interact with aluminum, forming a black precipitate.
• Monitor the patient's vital signs during infusion. If anaphylaxis occurs, treat symptomatically.
• No specific antidote for overdose exists. Treat hepatic and hematologic toxicity symptomatically.
• Nausea and vomiting may be severe enough to discontinue treatment. Nausea usually begins 1 to 6 hours after administration and may last 24 hours or more.
• Perform regular neurologic examinations. Discontinue the drug if neurotoxicity occurs.
• Maintain a urine output of 100 to 200 ml/hour for 18 to 24 hours after therapy.

• Monitor complete blood count (CBC) and platelet count weekly; myelosuppression may be cumulative. Leukocyte and platelet nadirs usually occur 18 to 23 days after a single dose and return to baseline within 13 to 62 days. Don't repeat the dose unless the platelet count exceeds 100,000/mm^3, white blood cell (WBC) count exceeds 4,000/mm^3, creatinine level falls below 1.5 mg/dl, or BUN level is less than 25 mg/dl.
• Monitor liver and kidney function. Renal insufficiency (usually reversible) may occur within 4 weeks. Patients with mild to moderate renal impairment may receive 50% to 75% of the recommended dose. Regimens of I.V. hydration, diuresis, and 6- to 8-hour infusions reduce the incidence and severity of nephrotoxicity.
• Cisplatin increases serum uric acid levels. Patients receiving antigout medications may need dosage adjustment.
• Advise women of childbearing age to avoid becoming pregnant during therapy.

• Warn the patient that this drug usually causes toxic effects.
• Give antiemetics to control nausea and vomiting, as ordered. If anaphylaxis occurs, give vasopressor agents, adrenocorticoids, antihistamines, or volume expanders, as ordered.
• Monitor CBC at least weekly. Monitor WBC count and platelet count closely, especially during expected nadir days (days 7 to 14 for WBC and days 9 to 16 for platelet count).

• Monitor the patient for signs and symptoms of infection, such as fever, sore throat, or chills.
• If the patient has thrombocytopenia, monitor for signs of bleeding, such as spontaneous epistaxis, hematuria, and easy bruising.
• Notify the doctor if stomatitis persists or worsens.
• The drug may contain benzyl alcohol.

• Use plastic I.V. containers to administer continuous infusions because the solution is more stable in plastic I.V. bags than in glass bottles.
• Examine the patient's mouth for ulcers before each dose.
• Monitor CBC, platelet count, and liver and kidney function. If WBC count rapidly declines or falls below 3,500/mm^3 or if platelet count falls below 100,000/mm^3, discontinue the drug, as ordered. WBC nadir usually occurs 9 to 14 days after treatment, possibly up to day 25; recovery occurs by day 30.
• Warn the patient of expected adverse effects.

• Give antiemetics, as ordered, for anorexia and nausea. Discontinue the drug, as ordered, if intractable vomiting or diarrhea or GI bleeding occurs.
• If infection occurs in a patient with myelosuppression, administer antibiotics, as ordered.
• Inspect the patient's skin regularly for signs of dermatologic reactions, such as rash, pruritus, erythema, increased pigmentation, or darkening of veins.
• Instruct the patient to avoid exposure to people with infections and to report any unusual bleeding or bruising.
• Advise women of childbearing age not to become pregnant during therapy. Advise mothers of infants not to breast-feed.

How peritoneal dialysis works

Peritoneal dialysis works by a combination of diffusion and osmosis.

Diffusion
In this process, particles pass through a semipermeable membrane from an area of high solute concentration to one of low solute concentration.

In peritoneal dialysis, the water-based dialysate contains glucose, sodium chloride, calcium, magnesium, acetate or lactate, and no waste products. Therefore, waste products and excess electrolytes in the blood cross through the semipermeable peritoneal membrane into the dialysate (see illustration). Removing the waste-filled dialysate and replacing it with fresh solution keeps waste concentration low and promotes further diffusion. Potassium may be added occasionally to maintain adequate serum levels. However, because failing kidneys can't excrete potassium, you'll need to monitor your patient's serum potassium level closely and adjust it as needed.

Osmosis
In this process, fluids move through a semipermeable membrane from an area of low solute concentration to one of high solute concentration.

In peritoneal dialysis, osmosis removes excess water from the patient's blood (see illustration). Dextrose in the dialysate promotes fluid movement by giving dialysate a higher solute-particle concentration than the blood.

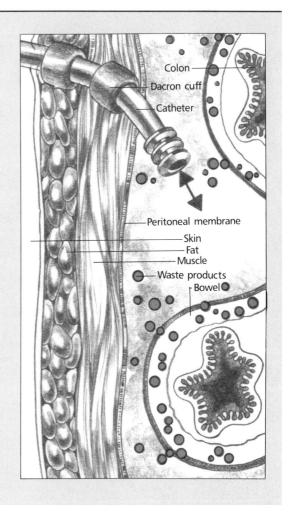

can roll up the empty bag, place it under his clothing, and perform normal activities. Six to 8 hours later, he drains the used solution into the bag and discards the bag. Then he attaches a new dialysate bag and instills the solution. He repeats this process 24 hours a day, 7 days a week.

Some patients combine CAPD and automatic cycling—a treatment called continuous-cycling peritoneal dialysis. The patient uses the CAPD pump during the day, and the cycler performs dialysis at night.

Although peritoneal dialysis isn't as effective as hemodialysis, it's safer, less expensive and stressful, and easier to perform. However, peritonitis can occur if bacteria (usually *Staphylococcus* or *Pseudomonas* organisms) enter the peritoneal cavity through the catheter or insertion site. Peritonitis can scar the peritoneum, causing it to thicken so it can't be used in dialysis. For this reason, peritoneal dialysis is usually contraindicated in patients who've had extensive abdominal surgery or abdominal trauma.

Intraperitoneal antibiotics

Typically, antibiotics are given intraperitoneally to patients with peritonitis caused by peritoneal dialysis. They're mixed in a solution, administered through a catheter, then drained after a specified dwell period. This technique produces high drug concentrations while avoiding the usual systemic adverse effects.

Equipment

The most common intraperitoneal access devices are a semipermanent indwelling catheter (such as the Tenckhoff catheter) and an implantable port (such as the PortaCath). A temporary indwelling catheter may also be placed percutaneously.

The Tenckhoff catheter is a soft, Silastic, semipermanent indwelling catheter with a Dacron cuff. One end goes in the peritoneal cavity and the other end protrudes externally. The cuff, secured in subcutaneous tissue, keeps the catheter in place and helps protect its inner portion from external contamination.

The PortaCath is a soft, Silastic, semipermanent catheter attached to a metal dome or portal. The doctor sutures the dome to subcutaneous tissue above the umbilicus, in the left upper abdominal quadrant. For transcutaneous entry, the doctor inserts a right-angle, 19G to 21G Huber needle through a silicone septum at the top of the port. Using a large-gauge needle expedites the infusion.

Insertion of access device

The doctor inserts the catheter at the patient's bedside or in the operating room. If you're the nurse assisting with the insertion, wash your hands and then gather the following equipment: antiemetic or sedative agent, if ordered; sterile face mask; sterile gloves; povidone-iodine solution; sterile fenestrated drape; 1% or 2% lidocaine; 3-ml syringe with a 25G 1" needle; scalpel with #11 blade; peritoneal stylet; appropriate catheter; sutures or nonallergenic tape; protective catheter cap, if needed; precut drain dressings; sterile gauze pads; and tape. (Commercial peritoneal dialysis kits or trays contain all the equipment needed for catheter placement and dressing changes.)

Give the patient an antiemetic or sedative to control nausea and anxiety, if ordered. Then help him into a supine position. Assist the doctor with catheter insertion by handing him equipment and supplies.

After putting on a sterile mask and gloves, the doctor cleans the patient's abdomen with povidone-iodine solution, then drapes it with a sterile drape.

Wipe the stopper of the lidocaine vial with povidone-iodine solution and let it dry. Invert the vial and hand it to the doctor so he can withdraw the lidocaine, using the 3-ml syringe with the 25G 1" needle.

The doctor anesthetizes a small area of the patient's abdomen below the umbilicus. After making a small incision with the scalpel, he inserts the catheter into the peritoneal cavity, using the stylet for guidance. Then he sutures or tapes the catheter in place.

Put on sterile gloves and apply the precut drain dressings around the catheter. Cover them with gauze pads and tape them securely.

Monitor the patient's vital signs and check the insertion site for bleeding. If a Tenckhoff catheter was inserted, assess the patient's tolerance for fluid exchange and help prevent fibrin clot formation by performing repeated fluid exchanges until intraperitoneal drainage appears clear. Then cap the catheter until it's ready for use.

Drug administration

The intraperitoneal route may be used to administer chemotherapeutic agents, dialysate, or antibiotics.

Administering chemotherapy

A specially trained oncology nurse can administer chemotherapeutic agents, following the steps below.

If ordered, insert an indwelling urinary catheter to promote patient comfort and to measure urine output during treatment.

Before starting intraperitoneal administration, insert a peripheral I.V. line and administer ordered fluids and electrolytes. The doctor may also order I.V. medications, such as analgesics or antiemetics. If your patient will receive intraperitoneal cisplatin, expect the doctor to order

I.V. sodium thiosulfate simultaneously. A neutralizing agent, sodium thiosulfate reduces cisplatin toxicity in the plasma without impeding its antitumor effects in the peritoneal cavity.

Assemble the following sterile equipment: 2 liters of 0.9% sodium chloride solution; preservative-free saline solution; warmer, heating pad, or water bath; two pairs of gloves; antiseptic solution, such as povidone-iodine; 1% lidocaine; Huber needle; transparent dressing; I.V. infusion pump; I.V. pole; ordered chemotherapeutic drug; syringes; heparinized saline flush solution; protective catheter cap or p.r.n. adapter, if needed; precut drain dressings; gauze pads; tape; and impervious container labeled CAUTION: CHEMOTHERAPY or CAUTION: BIOHAZARD for disposal of unused drugs or equipment.

Warm the 0.9% sodium chloride solution to body temperature, using the warmer, heating pad, or water bath. Obtain the patient's vital signs. Then wash your hands and put on gloves. Using aseptic technique, add the ordered dose of chemotherapeutic agent to the 0.9% sodium chloride solution.

If the patient has an implantable port, clean around the insertion site with antiseptic solution. Inject 0.2 ml of 1% lidocaine near the site. Then insert the Huber needle into the catheter until it touches the bottom of the port. Secure the needle with a transparent dressing.

If the patient has a Tenckhoff catheter, remove the protective cap or p.r.n. adapter and clean the end of the catheter with antiseptic solution.

With either an implantable port or a Tenckhoff catheter, check patency of the device by trying to aspirate fluid or by flushing it with 10 to 20 ml of heparinized saline solution. Place your stethoscope over the patient's lower abdominal quadrant. If you hear the sound of fluid, you can assume the device is patent.

Prime the I.V. tubing and attach it to the end of the Huber needle or Tenckhoff catheter. Instill the chemotherapeutic solution by gravity as rapidly as possible. (However, if the patient feels uncomfortable, slow the infusion rate.)

If the flow is sluggish, help the patient roll gently from side to side. If this doesn't speed the flow, irrigate the catheter with 0.9% sodium chloride solution. If the flow rate still doesn't improve and you're sure the catheter isn't blocked, attach an I.V. infusion pump.

During the infusion, monitor the patient for signs and symptoms of hypersensitivity to the drug. When 2 liters of solution have been instilled, clamp the drainage tubing. Let the solution remain in the peritoneal cavity for 4 hours. To move the solution around and enhance absorption, help the patient change position every 10 to 15 minutes for at least 1 hour after the infusion.

After the 4-hour dwell time, unclamp the drainage bag. To start outflow, aspirate fluid with a syringe and help the patient turn to the opposite side every 30 minutes. If drainage isn't adequate, ask him to perform the Valsalva maneuver while you apply pressure to his abdomen. However, be aware that incomplete drainage poses no real danger because intraperitoneal drugs are metabolized and excreted the same way as systemic drugs.

After 2 hours of drainage, flush the catheter with preservative-free saline solution, then heparinized saline solution. If the patient has an implantable port, remove the needle. If he has a Tenckhoff catheter, apply a new cap or p.r.n. adapter to the catheter end.

Put on a new pair of gloves, then apply the precut drain dressings around the catheter. Cover them with gauze pads and tape them securely.

Place all disposable equipment and unused drugs in impervious labeled containers. To prevent aerosol drug dispersion, don't clip needles. Place needles intact in the container for incineration. Even though you used gloves, wash your hands thoroughly with warm water and soap after giving any chemotherapeutic agent.

Administering dialysate

A specially trained nurse may perform the dialysis procedure, following the steps below.

Wash your hands and assemble the following sterile equipment: face masks; heating pad, warmer, or water bath; prescribed dialysate in 1- or 2-liter bottles or bags; any other prescribed medications, such as heparin or an antibiotic; dialysis administration set with drainage bag; I.V. pole; gloves; povidone-iodine sponges; gauze pads; tape; swab for specimen and labeled container, if needed; precut drain dressings; and 4" × 4" gauze pads.

Help the patient into the supine position and have him put on a sterile face mask. Inspect the dialysate, which should be clear and colorless. Then warm it to body temperature, using the heating pad, warmer, or water bath, to promote patient comfort during instillation and help dilate peritoneal capillaries. (Dilated capillaries enhance blood flow to the peritoneal membrane surface, helping to move wastes into the peritoneal cavity.)

Put on a sterile face mask. Add any prescribed medication to the dialysate, using strict aseptic technique to avoid contaminating the solution. (Heparin is commonly added to prevent fibrin accumulation in the catheter. If your patient has peritonitis, the doctor may want to add an antibiotic.)

Prepare the dialysis administration set. Close the clamps on all lines. You'll note that two lines merge to allow simultaneous infusion of two 1-liter dialysate containers. The lines then split, one going to the patient and the other to the drainage bag. Clamp all of these tubing segments.

Place the drainage bag below the patient to promote gravity drainage, then connect it to the drainage line. Connect the dialysate infusion lines to the dialysate bottles or bags. Next, hang the dialysate on the I.V. pole at the patient's bedside and prime the tubing by opening the infusion lines and letting the solution flow until all lines are primed. Close all clamps.

Put on sterile gloves and place a povidone-iodine sponge on the port of the dialysate container. Cover the port with a dry gauze pad and secure the pad with tape.

Saturate four gauze pads with povidone-iodine solution. Remove the dressing over the catheter and discard it, taking care not to touch the catheter or the patient's skin.

Check skin integrity at the catheter site. If you see drainage, obtain a swab specimen and place it in a labeled container. If the patient has drainage, tenderness, or pain at the cathe-

ter site, notify the doctor and don't proceed with the infusion until he tells you to.

Wrap one saturated gauze pad around the distal end of the catheter and leave it in place for 5 minutes. Clean the catheter and insertion site with two saturated gauze pads, moving in circles away from the site. Use a clean gauze pad with each wipe. Use straight strokes to clean the catheter, moving from the insertion site upward. Continue cleaning the catheter for another minute, using the remaining gauze pad.

Remove the povidone-iodine sponge from the catheter cap. Then remove the cap and use the last saturated gauze pad to clean the end of the catheter hub.

Connect the catheter to the administration set, using strict aseptic technique to prevent contaminating the catheter and solution (which could cause peritonitis).

Next, open the package of precut drain dressings and 4" × 4" gauze pads. Put on a new pair of sterile gloves. Apply the precut drain dressings around the catheter, cover them with gauze pads, and tape them securely.

To test catheter patency, unclamp the I.V. lines to the patient and rapidly instill 500 ml of dialysate into the peritoneal cavity. Next, clamp the I.V. lines to the patient, then immediately unclamp the lines to the drainage bag to allow fluid to drain into the bag. If the catheter's patent, you should see brisk outflow.

Once you've established patency, clamp the drainage bag lines and unclamp the lines to the patient. Infuse the prescribed volume of dialysate over 5 to 10 minutes.

Help the patient roll from side to side to distribute the dialysate equally throughout the peritoneum. As soon as the dialysate container empties, clamp the lines to the patient to prevent air from entering the tubing.

Let the solution dwell in the peritoneal cavity for the prescribed time (10 minutes to 4 hours). The solution will draw excess fluid, electrolytes, and accumulated wastes from the blood through the peritoneal membrane and into the dialysate. At the end of the dwell time, unclamp the drainage bag line and let the solution drain from the peritoneal cavity into the drainage bag.

When outflow ends, repeat the infusion-dwell-drain cycle for the prescribed number of times. Then clamp the catheter and put on a third pair of sterile gloves. Disconnect the administration set from the peritoneal catheter and place the sterile protective cap over the catheter's distal end.

Administering antibiotics

To administer intraperitoneal antibiotics, follow the same steps as for administering chemotherapeutic agents. (For a dialysis patient with peritonitis, add antibiotics to the dialysate, as ordered.)

Complications

Diarrhea may occur after any type of intraperitoneal therapy, from increased intra-abdominal pressure.

Cisplatin-induced hypomagnesemia, a serious complication of intraperitoneal chemotherapy, probably results from severe proximal tubular dysfunction. It causes such signs and symptoms as weakness, tremor, muscle twitching, paresthesia, ventricular arrhythmias, refractory hypocalcemia and hypokalemia, positive Chvostek's sign, and mental status changes.

Peritonitis is the most common complication of peritoneal dialysis. It usually results from a contaminated dialysate or leakage of solution from the catheter exit site back into the catheter tract. Bacterial infection at the catheter site may also cause peritonitis after intraperitoneal chemotherapy. However, aseptic technique usually prevents this complication. Signs and symptoms of peritonitis include fever, chills, rebound abdominal tenderness, labored respirations, nausea, and cloudy peritoneal drainage.

During the dwell phase of dialysis, severe respiratory distress may occur if the abdominal cavity becomes too full and the peritoneum presses against the lungs. If this happens, drain the peritoneal cavity. To help prevent respiratory distress, promote lung expansion through turning and deep-breathing exercises.

In a dialysis patient, protein depletion may occur if plasma protein diffuses into the dialysate through the peritoneal membrane. The patient may lose up to ½ oz (15 g) of protein daily — more if he has peritonitis.

In a patient with fluid retention, high-concentration (4.25%) dialysate can cause excessive fluid loss, leading to hypovolemia, hypotension, and shock. Fluid retention, another potential complication, may lead to blood volume expansion, hypertension, peripheral edema, pulmonary edema, or congestive heart failure.

Other complications of intraperitoneal administration include electrolyte imbalance and hyperglycemia (which serial blood glucose tests can identify).

Nursing considerations

• Make sure your patient is well hydrated before chemotherapy to help reduce adverse effects.

• Keep in mind that the doctor may order a perfusion scan before and after chemotherapy to confirm uniform drug distribution throughout the peritoneal cavity. The scan also identifies metastatic disease sites, loculations, and adhesions and can help gauge the effectiveness of treatment.

• Carefully monitor your patient's vital signs — especially respirations — during chemotherapy. A sudden rise in intra-abdominal pressure can limit diaphragmatic movement, causing respiratory distress. To reduce this risk, elevate the head of the bed and keep nasal oxygen nearby.

• If your patient has an implantable port, keep him in bed to prevent needle dislodgment, which may lead to infiltration and irritation of subcutaneous tissue.

• Maintain sterile technique to prevent infection or peritonitis, especially during dialysis. The high glucose concentration of dialysate enhances bacterial growth; frequent, long-term catheter access further increases the risk of infection.

• To help prevent infection and skin excoriation, change catheter dressings at least every 24 hours or whenever they become wet or soiled.

• During dialysis, monitor your patient's vital signs every 10 to 15 minutes for the first 1 to 2 hours of exchanges, then every 2 to 4 hours, or as needed. Notify the doctor if your

patient's condition changes abruptly.
• Check the color and clarity of dialysate outflow. It should be yellow and clear. During the first three or four cycles, it may be pink-tinged. If it remains pink-tinged or if you see gross blood, notify the doctor. If outflow contains feces (suggesting bowel perforation) or appears cloudy (suggesting peritonitis), notify the doctor, then obtain a sample for culture and Gram stain and send it to the laboratory for analysis.
• Expect your patient to have some discomfort or pain when dialysis begins. If he continues to feel pain later, document when it occurs, its quality and duration, and whether it radiates to other areas. Then notify the doctor. Pain during infusion usually results from too-rapid dialysate inflow or dialysate that's too cool or acidic. Severe, diffuse pain with rebound tenderness and cloudy effluent may signal peritoneal infection. Air accumulation under the diaphragm may cause pain that radiates to the shoulder. Incorrect catheter placement may cause severe, persistent perineal or rectal pain.
• Assess your patient's fluid balance at the end of each infusion-dwell-drain cycle. If the amount of fluid infused exceeds the amount recovered, he has a positive fluid balance. If the amount recovered exceeds the amount infused, he has a negative fluid balance. Notify the doctor if your patient retains 500 ml or more of fluid per cycle for three consecutive cycles or if he loses at least 1 liter of fluid per cycle for three consecutive cycles.
• Document the dialysate and any other medication given, the date and time, amount of dialysate infused and drained, how well the patient tolerated the procedure, and the appearance of the access device.
• If your patient's receiving dialysis, be aware that inflow-outflow problems can cause constipation. Be prepared to give a laxative or stool softener, as ordered.
• Provide a high-protein diet or protein supplement, if ordered, to prevent protein depletion in the dialysis patient. Also monitor periodic serum albumin levels.
• Weigh the dialysis patient daily to help determine the amount of fluid being removed. Document the time and any variation in weighing technique.

Patient teaching
Describe the catheter insertion and drug administration procedure to the patient and his family. Discuss benefits of the procedure, what's expected of the patient during the procedure, cosmetic concerns, activity restrictions, and possible complications.

To reduce the patient's anxiety and improve compliance, teach him about the prescribed drug and its regimen. Discuss possible adverse effects and how to manage them. Make sure the patient and his family have realistic expectations about dialysis or chemotherapy.

For home dialysis or chemotherapy, teach the patient or a family member how to perform the procedure, care for the catheter, and change dressings, using sterile technique. (See *Intraperitoneal chemotherapy: A simpler method*, pages 200 and 201.)

Inform the patient that intraperitoneal infusion usually causes temporary abdominal distention. Suggest that he wear loose-fitting clothing after therapy to promote comfort.

Teach the patient about the signs and symptoms of infection at the catheter site (redness, tenderness, or swelling) and of peritonitis (fever, persistent abdominal pain, slow or cloudy dialysis drainage, and swelling and tenderness around the catheter). Also teach him about the signs and symptoms of fluid imbalance. Tell him to call the doctor immediately if any of these problems occur.

Advise the patient to wear a medical alert bracelet or carry a card identifying him as a dialysis or chemotherapy patient. Instruct him to keep the doctor's or clinic's phone number with him at all times.

Intrapleural administration

An intrapleural drug is injected through the chest wall into the pleural space or instilled through a chest tube placed intrapleurally for

Intraperitoneal chemotherapy: A simpler method

If your patient is receiving intraperitoneal chemo-therapy at home through a Tenckhoff catheter, a family member or another caregiver may adminis-ter it. The method described here uses common supplies, such as an I.V. bag and administration set, instead of expensive dialysis equipment for both in-fusion and drainage. It also requires only clean technique instead of face masks and a sterile field.

Teach these steps to your patient's caregiver:
• Gather the following equipment: catheter clamp; two pairs of latex gloves; I.V. tubing; 50-ml bag of dextrose 5% in water (D_5W); chemotherapy solu-tion; povidone-iodine solution; 4" × 4" gauze pads; specimen container filled with povidone-iodine solution; 2" silk tape; p.r.n. adapter; sterile needle; povidone-iodine sponge; and heparinized saline flush solution, made by combining 3 ml hep-arin (1,000 units/ml) and 27 ml of 0.9% sodium chloride solution in a 30-ml syringe.
• Wash your hands and close the clamp on the Tenckhoff catheter. Put on two pairs of latex gloves.
• Prime the I.V. tubing with D_5W. Then remove the tubing from the D_5W bag and use it to spike the bag of chemotherapy solution. Discard the D_5W bag.
• Using 4" × 4" gauze pads soaked with povi-done-iodine solution, clean the connection site be-tween the p.r.n. adapter and the Tenckhoff catheter for 1 full minute.
• Remove the cap from the end of the catheter and submerge the catheter's open end into a spec-imen container filled with povidone-iodine solution.

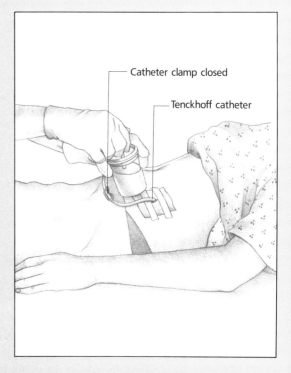

Catheter clamp closed

Tenckhoff catheter

• Leave it in for 3 to 4 minutes. Discard the used cap.
• Remove the catheter from the solution. Attach the I.V. tubing from the chemotherapy bag directly to the open end of the Tenckhoff catheter. Wrap the connection site with a 4" × 4" gauze pad soaked in povidone-iodine solution and tape it se-curely with 2" silk tape. Unclamp the catheter.

drainage. Intrapleural administration provides superior chemotherapeutic effects, reduces drug toxicity, and maintains higher and longer-lasting pleural drug concentrations. Increasingly, doctors are using it to promote analgesia, treat spontaneous pneumothorax, resolve pleural ef-fusions, and administer chemotherapy.

Reviewing chest anatomy will help you un-derstand how intrapleural administration works. The pleura, a serous membrane, encloses the lungs. It has two layers: the visceral pleura, which covers the lungs directly, and the pari-etal pleura, which lines the inner thoracic cav-ity. The pleural space — actually a potential space between the two pleural layers — contains a thin film of fluid.

The posterior intercostal arteries, arising in the aorta, supply blood to the posterior tho-racic wall. The intercostal nerves, which arise from the thoracic spinal nerves, innervate the thoracic wall and intercostal muscles. Intercos-tal nerves, arteries, and veins lie beneath the

Open the roller clamp on the I.V. tubing and infuse the chemotherapy solution at the prescribed rate.

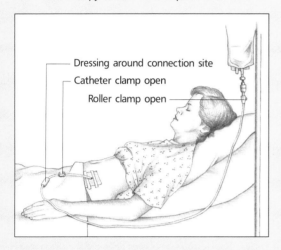

- Dressing around connection site
- Catheter clamp open
- Roller clamp open

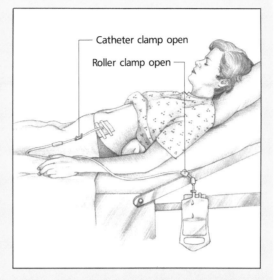

- Catheter clamp open
- Roller clamp open

• After infusing the chemotherapy solution, close the roller clamp on the I.V. tubing, then close the clamp on the catheter. To move the solution around in the peritoneal cavity, encourage the patient to change position every 10 to 15 minutes for at least 1 hour after the infusion.
• After the prescribed dwell time, lower the empty I.V. bag below the patient's abdomen. Open the roller clamp on the I.V. tubing; then open the clamp on the catheter. Allow fluid to drain into the I.V. bag, as shown in the third illustration, until you've accumulated the prescribed amount or drained for the prescribed period. Encourage the patient to change position frequently to promote drainage.

• When drainage is complete, close the roller clamp on the I.V. tubing. Then close the clamp on the catheter. Disconnect the I.V. tubing from the catheter and attach a capped needle securely to the end of the tubing. Apply a new p.r.n. adapter to the open end of the catheter. Remove your gloves and wash your hands.
• After the procedure, you must flush the catheter. To do this, open the clamp and clean the p.r.n. adapter with a povidone-iodine sponge. Flush the catheter with heparinized saline solution; then close the clamp. Measure the amount of fluid drainage by using the markings on the I.V. bag. Document the procedure and the patient's response.

ribs. The thoracic sympathetic nerve trunks and ganglia lie paravertebrally over the ribs, in front of the posterior intercostal vessels and nerves.

Researchers believe intrapleurally administered drugs diffuse across the parietal pleura and innermost intercostal muscles to affect the intercostal nerves. During an intrapleural injection, the needle passes through the intercostal muscles and parietal pleura on its way to the pleural space. The internal intercostal muscle is a key landmark for needle placement. It resists

the advancing needle, becoming the posterior intercostal membrane in the posterior chest region.

Unilateral sympathetic blockade may occur when an intrapleural anesthetic spreads across the posterior portion of the parietal pleura, affecting the upper sympathetic nerve chain and ganglia. To create a unilateral sympathetic blockade, such as to treat upper back pain, the doctor will position the patient with the affected side up, in a 20-degree Trendelenburg position, during anesthesia injection. By partially blocking the brachial plexus, this position causes shoulder and arm anesthesia. To block the lower intercostal and splanchnic nerves, such as to treat pancreatic pain, the doctor will have the patient sit during anesthesia injection.

Drugs commonly given by intrapleural injection include tetracycline, streptokinase, anesthetics, and chemotherapeutic agents (to treat malignant pleural effusion or lung adenocarcinoma). (See *Reviewing common intrapleural drugs,* pages 204 and 205.)

Intrapleural tetracycline helps prevent recurrent spontaneous pneumothorax by creating a chemical pleurodesis, which stops the pleural space from enlarging by making the two pleural layers adhere. In a patient with bacterial pneumonia, the doctor may administer intrapleural streptokinase to prevent pleural effusion by promoting drainage of inadequately evacuated empyema (pus accumulation in the pleural space). This intervention eliminates the need for further invasive procedures and improves the patient's prognosis.

Intrapleural anesthetics provide effective postoperative analgesia without the respiratory depression or sedation associated with opioids. For instance, the doctor may administer bupivacaine to treat postoperative pain from cholecystectomy, renal surgery, breast surgery, or rib fracture as well as to treat pain caused by thoracic injuries, cancerous chest metastases, or pancreatic cancer.

Contraindications to intrapleural administration include pleural fibrosis or adhesions, which impede drug diffusion to the intended site; pleural inflammation; sepsis; and infection at the puncture site. Patients with bullous emphysema and those receiving respiratory therapy using positive end-expiratory pressure also shouldn't have intrapleural injections because the injections may exacerbate an already compromised pulmonary condition.

Equipment

An intrapleural drug is given through an inserted catheter or a chest tube. Accessory equipment depends on which type of access device the doctor uses.

Insertion of access device

One of two access devices is used for an intrapleural injection: a #16 to #20 or #28 to #40 chest tube, or a 16G to 18G blunt-tipped intrapleural (epidural) needle and catheter. The doctor will use a chest tube for a patient with empyema, pleural effusion, or pneumothorax and an intrapleural catheter for any other patient.

Intrapleural catheter insertion

The doctor inserts the intrapleural catheter at the patient's bedside, with the nurse assisting.

Gather the following sterile equipment: gloves; gauze; antiseptic solution, such as povidone-iodine; drape; local anesthetic, such as 1% lidocaine; 3-ml and 5-ml syringes with 22G 1" and 25G ⅝" needles; 18G needle or scalpel; 16G to 18G blunt-tipped intrapleural needle and catheter; saline-lubricated glass syringe; dressings; sutures; and tape.

Position the patient with the affected side up. The doctor will insert the catheter into the fourth to eighth intercostal space, 3" to 4" (8 to 10 cm) from the posterior midline. (See *Intrapleural administration,* page 206.)

The doctor puts on sterile gloves, cleans around the puncture site with antiseptic-soaked gauze, then covers the area with a sterile drape. Next, he fills the 3- to 5-ml syringe with local anesthetic and injects it into the patient's skin and deep tissues.

The doctor punctures the skin with the 18G needle or scalpel, which helps the blunt-tipped intrapleural needle penetrate the skin over the superior edge of the lower rib in the chosen interspace. Keeping the bevel tilted upward, he directs the needle medially at a 30- to 40-degree angle to the skin. When the needle tip punctures the posterior intercostal membrane, he removes the stylet and attaches a saline-lubricated glass syringe containing 2 to 4 cc of air to the needle hub.

During puncture, tell the patient to hold his breath (or momentarily disconnect him from mechanical ventilation) until the needle's removed. This helps prevent the needle from injuring lung tissue.

The doctor advances the needle slowly, taking care not to apply pressure to the plunger. When the needle punctures the parietal pleura, negative intrapleural pressure moves the plunger outward. The doctor then removes the syringe from the needle and threads the intrapleural catheter through the needle until he's advanced it about 2" (5 cm) into the pleural space. Without removing the catheter, he carefully withdraws the needle.

Tell the patient he can breathe again (or reconnect mechanical ventilation).

After the catheter's inserted, the doctor coils it to prevent kinking, then sutures it securely to the patient's skin. He confirms catheter placement by aspirating. Resistance indicates correct placement in the pleural space. Aspirated blood means the catheter's probably in a blood vessel; aspirated air means it's probably in a lung. The doctor will order a chest X-ray at this time to detect pneumothorax.

Apply a sterile dressing over the insertion site to prevent catheter dislodgment. Take the patient's vital signs every 15 minutes for the first hour after the procedure, then as needed.

Chest tube insertion
The doctor inserts the chest tube, with the nurse assisting.

Gather the following sterile equipment: towels; gloves; gauze; antiseptic solution, such as povidone-iodine; 3- to 5-ml syringe; anesthetic, such as 1% lidocaine; 18G needle or scalpel; chest tube with or without trocar (#16 to #20 catheter for air or serous fluid, #28 to #40 for blood, pus, or thick fluid); two rubber-tipped clamps; sutures; drain dressings; tape; and thoracic drainage system and tubing.

Position the patient with the affected side up and drape him with sterile towels.

The doctor puts on gloves and cleans the appropriate site with gauze-soaked antiseptic solution. If the patient has a pneumothorax, the doctor uses the second intercostal space as the access site because air rises to the top of the pleural space. If the patient has a hemothorax or pleural effusion, the doctor uses the sixth to eighth intercostal space because fluid settles to the bottom of the pleural space.

The doctor fills the syringe with a local anesthetic and injects it into the site. He makes a small incision with the needle or scalpel, then inserts the appropriate-sized chest tube and immediately connects it to the thoracic drainage system or clamps it close to the patient's chest. He sutures the tube to the skin.

Tape the chest tube to the patient's chest distal to the insertion site to help prevent accidental dislodgment. Also tape the junction of the chest tube and drainage tube to prevent their separation. Apply sterile drain dressings and tape to the site.

After insertion, the doctor checks tube placement with a chest X-ray. Take the patient's vital signs every 15 minutes for 1 hour, then as needed. Auscultate his lungs at least every 4 hours to assess air exchange in the affected lung. Diminished or absent breath sounds mean the lung hasn't reexpanded.

Drug administration
The doctor injects medication through the intrapleural catheter or chest tube, with the nurse assisting.

If the patient will receive chemotherapy, the doctor will probably ask you to give an antiemetic at least ½ hour beforehand.

Gather the following sterile equipment: gloves; gauze pads; povidone-iodine solution; ordered medication; appropriate-sized needles and syringes; 1% lidocaine, if necessary; dressings; and tape.

Position the patient with the affected side up. Help the doctor move the dressing away from the intrapleural catheter or chest tube and clamp the drainage tube, if present.

The doctor disinfects the access port of the catheter or chest tube with antiseptic-soaked gauze. Draw up the appropriate medication dose and hand it to the doctor with the vial so he can verify the correct dose.

The doctor injects the medication. If it's an anesthetic, he gives a bolus or loading dose initially, then changes to continuous infusion. If it's tetracycline, he mixes it with an anesthetic, such as lidocaine, to alleviate pain during injection.

Reapply the dressings around the catheter. Monitor the patient closely during and after drug administration to gauge the effectiveness

(Text continues on page 206.)

Reviewing common intrapleural drugs

The intrapleural route may be used to administer an anesthetic, chemotherapeutic agent, antibiotic, or thrombolytic enzyme. This chart presents important information about drugs commonly given by this route.

DRUG	INDICATIONS AND DOSAGE	MECHANISM OF ACTION
bleomycin (Blenoxane)	Treatment of testicular carcinoma; squamous cell carcinoma of the head, neck, esophagus, skin, and GI tract; lung cancer; Hodgkin's lymphoma; and malignant lymphoma *Adult dosage:* 150 units by intrapleural injection. Lifetime dosage not to exceed 400 units (to prevent pulmonary toxicity)	Drug may inhibit synthesis of deoxyribonucleic acid (DNA), ribonucleic acid, and proteins by binding directly with DNA; may also break single- and double-stranded DNA. When injected into pleural space to treat malignant effusion, 50% of drug is absorbed. Distributed rapidly and extensively, bleomycin concentrates in skin and lungs (which may explain some toxicities resulting from lack of inactivating enzymes in these tissues). It undergoes significant tissue inactivation, especially in the liver and kidneys. Up to 50% of dose is excreted in the urine within 24 hours, 20% to 40% as active drug.
bupivacaine (Marcaine)	Infiltration, spinal, or epidural anesthesia; peripheral or sympathetic nerve block *Adult dosage:* dosage not to exceed 175 mg when administered alone or 225 mg when administered with epinephrine. Daily dosage not to exceed 400 mg of solution without preservatives. Usually, dose shouldn't be repeated more than once every 3 hours.	Like other local anesthetics, bupivacaine blocks nerve impulses at the point of contact. It accumulates and causes the nerve cell membrane to expand. As the membrane expands, the cell loses its ability to depolarize, and therefore its ability to transmit impulses. Absorption rate varies with dosage and administration site. Bupivacaine is distributed throughout the body, including the central nervous system (CNS). Little drug transfers to the placenta. Direction of drug's route depends on patient position, movement, spinal curvature, dose, and specific gravity and volume of solution. Bupivacaine is metabolized by microsomal enzymes in the liver and is excreted by the kidneys.
streptokinase (Kabikinase, Streptase)	Treatment of pleural effusion and pulmonary embolism *Adult dosage:* Loading dose of 250,000 units: maintenance dose of 100,000 units/hour.	Promotes thrombolysis by converting residual plasminogen to plasmin, which degrades fibrin clots, fibrinogen, and precoagulant Factors V and VII. Drug decreases blood and plasma viscosity and reduces the tendency of erythrocytes to form aggregates, thereby increasing perfusion of collateral blood vessels. The plasminogen activation system begins promptly after infusion; response occurs in 3 to 4 hours. Antibodies and the reticuloendothelial system remove the drug from the body.
tetracycline (Achromycin, Tetracyn)	Treatment of recurrent spontaneous pneumothorax *Adult dosage:* one-time dose of 1,500 mg	Tetracycline is a broad-spectrum antibiotic, bacteriostatic, and antiprotozoal agent that inhibits protein synthesis by binding to the 30S ribosomal subunit of microorganisms. The drug is readily distributed throughout body tissues and fluids (except in the CNS). It binds variably to plasma proteins and localizes in bone, liver, spleen, tumors, and teeth. Tetracycline isn't metabolized but is excreted unchanged in urine and feces in high concentrations. It appears in breast milk.

NURSING CONSIDERATIONS

• Because 1% of lymphoma patients have an anaphylactic reaction to bleomycin, these patients should receive two test doses of 2 to 5 units before the initial dose.
• Assess respiratory function carefully before each treatment, especially in patients at high risk for pulmonary toxicity. Signs of toxicity include dyspnea, bibasilar crackles, and a nonproductive cough.
• Monitor blood urea nitrogen level, creatinine clearance, and pulmonary function. Arrange for chest X-rays before and during treatment.
• Monitor the patient closely for 1 hour after treatment.
• Reduce dosage in patients with renal failure, as ordered.
• Warn the patient about possible hair loss (usually temporary).
• As part of combination therapy, this drug may enhance anticancer effects without increasing bone marrow toxicity.

• Administer cautiously to patients with hepatic dysfunction.
• Observe for adverse CNS reactions, including dizziness, disorientation, blurred vision, drowsiness, and seizures. Take safety measures, such as constant patient supervision and seizure precautions. If reactions occur, notify the doctor.

• Contraindicated in patients with ulcerative wounds, active internal bleeding, recent trauma with possible internal injuries, visceral or intracranial cancer, ulcerative colitis, diverticulitis, severe hypertension, acute or chronic hepatic or renal insufficiency, uncontrolled hypocoagulation, chronic pulmonary disease with cavitation, subacute bacterial endocarditis, rheumatic valvular disease, recent cerebral embolism, thrombosis or hemorrhage, and diabetic hemorrhagic retinopathy (because excessive bleeding may occur).
• Use with extreme caution in pregnant patients and in patients up to 10 days postpartum; after any intracranial, intraspinal, or intra-arterial diagnostic procedure; and after any surgery, including liver or kidney biopsy, lumbar puncture, thoracentesis, paracentesis, and extensive or multiple cutdowns.
• Use with caution in patients with arterial emboli arising from the left side of the heart because of the risk of cerebral infarction.
• Monitor for minor allergic reaction, manifested by fever and chills; as ordered, give antihistamines, acetaminophen, or corticosteroids.
• Apply local pressure to treat minor bleeding.

• Obtain specimen for culture and sensitivity tests before therapy.
• Be aware that the intrapleural route is painful. As ordered, administer a local anesthetic with the drug.
• Advise the patient to avoid sun exposure because photosensitivity can occur.
• If diarrhea persists during therapy, obtain specimens for stool culture to rule out pseudomembranous colitis.
• With long-term therapy, monitor hematopoietic, renal, and hepatic studies.
• For a patient with diabetes mellitus, monitor the blood glucose level.
• Tetracycline is incompatible with most other drugs. Before administering, find out what other drugs the patient is taking.

Intrapleural administration

In intrapleural administration, the doctor injects a drug into the pleural space using a catheter.

Help the patient lie on one side with the affected side up. The doctor inserts a needle into the fourth to eighth intercostal space, 3" to 4" (8 to 10 cm) from the posterior midline. He then advances the needle medially over the superior edge of the patient's rib through the intercostal muscles until it tangentially penetrates the parietal pleura, as shown. The catheter is advanced into the pleural space through the needle, which is then removed.

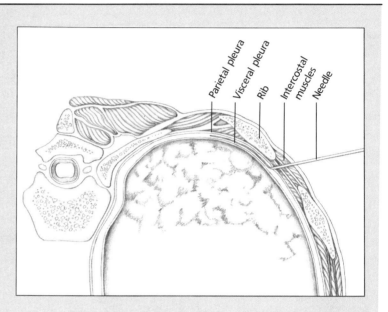

of drug therapy and to check for complications and adverse effects.

Complications
Pneumothorax or tension pneumothorax may occur if the doctor accidentally injects air into the pleural cavity. These complications are more likely in a patient who's on mechanical ventilation.

Accidental catheter placement in the lung can lead to respiratory distress; catheter placement within a vessel can increase the medication's effects. With catheter fracture, lung puncture may occur.

Laceration of intercostal vessels can cause bleeding.

Local anesthetic toxicity can lead to tinnitus, metallic taste, light-headedness, somnolence, visual and auditory disturbances, restlessness, delirium, slurred speech, nystagmus, muscle tremor, seizures, arrhythmias, and cardiovascular collapse. A local anesthetic containing epinephrine can cause tachycardia and hypertension.

Intrapleural chemotherapeutic drugs can ir-

ritate the pleura chemically and cause such systemic effects as neutropenia and thrombocytopenia. Administering intrapleural tetracycline without an anesthetic causes pain.

The insertion site can become infected. However, meticulous skin preparation, strict aseptic technique, and sterile dressings usually prevent infection.

Nursing considerations
• Make sure the patient has signed a consent form.
• Before catheter insertion, ask the patient to urinate to reduce the risk of bladder perforation and promote comfort.
• If the patient's receiving a continuous infusion, label the solution bag clearly. Cover all injection ports so other drugs aren't injected into the pleural space accidentally.
• If the chest tube accidentally dislodges, cover the site at once with a sterile gauze pad and tape it in place. Stay with the patient, monitor his vital signs, and observe carefully for signs and symptoms of tension pneumothorax: hypotension; distended neck veins; absent breath

sounds; tracheal shift; hypoxemia; weak, rapid pulse; dyspnea; tachypnea; diaphoresis; and chest pain. Have another nurse call the doctor and gather the equipment needed to reinsert the tube.

• Keep rubber-tipped clamps at the bedside. If a commercial chest-tube system cracks or a tube disconnects, use the clamps to clamp the chest tube close to the insertion site temporarily. However, be sure to observe the patient closely for signs of tension pneumothorax because no air can escape from the pleural space while the tube's clamped.

• You can wrap a piece of petroleum gauze around the chest tube at the insertion site to make an airtight seal, then apply the sterile dressing. After the chest tube's removed, use the petroleum gauze to dress the wound, then cover it with a new piece of sterile gauze.

• After the catheter's removed, inspect the skin at the entry site for signs of infection, then cover the wound with a sterile dressing.

• After removing the catheter, document that you saw the mark at the tip that indicates the catheter was removed intact.

Patient teaching
Explain the purpose and benefits of the intrapleural catheter or chest tube to the patient and his family. Describe the procedure and possible adverse effects, and allow time for them to ask questions.

If the patient's receiving chemotherapy, describe the drugs and drug regimen. Discuss possible adverse effects and how to manage them.

Warn the patient to use care to prevent the chest tube or catheter from dislodging. Show him how to apply rubber-tipped clamps in case the tube or drain should dislodge or separate, and tell him to call you if this happens.

Gastrostomy button

The gastrostomy button serves as an alternative to a gastrostomy tube for an ambulatory patient receiving long-term enteral nutrition.

Inserted into an established stoma, it can remain implanted for up to 6 months. The button has a mushroom-shaped dome at one end and two wing tabs and a flexible safety plug at the other end. The button lies almost flush with the skin, with only the top of the safety plug visible.

The gastrostomy button has several advantages. Usually, it can be inserted into a stoma in less than 15 minutes. Compared to an ordinary feeding tube, the device has cosmetic appeal, reduces skin irritation and breakdown, is easy to maintain, and is less likely to become dislodged and migrate.

A one-way antireflux valve mounted just inside the mushroom dome prevents leakage of gastric contents. The button usually requires just one replacement — after 3 to 4 months — typically because the antireflux valve wears out.

A drug delivered by gastrostomy button is absorbed through the gastric mucosa the same way as an oral drug. After absorption, it passes through the liver and is distributed systemically. However, because it bypasses the mouth, where the breaking down of ingested substances begins, it must be given in liquid form. So you'll need to either reconstitute liquid or powder medications or crush pills finely and dissolve them in water. Check with the pharmacist and manufacturer's guidelines before crushing medications because some enteric-coated and long-acting tablets shouldn't be crushed.

Equipment
Gastrostomy buttons come in three sizes. If you don't know what size your patient needs, take all three sizes to the bedside. You also may need a mortar and pestle.

Insertion of access device
Although the doctor initially inserts the gastrostomy button with a nurse's assistance, you or the patient will have to reinsert it if it pops out. The insertion and reinsertion procedures are essentially the same. (See *Reinserting a gastrostomy button,* page 208.)

Reinserting a gastrostomy button

If your patient's gastrostomy button pops out (such as from coughing), you or the patient will need to reinsert it. Here are the steps to follow.

Gather gloves, the gastrostomy button (shown at right), mild soap and water or povidone-iodine solution, an obturator, water-soluble lubricant and, if necessary, the ordered medication, a catheter adapter, and a catheter.

    Before reinsertion, wash your hands and put on gloves, then wash the button with soap and water and rinse it thoroughly.

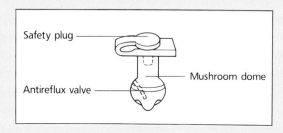

Check the depth of the stoma to make sure you have a button of the correct size. Then clean around the stoma with soap and water or povidone-iodine solution and let it air dry.

    Lubricate the obturator with a water-soluble lubricant and distend the button several times to ensure patency of the antireflux valve. Lubricate the mushroom dome and stoma. Gently push the button through the stoma into the stomach, as shown at right.

    Remove the obturator by rotating it gently as you withdraw it to keep the antireflux valve from adhering. If the valve sticks nonetheless, gently push the obturator back into the button until the valve closes.

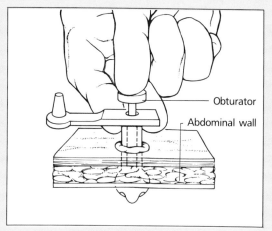

After removing the obturator, check the valve to make sure it's closed. Then close the flexible safety plug, which should be relatively flush with the skin surface, as shown at right.

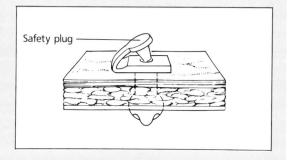

If you need to administer the drug right away, open the safety plug and attach the adapter and catheter, as shown here. Deliver the drug as ordered.

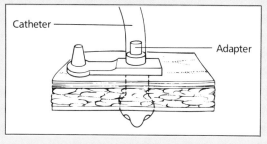

Drug administration

You'll administer medications through the gastrostomy button.

Gather sterile equipment: gloves, ordered medication, lukewarm water for mixing and flushing, 5- to 30-ml syringe, syringe for flushing, and a cotton-tipped applicator.

Wash your hands and put on gloves. Prepare the medication by reconstituting the ordered powder or liquid or by crushing the ordered tablet and dissolving it in lukewarm water. Draw up the medication into a 5- to 30-ml syringe, then inject it directly into the gastrostomy button opening. (The button is made to accommodate to standard syringes so that they fit exactly.)

Flush the button with a syringe filled with 10 ml of water. Then clean the inside of the button with a cotton-tipped applicator and water to preserve its patency and dislodge any medication particles. Snap the safety plug in place to keep the lumen clean and prevent leakage if the antireflux valve fails.

Nursing considerations

• If the gastrostomy button pops out during drug administration, reinsert it. If you're not sure how much drug was delivered, check with the doctor before repeating the dose.
• Document the medication and time administered. Maintain intake and output records, as necessary. Record the appearance of the stoma and surrounding skin.
• Clean peristomal skin once a day with mild soap and water or povidone-iodine solution. To help prevent skin irritation, let the skin air dry for 20 minutes. Be sure to clean the site whenever spills occur.

Patient teaching

Explain the purpose of the button, the insertion procedure, and the medication administration to the patient and his family. Discuss benefits and potential adverse effects and answer any questions.

Before discharge, make sure the patient or a family member can care for the button, administer medications, and reinsert the button if it pops out. Provide written instructions and information about replacement supplies.

Intraocular administration

Intraocular drugs can be given through an eye medication disk — a small, flexible oval consisting of two soft, outer layers and a middle layer containing medication. The disk is inserted somewhat like a contact lens, except that it's placed in the conjunctival sac and floats on the sclera between the iris and lower eyelid. When moistened by ocular fluid, it releases medication for up to 1 week before needing replacement.

Eye medication disks are especially useful for administering pilocarpine to patients with chronic open-angle or acute narrow-angle glaucoma. A cholinergic and miotic agent, pilocarpine stimulates and contracts the sphincter muscle of the iris, contracting the pupil. It also makes the ciliary muscle contract, causing accommodation with anterior chamber deepening and dilation of the conjunctival vessels of the outflow tract.

The disks have several advantages. Unlike eyedrops, they don't require frequent insertion. The patient can wear them when sleeping, swimming, and engaging in sports and when using contact lenses. Eye moisture doesn't affect the disks. And because they release medication continuously, at a rate tailored to each patient, doses are significantly lower than with conventional eyedrops. Disadvantages include mild tearing or redness of the sclera and eyelid, increased mucus discharge, itchiness, and cost.

All eye medication disks are contraindicated in patients with inflammatory eye conditions (such as conjunctivitis and keratitis), retinal detachment, and whenever pupil constriction should be avoided. Pilocarpine disks are contraindicated in patients receiving carbachol, atropine, scopolamine, or phenylephrine. They should be used cautiously in patients with acute cardiac failure, bronchial asthma, urinary tract obstruction, GI spasm, peptic ulcer, hyperthyroidism, and parkinsonism.

How to insert and remove an eye medication disk

You'll find that inserting and removing an eye medication disk is easy. However, the inner eye is an extremely sensitive area, and most people are squeamish about having it touched. So you need to know how to perform this procedure quickly and precisely to reduce patient anxiety. Follow these guidelines.

Inserting the disk
• Wash your hands and don gloves.
• Press your fingertip against the oval disk so it lies lengthwise across your fingertip. It should stick to your finger. Lift the disk out of its packet.
• Gently pull the patient's lower eyelid away from the eye and place the disk in the conjunctival sac, as shown below. The disk should lie horizontally, not vertically. It will adhere to the eye naturally.

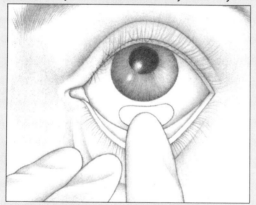

• Pull the lower eyelid out, up, and over the disk. Tell the patient to blink several times. If the disk is still visible, pull the lower lid out and over the disk again. Tell the patient that once the disk is in place, he can adjust its position by gently pressing his finger against his closed lid. But caution him against rubbing his eye or moving the disk across the cornea.
• If the disk falls out, wash your hands, rinse the disk in cool water, and reinsert it. If it appears bent, replace it.
• If both of the patient's eyes are being treated with medication disks, replace both disks at the same time so that both eyes receive medication at the same rate.
• If the disk repeatedly slips out of position, reinsert it under the upper eyelid. To do this, gently lift and evert the upper eyelid and insert the disk in the conjunctival sac. Gently pull the lid back into position and tell the patient to blink several times. The patient may press gently on the closed eyelid to reposition the disk. The more he uses the disk, the easier he'll be able to retain it. If he can't, notify the doctor.
• If the patient will continue using an eye medication disk after discharge, teach him to insert and remove it himself. To check his mastery of these skills, have him demonstrate insertion and removal for you.
• Teach the patient about possible adverse reactions. Eye medication disks can cause foreign-body sensation in the eye, mild tearing or redness, increased mucus discharge, eyelid redness, and itchiness. A pilocarpine disk can cause blurred vision, stinging, swelling, and headaches. Inform the patient that mild symptoms are common but should subside within the first 6 weeks. Tell him to report persistent or severe symptoms to his doctor.

Removing the disk
• You can remove an eye medication disk with one or two fingers. To use one finger, wash your hands, put on gloves, and evert the lower eyelid to expose the disk. Then use the forefinger of your other hand to slide the disk onto the lid and out of the patient's eye.

To use two fingers, evert the lower lid with one hand to expose the disk. Then pinch the disk with the thumb and forefinger of your other hand and remove it from the eye.
• If the disk migrates to the upper eyelid, apply long circular strokes to the patient's closed eyelid with your finger until you can see the disk in the corner of the eye. Once the disk is visible, place your finger directly on it and move it to the lower sclera. Then remove it as you would a disk lodged in the lower lid.

Equipment
The eye medication disk is the only specialized equipment needed.

Drug administration
You'll insert the eye medication disk the first time. After discharge, the patient can insert it himself once you've taught him how. (See *How to insert and remove an eye medication disk.*)

Complications
Eye infection can occur from poor hygiene during disk insertion or from difficulty removing the disk.

With a pilocarpine disk, complications include blurred vision, nausea, vomiting, increased salivation, bronchospasm, brow pain, and myopia. The last two problems usually disappear in 10 to 14 days.

Nursing considerations
After inserting the disk, document the procedure, the medication inserted, the eye or eyes treated, and the date, time, and dosage. Also record the patient's response, including any adverse affects.

Patient teaching
If the patient will be using the disk at home, teach him or a family member how to insert and remove it. To check skill mastery, have him do a return demonstration. Stress the importance of thorough hand washing before disk insertion or removal.

Instruct the patient to insert the disk before he goes to bed to minimize the blurring that immediately follows disk insertion.

Warn the patient to expect mild tearing and scleral redness, increased mucus discharge, eyelid redness, and itchiness.

If the patient has a pilocarpine disk, instruct him to check with you or the doctor before taking other prescribed or over-the-counter drugs. Many drugs, including antihistamines and sleep preparations, have anticholinergic effects. Inform him that adverse reactions might occur, especially temporarily blurred vision. Tell him to report any persistent or severe symptoms to the doctor.

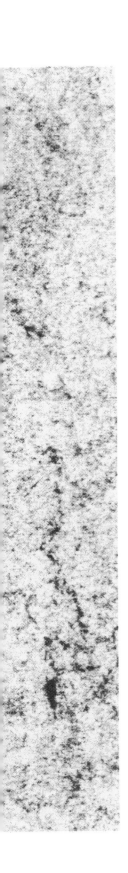

Suggested readings

Baer, W., and Williams, B. *Clinical Pharmacology and Nursing,* 2nd ed. Springhouse, Pa.: Springhouse Corp., 1992.

Belcher, A.E. *Cancer.* Clinical Nursing Series, vol. 8. St. Louis: Mosby-Year Book, 1992.

Bragg, C. "Interpleural Analgesia," *Heart and Lung* 20(1):30-38, January 1991.

Camp-Sorrell, D. "Advanced Central Venous Access," *Journal of Intravenous Nursing,* 13(6):361-69, November-December 1990.

Collins, J., and Lutz, R. "In Vitro Study of Simultaneous Infusion of Incompatible Drugs in Multilumen Catheters," *Heart and Lung* 20(3):271-77, May 1991.

DiPero, T., et al., eds. *Pharmacotherapy: A Pathophysiologic Approach,* 2nd ed. New York: Elsevier, 1992.

Doane, L., et al. "How to Give Peritoneal Chemotherapy," *American Journal of Nursing* 90(4):58-66, April 1990.

Drug Information 88. Bethesda: American Society of Hospital Pharmacists, Inc., 1988.

Economou, S., et al. *Adjuncts to Cancer Surgery.* Philadelphia: Lea and Febiger, 1991.

Ferrante, M.F., et al. *Patient-controlled Analgesia.* Cambridge, Mass.: Blackwell Scientific Publications Inc., 1990.

Gilman, A., et al. *Goodman & Gilman's The Pharmacological Basis of Therapeutics,* 8th ed. New York: McGraw-Hill Book Co., 1990.

Groenwald, S., et al. *Cancer Nursing: Principles and Practice,* 2nd ed. Boston: Jones and Bartlett, 1990.

Harrington, D. "The Advantages and Disadvantages of Adding Drugs to Total Parenteral Nutrition Solutions," *Infusion* 13(2):9-11, 1989.

Illustrated Manual of Nursing Practice. Springhouse, Pa.: Springhouse Corp., 1991.

I.V. Therapy. Clinical Skillbuilders Series. Springhouse, Pa.: Springhouse Corp., 1991.

Johnston, J.B., and Messina, M. "Erroneous Laboratory Values Obtained from Central Catheters," *Journal of Intravenous Nursing* 14(1):13-15, January/February 1991.

Koda-Kimble, M., ed. *Applied Therapeutics: The Clinical Use of Drugs,* 5th ed. Vancouver, Wash.: Applied Therapeutics, Inc., 1992.

Kwan, J.W. "High-technology I.V. Infusion Devices," *American Journal of Hospital Pharmacy* 48(Suppl. 1):S36-S51, October 1991.

Light, R., et al. "Intrapleural Tetracycline for the Prevention of Recurrent Spontaneous Pneumothorax: Results of a Department of Veterans Affairs Cooperative Study," *JAMA* 264(17):2224-30, November 7, 1990.

Long-term Central Venous Catheters, Procedures Video Series. Springhouse, Pa.: Springhouse Corp., 1992.

McCaffery, M., and Beebe, A. *Pain: Clinical Manual for Nursing Practice.* St. Louis: Mosby-Year Book, 1989.

Miaskowski, C., et al., eds. "Advances in Oncology Nursing," *Nursing Clinics of North America* 25(2), June 1990.

Montaldo, P., et al. "Pharmacokinetics of Intrapleural Versus Intravenous Etoposide and Teniposide in Patients with Malignant Pleural Effusion," *Oncology* 47(1):55-61, 1990.

Nursing93 Drug Handbook. Springhouse, Pa.: Springhouse Corp., 1993.

Nursing Procedures. Springhouse, Pa.: Springhouse Corp., 1992.

Owen, D., Jr., et al. "When to Aspirate and Inject Joints," *Patient Care* 24(14):128-45, September 1990.

Photoguide to Drug Administration. Springhouse, Pa.: Springhouse Corp., 1992.

Piascik, M. "Research and Development of Drugs and Biologic Entities." *American Journal of Hospital Pharmacy* 48(Suppl. 1):S4-S13, 1991.

Plumer, A.L. *Principles and Practice of Intravenous Therapy,* 4th ed. Boston: Little Brown, 1987.

Robinson, D., and Mauger, J. "Drug Delivery Systems," *American Journal of Hospital Pharmacy* 48(Suppl. 1):S14-S23, 1991.

Renneker, M. *Understanding Cancer,* 3rd ed. Menlo Park, Calif.: Bull Publishers, 1988.

Ryder, E. "All about Patient-Controlled Analgesia," *Journal of Intravenous Nursing,* 14(6):371-82, November/December 1991.

St. Marie, B. "Narcotic Infusions—A Changing Scene," *Journal of Intravenous Nursing,* 14(5):334-44, September/October 1991.

Simonson, G., et al. "Re-establishing Patency in the Occluded Implanted Central Venous Access Device," *Critical Care Nurse* 9(9):13-21, October 1989.

Symreng, T., et al. "Intrapleural Bupivacaine—Technical Considerations and Intraoperative Use," *Journal of Cardiothoracic Anesthesia* 3(2):139-43, April 1989.

Tenenbaum, L. *Cancer Chemotherapy.* Philadelphia: W.B. Saunders Co., 1989.

Viall, C.D. "Your Complete Guide to Central Venous Catheters,'" *Nursing90* 20(2):34-41, February 1990.

Wheeler, C. "Pediatric Intraosseous Infusion," *Journal of Intravenous Nursing* 12(6):371-76, November/December 1989.

Willsie, E., et al. "The Use of Intrapleural Streptokinase in the Treatment of Thoracic Empyema," *American Journal of Medical Science* 300(5):296-300, November 1990.

Wilson, T., et al., eds. *Harrison's Principles of Internal Medicine,* vols. I and II, 12th ed. New York: McGraw-Hill Book Co., 1991.

Winters, V., et al. "A Trial with a New Peripheral Implanted Vascular Access Device," *Oncology Nursing Forum* 17(6):891-96, November/December 1990.

Advanced skilltest

You can test your knowledge of advanced drug administration by answering the following multiple-choice questions. The answers, along with rationales, appear on pages 219 to 221.

1. What's the main advantage of the transdermal route?

    a. It makes drug administration easier.

    b. It helps improve patient compliance.

    c. It can be used on a patient with abnormal skin.

    d. It provides a rapid onset of action.

2. The drugs developed by biotechnology:

    a. remain more stable than other drugs.

    b. require relatively few human subjects during drug testing and receive quick approval from the Food and Drug Administration (FDA).

    c. have a longer shelf life than other drugs.

    d. need special storage facilities and have a short shelf life.

3. A patient who has a unique, unpredictable reaction to a drug — other than an allergic reaction — is experiencing:

    a. anaphylactic shock.

    b. a hypersensitivity reaction.

    c. an idiosyncratic response.

    d. a pharmacodynamic effect.

4. The most dangerous result of the precipitate that can form from the infusion of incompatible drugs is:

    a. a block in the I.V. tubing.

    b. an unpredictable drug effect.

    c. thrombophlebitis and emboli.

    d. pain.

5. The peripheral I.V. route allows what percentage of a drug to reach the systemic circulation?

    a. 60%

    b. 80%

    c. 90%

    d. 100%

6. Although selection of a venipuncture site depends on several factors, the best sites include:

    a. dorsal veins of the hand and the cephalic and basilic veins in the lower arm.

    b. veins in the leg and foot.

    c. antecubital veins.

    d. veins in the upper arm.

7. What systemic complication of I.V. therapy can cause signs of congestive heart failure, such as increased blood pressure, crackles, neck vein distention, and shortness of breath?

    a. Dyspnea

    b. Hypovolemic shock

    c. Circulatory overload

    d. Pulmonary edema

8. If a patient who receives a bolus dose of a drug develops a headache, syncope, flushed face, tightness in the chest, and an irregular pulse rate, and his plasma studies show a toxic drug level, what would you suspect?

    a. Speed shock

    b. Circulatory overload

    c. Anaphylactic shock

    d. Hypersensitivity

9. A patient who receives several blood transfusions may develop antibodies against leukocytes. To prepare a unit of blood for such a patient, you would:

    a. run it through a blood filter.

    b. run it through a blood warmer.

    c. add a leukocyte-removal filter to the blood bag.

    d. run it through an infusion pump.

10. What's the most important advantage of patient-controlled analgesia (PCA)?

    a. It frees both patient and nurse from the frequent administration of pain medication.

    b. It tends to decrease the amount of pain and sedation the patient experiences.

    c. It gives the patient more control over his pain.

    d. It allows the safe administration of narcotics.

11. The veins most commonly used for a central venous (CV) line are the subclavian and the:

    a. internal jugular.

    b. femoral.

    c. external jugular.

    d. superior vena cava.

12. Some health care facilities prohibit the administration of amphotericin B through a CV line because:

    a. the drug may extravasate into the surrounding tissue.

    b. this caustic drug must be greatly diluted, thereby increasing the risk of fluid overload.

    c. the drug may lower potassium levels, triggering cardiac arrhythmias.

    d. the rapid absorption and high blood concentration that result from infusion through a CV line may lead to drug toxicity.

13. Care of a CV catheter includes all of the following *except:*

    a. placing the patient in Trendelenburg's position before the insertion of a CV line.

    b. drawing blood back through each lumen to prevent air embolism after insertion of a multilumen catheter.

    c. changing the dressing on the catheter every 48 to 72 hours.

    d. flushing a Groshong catheter with 3 to 5 ml of heparinized solution every 7 days.

14. Which implanted vascular access port (VAP) allows side entry instead of top entry?

    a. Med-i-Port

    b. Port-A-Cath

    c. S.E.A. Port

    d. Infuse-A-Port

15. For a patient who needs frequent magnetic resonance imaging (MRI), the doctor may consider implanting a VAP made with any of the following materials *except:*

    a. plastic.

    b. titanium.

    c. stainless steel.

    d. Silastic.

16. Parenteral nutrition solution should contain what electrolytes?

    a. Glucose and lipids

    b. Sodium, potassium, magnesium, calcium, and phosphorus

    c. Carbohydrates and protein

    d. Vitamins D, B, and C

17. What's the highest percentage of dextrose that a solution of peripheral parenteral nutrition (PPN) should contain?

    a. 50%

    b. 40%

    c. 10%

    d. 5%

18. How often do most patients receiving parenteral nutrition need blood work performed?

    a. Once weekly

    b. Daily

    c. Every other week

    d. Three times a week

19. What ranks as the most serious complication of parenteral nutrition?

    a. Catheter-related sepsis

    b. Hyperglycemia

    c. Thrombophlebitis

    d. Fluid and electrolyte imbalances

20. A patient receiving parenteral nutrition may also need a lipid emulsion to provide:

    a. ascorbic acid.

    b. added nutrients.

    c. calories and essential fatty acids.

    d. additional vitamins and electrolytes.

21. Which of the following cancers responds most readily to chemotherapy?

    a. Colon cancer

    b. Prostate cancer

    c. Lung cancer

    d. Acute leukemia

22. Which of the following signs and symptoms suggest an adverse reaction to bone marrow suppression?

    a. Weight loss and nausea

    b. Fever, chills, and hypotension

    c. Hypertension, anxiety, and diaphoresis

    d. Anorexia, mouth ulcers, and bruising

23. A patient receiving chemotherapy may need leucovorin calcium rescue when receiving high doses of:

    a. cyclophosphamide.

    b. cisplatin.

    c. plicamycin.

    d. methotrexate.

24. The Occupational Safety and Health Administration (OSHA) has established guidelines for health care workers who handle chemotherapeutic drugs. Their two most important recommendations call for special training for those who work with chemotherapeutic drugs and which of the following:

    a. a ban on food and drink in areas where these drugs are mixed.

    b. the use of biological safety cabinets for mixing these drugs.

    c. strict adherence to the manufacturer's instructions for preparing the drugs.

    d. the use of clean, plastic absorbent pads to cover surfaces where drug preparation takes place.

25. Who is responsible for inserting an epidural catheter?

    a. The nurse

    b. The doctor's assistant

    c. The anesthesiologist

    d. The neurologist

26. If the dura is torn during or after epidural catheterization, spinal fluid will leak out of the subarachnoid space, causing a post-spinal puncture headache. If this occurs, you would:

    a. increase the patient's fluid intake and help him to lie down.

    b. administer narcotics, as ordered, until the headache subsides.

    c. inject 10 ml of 0.9% sodium chloride solution, as ordered, into the epidural space.

    d. inject 15 to 20 ml of the patient's own blood, as ordered, into the epidural space.

27. What structure prevents or slows the passage of water-soluble drugs into the central nervous system (CNS)?

    a. The blood-brain barrier

    b. Cerebrospinal fluid

    c. The dura mater

    d. The Ommaya reservoir

28. To achieve the same effect as an intrathecal dose, the anesthesiologist must administer an epidural dose that's:

    a. five times as great.

    b. ten times as great.

    c. one-third as great.

    d. one-tenth as great.

29. After completely inhaling a drug from a metered-dose inhaler, the patient should:

    a. hold his breath for several seconds and then exhale slowly.

    b. hold his breath for at least 1 minute and then exhale quickly.

    c. exhale slowly.

    d. take two more short breaths, hold his breath as long as he can, and exhale.

30. You can administer all of the following emergency drugs endotracheally *except:*

    a. atropine.

    b. epinephrine.

    c. dopamine.

    d. lidocaine.

31. In the lungs, gas exchange occurs in the:

    a. bronchioles.

    b. alveoli.

    c. pulmonary capillaries.

    d. pleura.

32. Which of the following is *not* an advantage of the mini-nebulizer?

    a. It is compact and disposable.

    b. It works with any compressed gas system.

    c. It provides both oxygen and aerosol therapy.

    d. It helps maximize medication distribution when the patient inhales correctly.

33. What controls the absorption rate of a drug given transdermally or subdermally?

    a. The delivery system, application site, and the skin integrity at that site

    b. The preparation of the application site

    c. The patient's metabolism

    d. The patient's activity level

34. The flexible capsules used in subdermal implants are made of:

    a. plastic.

    b. rubber.

    c. liposomes.

    d. Silastic.

35. What is the most common adverse effect of a transdermal patch?

    a. Excessively high serum drug levels

    b. Dependency and increased drug tolerance

    c. Pruritic rash

    d. An increase in noncompliance

36. When caring for a patient with a radiation implant, what general principles should you always follow?

    a. Wear a lead apron and use a lead shield and lead-lined containers.

    b. Wear a film badge and use a pocket dosimeter and long-handled forceps.

    c. Follow radiation precautions and heed all RADIATION PRECAUTION signs and warning labels.

    d. Maintain your distance, use the appropriate shielding, and deliver care in the shortest time possible.

37. Intrapleural drug administration can lead to:

    a. pleural effusion.

    b. pleural fibrosis.

    c. pleural inflammation.

    d. pneumothorax.

38. Which of the following is *not* true of intraperitoneal chemotherapy?

a. It keeps drug levels in the portal vein high, thus helping to prevent liver metastasis.

b. It allows the liver to detoxify drugs before they reach systemic circulation.

c. It decreases the risk of bone marrow suppression compared with I.V. chemotherapy.

d. It results in high systemic drug levels, thus helping to prevent extraperitoneal metastases.

39. Adults usually don't receive drugs through the intraosseous route because:

a. this method of administration causes too much pain.

b. they have too much adipose tissue.

c. their bone marrow isn't vascular enough.

d. they may develop osteomyelitis.

40. All of the following contraindicate intra-articular injections *except:*

a. a septic joint.

b. osteoporosis.

c. an intra-articular fracture.

d. rheumatoid arthritis.

Answers and rationales

1. b. The transdermal route improves compliance by relieving the patient's responsibility for taking medication. It doesn't make drug administration significantly easier. A transdermal patch shouldn't be applied to abnormal skin. Drugs given by this route have a comparatively slow onset of action.

2. d. These drugs commonly have a shorter shelf life than other drugs, and some of them—especially protein and peptide drugs—require special storage facilities. They're no more stable than other drugs and must follow the same testing and FDA approval guidelines.

3. c. An idiosyncratic response can result in any number of unpredictable patient-specific symptoms, such as nervousness from a tranquilizer. Anaphylactic shock and hypersensitivity are allergic reactions. The pharmacodynamic effect is the expected one that the drug will have on the patient.

4. c. Thrombophlebitis and emboli can be life-threatening, posing the greatest risk to the patient's well-being.

5. d. When administered directly into any vein, a drug is completely absorbed.

6. a. Best for long-term therapy, the dorsal veins of the hand leave more proximal sites as therapy progresses. The patient is more comfortable when veins in the lower arm are used, so they're usually preferred for short-term therapy. After all lower sites have been used, veins in the upper arm are chosen. A venipuncture in the veins of the leg or foot may compromise circulation, leading to thrombophlebitis. The antecubital veins should only be used for a large-bore needle, to infuse drugs that require a large volume dilution.

7. c. Circulatory overload—the result of a rapid increase in I.V. flow rate—can trigger these signs. Dyspnea is shortness of breath that can stem from anxiety and certain cardiac disorders. Hypovolemic shock results from decreased intravascular volume caused by hemorrhage, trauma, burns, diarrhea, vomiting, or diuresis. Pulmonary edema—caused by elevated pulmonary venous and capillary hydrostatic pressures—represents a complication of cardiac disorders.

8. a. Speed shock, the result of giving a drug too quickly, causes these signs and symptoms and can lead to cardiac arrest. Circulatory overload causes signs of congestive heart failure. Anaphylactic shock and hypersensitivity result from an allergic reaction.

9. c. Only a leukocyte-removal, or pall, filter will take out the leukocytes, reducing the chance of a transfusion reaction.

10. b. Although PCA does give the patient more control over his pain, the most important advantage is the decrease in the amount of pain and sedation experienced.

11. a. Both the internal jugular and subclavian veins are large and lie close to the heart, allowing the insertion of a CV line directly into the superior vena cavae or right atrium.

12. c. Some health care facilities prohibit the administration of amphotericin B through a CV line because of the possibility of a rapid decrease in potassium, leading to cardiac arrhythmias.

13. d. You'd flush a Groshong catheter with 5 ml of sterile 0.9% sodium chloride solution, not heparin solution. The pressure-sensitive two-way valve eliminates the need for frequent heparin flushes.

14. c. The S.E.A. Port is the only one of these devices that allows side entry.

15. c. Stainless steel can distort the image produced by MRI.

16. b. Although parenteral solution can contain glucose and other carbohydrates, lipids, protein, and vitamins, only sodium, potassium, magnesium, calcium, and phosphorus are electrolytes.

17. c. A PPN solution that contains more than 10% dextrose can cause venous sclerosis.

18. d. Patients need monitoring three times a week to adequately monitor their progress, although patients who don't maintain therapeutic serum electrolyte levels may need daily blood work.

19. a. Catheter-related sepsis responds less readily to treatment than other complications and can lead to septic shock and death.

20. c. The extra calories and fatty acids provided by lipid emulsions help prevent essential fatty-acid deficiency and provide energy. The patient's major nutrients come from the parenteral nutrition solution, not the emulsion. Lipid emulsions don't contain ascorbic acid, vitamins, or electrolytes.

21. d. Because acute leukemia causes rapid cell division, it responds more readily to chemotherapy. In colon, prostate, and lung cancers, fewer cells undergo cell division at any one time, making these cancers less responsive to chemotherapy.

22. b. An adverse reaction to bone marrow suppression can cause fever, chills, bleeding gums, fatigue, and hypotension. Chemotherapy, not bone marrow suppression, can trigger the other signs and symptoms mentioned.

23. d. A derivative of folic acid, leucovorin calcium counteracts the effects of folic acid antagonists, such as methotrexate. The other drugs aren't folic acid antagonists.

24. b. Although OSHA also recommends the other measures, it stresses the importance of safety cabinets, which play a vital role in preventing accidents and minimizing exposure to these drugs.

25. c. Only the anesthesiologist has the necessary expertise for this procedure.

26. d. Epidural blood patch is the treatment of choice.

27. a. Formed by the tight junctions between endothelial cells in brain capillaries, the blood-brain barrier prevents most water-soluble drugs from passing into the CNS. Neither cerebrospinal fluid nor the dura mater prevents the passage of drugs. The Ommaya reservoir is a device inserted into the right frontal region of the brain that acts as a reservoir for medication.

28. b. Unlike an intrathecal dose, an epidural dose must pass through the dura mater. Therefore, the anesthesiologist needs to inject ten times the amount of drug to achieve the same effect.

29. a. By holding his breath for several seconds, the patient gives the drug a chance to reach all the alveoli — the terminal air sacs in the lungs. Exhaling slowly helps keep the distal bronchioles open, increasing drug absorption and diffusion and improving gas exchange.

30. c. Dopamine can only be administered by I.V. infusion.

31. b. The alveoli are surrounded by a capillary network, where oxygen from inhaled air diffuses into the bloodstream while carbon dioxide passes back into the lungs for exhalation. The bronchioles are passageways to the alveoli. Oxygen binds to hemoglobin in the pulmonary capillaries. The pleura is the serous membrane that lines the lungs.

32. c. Only the large-volume nebulizer provides both oxygen and aerosol therapy.

33. a. The delivery system, application site, and skin integrity at the site all affect the absorption rate of a transdermal or subcutaneous drug. Skin preparation and the patient's metabolism and activity level have no effect on the absorption rate.

34. d. Only Silastic has the necessary properties to control drug release in a subdermal implant.

35. c. The most common adverse effect of a transdermal patch is a pruritic rash. Because of its slow drug release, the patch doesn't cause high serum drug concentrations or increased drug tolerance and dependency. Because it's painless and simple to use, the patch can actually promote a patient's compliance.

36. d. Although any of these measures can take on particular importance in a specific situation, the final answer covers the general principles—time, distance, and shielding— that you should always follow.

37. d. Intrapleural drug administration can sometimes allow air into the pleural space, causing a pneumothorax. Pleural effusion—the collection of fluid in the interstitial and air spaces of the lungs—results from bacterial pneumonia. Pleural fibrosis and pleural inflammation prohibit intrapleural drug administration.

38. d. Because injecting a drug directly into the peritoneal cavity bypasses the circulatory system, intraperitoneal chemotherapy doesn't cause high systemic drug levels.

39. c. At about age 5, the vascular red bone marrow that carries drugs and fluids to the systemic circulation is replaced by less vascular yellow marrow that doesn't transport drugs or fluids.

40. d. Intra-articular corticosteroid injections actually help relieve the symptoms of rheumatoid arthritis. A septic joint, osteoporosis, and an intra-articular fracture all increase the risk of complications from an intra-articular injection.

Index

i refers to an illustration; t refers to a table

i refers to an illustration; t refers to a table